Modern Concepts in Gastroenterology
Volume 1

TOPICS IN GASTROENTEROLOGY

Series Editor: **Howard M. Spiro, M.D.**
Yale University School of Medicine

COLON
Structure and Function
Edited by Luis Bustos-Fernandez, M.D.

KEY FACTS IN GASTROENTEROLOGY
Jonathan Halevy, M.D.

MEDICAL ASPECTS OF DIETARY FIBER
Edited by Gene A. Spiller, Ph.D., and Ruth McPherson Kay, Ph.D.

MODERN CONCEPTS IN GASTROENTEROLOGY
Edited by Alan B. R. Thomson, M.D., L. R. DaCosta, M.D., and
William C. Watson, M.D.

NUTRITION AND DIET THERAPY
IN GASTROINTESTINAL DISEASE
Martin H. Floch, M.D.

PANCREATITIS
Peter A. Banks, M.D.

A Continuation Order Plan is available for this series. A continuation order will bring delivery of each new volume immediately upon publication. Volumes are billed only upon actual shipment. For further information please contact the publisher.

Modern Concepts in Gastroenterology
Volume 1

Edited by

Alan B. R. Thomson, M.D.

The University of Alberta
Edmonton, Alberta, Canada

L. R. DaCosta, M.D.

Queen's University
Kingston, Ontario, Canada

and

William C. Watson, M.D.

Victoria Hospital
London, Ontario, Canada

PLENUM MEDICAL BOOK COMPANY
NEW YORK AND LONDON

ISBN-13: 978-1-4612-9002-5   e-ISBN-13: 978-1-4613-1789-0
DOI: 10.1007/ 978-1-4613-1789-0

233 Spring Street, New York, N.Y. 10013

Plenum Medical Book Company is an imprint of Plenum Publishing Corporation

*Dedicated to our wives,
Jeannette, Judy, and Elspeth*

Contributors

Lawrence J. Brandt, Montefiore Hospital and Medical Center, Bronx, New York 10467

C. J. de Gara, The Intestinal Diseases Research Unit and Division of Gastroenterology, McMaster University Medical Centre, Hamilton, Ontario, Canada L8N 3Z5

Geoffrey C. Farrell, The University of Sydney and Gastroenterology Unit, Westmead Hospital, Westmead, NSW, Australia 2145

Daphna Fenyves, Clinical Research Centre, Saint-Luc Hospital, Montreal, Quebec, Canada H2X 3J4

Josef E. Fischer, Department of Surgery, University of Cincinnati Medical Center, Cincinnati, Ohio 45267

Hugh James Freeman, The University of British Columbia, Health Sciences Centre Hospital, Vancouver, British Columbia, Canada V6T 1W5

David Fromm, Department of Surgery, State University of New York–Upstate Medical Center, Syracuse, New York 13210

Grant Gall, Department of Medicine, University of Calgary, Calgary, Alberta, Canada T2N 1N4

Donald J. Glotzer, Departments of Surgery, Beth Israel Hospital and Harvard Medical School, Boston, Massachusetts 02115

J. Richard Hamilton, Division of Gastroenterology, Department of Pediatrics, University of Toronto and The Research Institute, The Hospital for Sick Children, Toronto, Ontario, Canada M5G 1X8

Walter J. Hogan, Froedtert Memorial Lutheran Hospital, Milwaukee, Wisconsin 53226

R. H. Hunt, The Intestinal Diseases Research Unit and Division of Gastroenterology, McMaster University Medical Centre, Hamilton, Ontario, Canada L8N 3Z5

D. B. Jones, The Intestinal Diseases Research Unit and Division of Gastroenterology, McMaster University Medical Centre, Hamilton, Ontario, Canada L8N 3Z5

Jutta K. Preiksaitis, University of Alberta, University Hospital, Edmonton, Alberta, Canada T6G 2C7

Roy M. Preshaw, Department of Surgery and Gastrointestinal Research Unit, University of Calgary Medical School, Calgary, Alberta, Canada T2N 4N1

Robert H. Riddell, McMaster University Medical Centre, Hamilton, Ontario, Canada L8N 3Z5

Fergus Shanahan, Division of Gastroenterology, University of California at Los Angeles School of Medicine, Los Angeles, California 90024

Howard M. Spiro, Section of Gastroenterology, Yale University School of Medicine, New Haven, Connecticut 06510

Giles W. Stevenson, McMaster University, Hamilton, Ontario, Canada L8N 3Z5

Stephan R. Targan, Division of Gastroenterology, University of California at Los Angeles School of Medicine, Los Angeles, California 90024

Bryce R. Taylor, Toronto General Hospital, Toronto, Ontario, Canada M5KG 1L7

Hillar Vellend, Departments of Medicine and Microbiology, Faculty of Medicine, University of Toronto, Toronto, Ontario, Canada M5G 2C4

Jean-Pierre Villeneuve, Clinical Research Centre, Saint-Luc Hospital, Montreal, Quebec, Canada H2X 3J4

W. C. Watson, Department of Gastroenterology, Victoria Hospital, London, Ontario, Canada N6A 4G5

Foreword

A fine team of state-of-the-art researcher/clinicians who know their fields, have contributed to the advancement of knowledge, and are in a position to judge what is truly important have here pooled their thoughts in a series of chapters on the cutting edges of gastroenterology. Four attributes render this volume superior to other update-oriented publications. The first striking feature, which is immediately evident upon scanning the table of contents, is the imaginative choice of subjects, ranging from traveler's diarrhea and sexually transmitted GI infections through TPN and interventional endoscopy to geriatrics and iatrogenic disease.

A second outstanding feature of this volume is its success in balancing basic pathophysiology with practical considerations of clinical management. This is achieved in the discussions of such diverse topics as acid-peptic diseases, infectious and other diarrheal syndromes, and hepatitis immunization. Throughout the book we are led smoothly from basic science principles to specific recommendations for diagnosis and therapy. This practical emphasis appears repeatedly and sometimes produces a delightful surprise, such as a chapter on radiology that is not technology-based but instead problem-oriented.

A third remarkable feature is the critically analytical perspective adopted by many of the authors. Not content merely to tabulate and review, survey and summarize, they have taken a hard evaluative look at their subjects. Ulcer medications, gallstone dissolution, invasive therapeutic endoscopy, nutritional support systems, pills and prophylaxis for traveler's diarrhea, new operations for inflammatory bowel disease, and other items in the gastroenterological armamentarium are assessed from personal viewpoints that are nourished by extensive experience and critical judgment. The results are stimulating and refreshing, as exemplified by the welcome infusion of science, common sense, and intellectual curiosity into the controversial arena of food allergy and intolerance.

Finally, and most notably, the entire volume is woven together with a rare sensitivity to ethics, economic and psychosocial concerns, and humanism. These issues are perhaps expected to be raised in considerations of functional bowel disease, reviews of GI disorders in the elderly, or special chapters like Howard Spiro's eloquent contribution on "Dilemmas and Decisions in Digestive Disease." It is particularly gratifying, however, to find humanistic attitudes also permeating discussion of interventional endoscopy, TPN, and surgical techniques. This attention to ethical issues is well exemplified by the inclusion of a chapter on "Iatrogenic Aspects of Gastroenterological Practice," in which W. C. Watson sensibly warns us, "Just because something *can* be done does not mean it *needs* to be done or *should* be done."

David B. Sachar, M.D.
Professor of Clinical Medicine
Director, Division of Gastroenterology
The Mount Sinai Medical Center
New York, New York

Preface

This work arises from submissions made at the first and second symposia on Recent Advances in Gastroenterology held by the Canadian Association of Gastroenterology. The proposed audience for this volume is the general internist and the general surgeon, as well as those in specialties in gastroenterology and hepatology. In addition, this publication will be of use and benefit to senior medical residents preparing for subspecialty examinations in internal medicine, general surgery, and gastroenterology.

The rate of change of medical practice and the growth of its scientific and information base are intimidating. This is particularly true of gastroenterology, which has major specialty divisions of its own. Through the generous support of Glaxo Canada Ltd., and with the organizational assistance of the Royal College of Physicians and Surgeons of Canada, the Canadian Association of Gastroenterology is pleased to undertake its commitment to the advancement of science and the improvement in the quality of the care of patients with diseases of the gastrointestinal tract. We are fortunate in having a distinguished group of contributors from North America. Their subjects are diverse, important, and topical.

It gives us special pleasure to acknowledge the considerable assistance from Glaxo Canada, and the support of its former president, the late Mr. Frank Burke.

We would also like to express our appreciation to Mr. Frank M. Sabatino of Glaxo Canada for his enthusiastic support of this project.

Alan Thomson
L. R. Da Costa
William C. Watson

Alberta and London

Contents

A Physiological Basis for the Rational Therapy of Peptic Ulcer

C. J. de Gara, D. B. Jones, and R. H. Hunt

1. INTRODUCTION

Peptic ulcer continues to present a significant clinical problem. Although the overall incidence and prevalence of the disease probably remain unchanged, dramatic improvements in medical therapy have markedly altered the patterns of referral in the last decade. Thus, surgical intervention for uncomplicated disease has become a relative rarity in most centers, the majority of effective therapies being administered by primary care physicians. An increasing number of potent ulcer-healing agents are now available to the physician demanding better understanding of the disease pathophysiology. The etiology and reason for relapse remain unknown, but continuing research into the cellular control mechanisms of acid and pepsin secretion and mucosal resistance is leading to a more logical and focused therapeutic approach.

2. AGGRESSIVE FACTORS

2.1. Acid

The normal human stomach contains approximately one billion parietal cells, which have the capacity to secrete 30 mmol of H^+ ion or

C. J. de Gara, D. B. Jones, and R. H. Hunt • The Intestinal Diseases Research Unit and Division of Gastroenterology, McMaster University Medical Centre, Hamilton, Ontario, Canada L8N 3Z5.

more per hour under maximal stimulation. Although the correlation between parietal cell mass, acid secretory state, and acid peptic disorders remains inconclusive, maximal acid output and nocturnal acid secretion tend to be increased in peptic ulcer patients compared with controls.[1,2] The adage "No acid, no ulcer"[3] is still pertinent, as testified to by the fact that acid suppression therapy, either pharmacologically or surgically, has proved highly effective in the management of peptic ulceration.

The studies of the mechanisms controlling acid secretion involve human or intact animal gastric aspiration with or without intragastric titration[4] and indicator dilution.[5] *In vitro* study includes Ussing chambered gastric mucosa,[6] isolated gastric gland preparations,[7] and the isolated purified parietal cell.[8] Within the limitations of *in vitro* preparations, valuable information may be obtained regarding receptor and intracellular function. However, the measurement of acid secretion remains indirect.

Acid secretion is regulated by chemical messengers which are targeted to the parietal cell (Fig. 1) by one of three *primary* modes: *neurocrine, endocrine,* or *paracrine.*[9] Subsequently, intracellular function is mediated by a group of *secondary* messengers (vide infra). Three substances are recognized as primary messengers on the parietal cell, viz., acetylocholine (neurocrine) released by postganglionic neurons, gastrin (endocrine) from the G cells of the antral mucosa, and histamine (paracrine) released locally from mast cells of the oxyntic mucosa. Parietal cell function is mediated through receptors for each of these systems. MacIntosh[10] and later Code[11] proposed histamine as the final common pathway for acid secretion by the parietal cell, but this has not been substantiated. The hypothesis proposed by Grossman and Konturek[12] and further developed by Soll[13] considers that each secretagogue acts at its own receptor site on the parietal cell and that their actions are parallel to, and facilitated by, one another. This action has been termed a "permissive effect" and represents the currently held view which allows for antagonists of one receptor to inhibit stimulation produced at another receptor.

2.2. Neurocrine Control (Muscarinic Receptors)

Stimulation of the vagus nerve either endogenously with insulin hypoglycemia or modified sham feeding or exogenously with bethanecol results in gastric acid secretion, an effect that can be blocked by the administration of an anticholinergic agent or by vagotomy. Histamine may potentiate this cholinergic stimulus both *in vivo* and *in vitro*. In addition, vagal stimulation may also promote gastric secretion by increasing

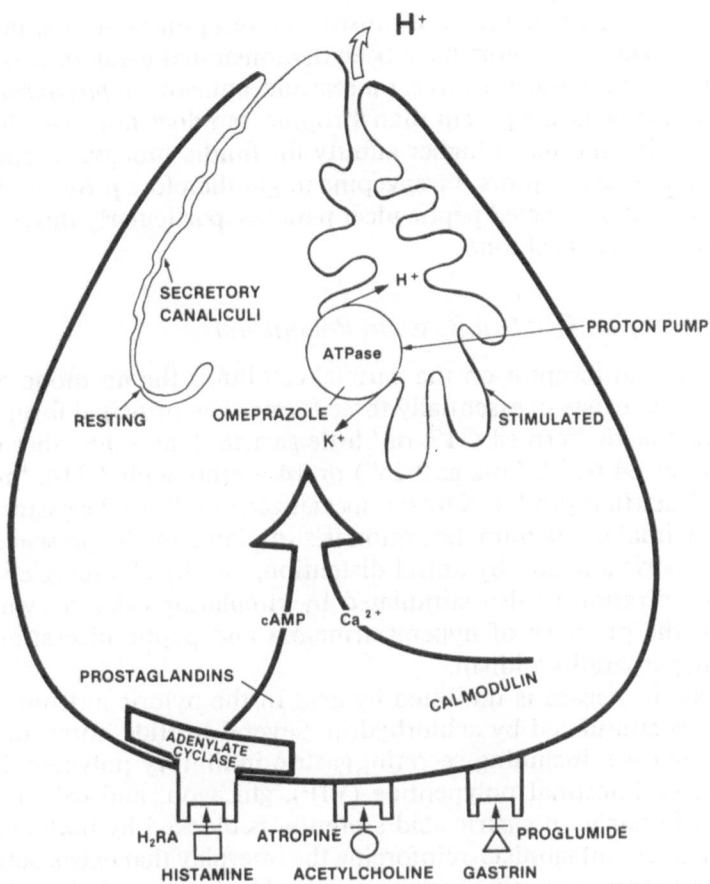

Figure 1. Schematic representation of the parietal cell showing the receptor systems (histamine, acetylcholine, gastrin), the second messengers (cyclic AMP and calcium ions), and the proton pump activated in the stimulated state. The postulated site of each antagonist—histamine receptor antagonist (H₂RA), atropine, proglumide, prostaglandins, and omeprazole—is as shown.

gastrin release.[14] It has been suggested that those patients who are relatively resistant to H₂ receptor antagonist therapy[15] may possess an increased vagal drive which may account for the success of vagotomy in healing duodenal ulcers in these patients.[16]

Recently, evidence has accumulated for the existence in the gastric mucosa of two populations of muscarinic receptor subtypes, termed M_1 and M_2.[17] These receptors have been demonstrated using *in vitro* binding techniques with the selective muscarinic antagonist *pirenzepine*. This anticholinergic is less potent than atropine, but does not cross the blood–brain barrier and has a higher affinity for fundic mucosa receptors than smooth muscle receptors. Pirenzepine might therefore prove useful in the management of selected peptic ulcer patients, particularly those who may have increased vagal tone.

2.3. Endocrine Control (Gastrin Receptors)

A second receptor on the parietal cell binds the hormone *gastrin*, a peptide that exists in essentially three forms. The principal form contains 17 amino acids (termed G17, or "little gastrin"), and the other two contain either 34 (G34, "big gastrin") or 14 amino acids (G14, "mini gastrin"). Gastrin is produced by the specialized G cells of the gastric antrum and proximal duodenum. Secretion is stimulated by the presence of food in the gastric antrum, by antral distention, and by cholinergic stimulus. Gastric secretion is also stimulated by circulating calcium, which may explain the presence of hypergastrinemia and peptic ulceration in primary hyperparathyroidism.

Gastrin release is inhibited by acid in the pyloric antrum and conversely is stimulated by achlorhydria. Several peptide hormones inhibit gastrin release, including secretin, gastric inhibitory polypeptide (GIP), vasoactive intestinal polypeptide (VIP), glucagon, and calcitonin. The action of gastrin on gastric acid secretion is blocked by both anticholinergics and H_2 antagonists, reinforcing the interplay that exists between the three receptors. A specific gastrin receptor blocking agent—proglumide—is available but has, as yet, no clinical value.

Hypergastrinemia is found in many disease states, e.g., pernicious anemia, chronic renal failure, and hyperparathyroidism. Gastrinoma (Zollinger–Ellison syndrome), antral G-cell hyperplasia, and postsurgical gastric antral retention are all associated with gastric acid hypersecretion and peptic ulcer diathesis. In Zollinger–Ellison syndrome, abnormally high and persistent levels of gastrin are released from tumors, usually of the pancreatic islet cells. In this condition, severe and intractable peptic ulceration is common. In antral G-cell hyperplasia, hypergastrinemic hyperchlorhydria occurs in the absence of a gastrin-producing tumor. The diagnosis is histological, the condition being similar to the Z–E syndrome in that the hypergastrinemia is not reversed by antral acidification. In antral G-cell hyperplasia, the hypergastrinemia may increase after a meal, remain unchanged after calcium, and decrease after secretin, whereas the hypergastrinemia associated with the Z–E syndrome is usually unchanged by meals and increased by secretin and calcium.

2.4. Paracrine Control (Histamine Receptors)

The discovery of a subclass of histamine H_2 receptors on the parietal cell[18] and the subsequent development of specific agonists and antagonists to this receptor stimulated major advances in the understanding of acid-related disorders. Histamine and the H_2 receptor agonist *impromidine*[19] are potent stimulators of acid secretion in isolated rabbit parietal cells and isolated gastric glands of man, rabbit, and dog. Conversely, this receptor may be blocked, with resultant inhibition of acid secretion, by specific H_2 receptor antagonists such as *cimetidine* or *ranitidine*.

2.5. Second Messengers in the Parietal Cell

The use of isolated gland and cell models has proved important for the determination of receptor and intracellular mechanisms of acid secretion. The currently held concept proposes ligand binding to the cell receptor, initiating changes in the plasma membrane with the generation of cyclic AMP or alteration in Ca^{2+} permeability. Subsequent changes in intracellular cyclic AMP or intracellular free Ca^{2+} produce an alteration in parietal cell function.[20]

2.5.1. Cyclic AMP

The H_2 receptor is coupled to adenylate cyclase and activation elevates parietal cell cyclic AMP.[21] Currently much work is attempting to elucidate the complex activation of adenylate cyclase and the biochemical mechanism whereby cyclic AMP activates the secretory canalicular apparatus.

2.5.2. Calcium Ions

Both the cholinergic response, in rabbit gastric glands and dog parietal cell, and the gastrin response, in gastric glands, require extracellular Ca^{2+}.[22,23] The regulation of intracellular Ca^{2+} depends on passive Ca^{2+} entry and active exit pathways across the basal–lateral membrane. Vesicles isolated from the gastric mucosa show the presence of an ATP-dependent, calmodulin-activated Ca^{2+} pump. Although the effects of intracellular Ca^{2+} changes have not been established for parietal cell, a gastric mucosal Ca^{2+}-dependent protein kinase has been described.[24] The physiological importance of Ca^{2+} in the regulation of acid secretion is becoming more apparent and has been shown to be required for membrane fusion events in other cell systems.[25]

2.5.3. The Proton Pump

The absolute dependence of acid secretion in the mammalian parietal cell on ATP, K^+ and Cl^- has been established in chambered preparations, isolated glands, and isolated gastric vesicles.[26] The system responsible for the generation of the proton gradient is a plasma-membrane-bound ATPase which requires the presence of luminal K^+ for its activity. This H^+/K^+-ATPase enzyme proton pump is situated at the acid secretory membrane. The substituted benzimidazoles are a group of compounds which have been shown to interfere with this pump and as a consequence inhibit gastric acid secretion.[27]

The discovery of this enzyme system represents a dramatic advance in the understanding of parietal cell physiology. The action of the benzimidazoles, unlike receptor antagonists which competitively inhibit basal membrane receptor systems, is noncompetitive, dose dependent, and long-lasting.[28] Omeprazole is the first compound of this group to be used in humans, and up to 98% acid reduction is seen with larger doses of 80 mg, while 30 mg produces 50–60% reduction for up to 5 days.[29]

Much remains to be investigated with regard to parietal intracellular function and the complex interrelationship between the membrane receptors, cyclic AMP, Ca^{2+}, and the proton pump, and no doubt newer agents will be targeted at these functions.

2.6. Pepsin

Pepsin, an acid protease secreted as several isoenzymes, was first described 150 years ago.[30] Pepsin is important to our understanding of the pathophysiology of peptic ulceration since this does not occur unless pepsin is present in addition to acid.[31-33] Surprisingly little is known about the control of pepsin in humans, but it has been generally assumed that the mechanisms are the same as those for acid.

Pepsin was first named and characterized by Schwann in 1836.[30] In 1933, Northrop crystallized pepsin from bovine gastric juice and found it to have a molecular weight of 35,000.[34] The unique properties of pepsin include optimal enzyme activity at pH 1.5–2.5 and inactivation at pH 7.[35] Pepsinogens are the inactive precursors of pepsins stored within zymogen granules of the chief cell, are secreted into the gastric lumen, and are converted into pepsin(s) by an autocatalytic mechanism in the presence of hydrogen ion.[35] One percent of the pepsinogens pass into the circulation by an unknown mechanism and subsequently undergo renal excretion as uropepsinogen.[36] The significance and importance of the pepsinogens in plasma is little understood, although many workers have attempted to relate serum pepsinogen heterogeneity to genotype and disease.[37-39]

It has been assumed that pepsin secretion varies pari passu with acid secretion, although there is now some evidence to suggest that this is not always the case. A philosophy propounded by Code[11] that "nature seldom issues monopolies in the control of important biological functions" applies not only to acid secretion but also to pepsin. His statement finds support on evolutionary grounds from species such as the chicken that has a single cell type responsible for the secretion of both acid and pepsin, while in other species, including humans, separate cell types have evolved.[40]

As with studies of acid secretion, the control of pepsin secretion has been investigated in isolated chief cell or mucosal gland preparations, and in both humans and animal models. Although a three-receptor system is accepted for parietal cell function, the presence of these receptors on the chief cell is not certain. The control mechanisms for pepsin secretion in humans have not been clearly worked out. Pepsin secretion appears to be predominantly under vagal control,[41] but the various receptor activating secretagogues may also be of importance. The control of secretion may be an interplay between the receptors, a final common mediator process or possibly a nonreceptor-mediated event governed by the intimate spatial relationship between chief and parietal cells, thus making intercellular communication possible. An alternate hypothesis of pepsin secretion control relates to the fact that topical acid is also known to stimulate pepsin secretion in both humans[42] and dogs.[43] A mucosal/cholinergic reflex has therefore been postulated whereby the back-diffusion of acid stimulates pepsin secretion to ensure maximal secretory rates only in the presence of sufficient acid to convert pepsinogen to pepsin. The physiological control of pepsin secretion is further complicated by the effects of gastrointestinal peptide hormones such as secretin, which administered exogenously cause an inhibition of acid secretion while stimulating pepsin secretion.[44]

2.7. Pepsin and the Neurocrine System

The primary stimulus to pepsin secretion by the chief cell is cholinergic[41] whether endogenous (insulin, 2-deoxyglucose, or shamfeeding) or exogenous (bethanecol or urecholine). The volume of gastric secretion is also believed to be predominantly under vagal control.[45] This vagal component of pepsin secretion is seen not only in the dog,[46] but also in humans.[47]

Gibson et al.[48] found that administration of an H_2 receptor antagonist during a background of cholinergic stimulation caused an increase in pepsin secretion. Conversely, Hirschowitz and Molina[49] found that cimetidine in the presence of bethanecol inhibited pepsin secretion whereas metiamide and ranitidine did not alter pepsin secretion. Studies in the cat have shown that an increased resistance to H_2RA blockade of gastric secretion develops with increasing degrees of vagal stimulation.[50] It seems, therefore, that the cholinergic drive to the chief cell can be inhibited, remain unchanged, or be enhanced by H_2RA.

The volume of gastric secretion is also predominantly under vagal control,[43] which may account for the higher duodenal ulcer healing rates achieved by vagotomy than medical therapy.[51] In a study in patients whose ulcers failed to respond to cimetidine there was an increase in pepsin output with cimetidine, 1 g/day, whereas atropine, 4.8 mg/day, decreased pepsin output, although neither change achieved statistical significance. When both drugs were combined, pepsin output was decreased significantly.[52] These observations suggest that patients with severe refractory ulcer disease may possess a higher vagal drive which not only gives rise to greater levels of intragastric pepsin but also produces a resistance to H_2 receptor blockade.

2.8. Pepsin and the Endocrine System

In humans, the observed effects of pentagastrin on pepsin secretion vary considerably between workers. Some quote pepsin concentration and others pepsin output. Pepsin output is a product of the volume of gastric secretion and pepsin concentration; therefore, agents affecting volume will alter pepsin output, while not necessarily affecting pepsin secretion. Interpreting Berstad and Petersen's work[53] in healthy volunteers, doses of pentagastrin ranging from 0.06 to 7.0 µg/kg per hr produced an initial rise in pepsin concentration followed by a return to basal levels. A similar effect occurred with pepsin output in a dose–response study by Aagaard et al.[54] in duodenal ulcer patients. Conversely, other workers[55,56] have shown that pepsin secretion is increased by pentagastrin.

2.9. Pepsin and the Paracrine System

Most conflict regarding pepsin secretion relates to histamine studies. In the dog[57] and the cat[58] pepsin secretion is stimulated by low doses of histamine and suppressed by increasing doses which stimulate gastric hydrogen ion secretion. This biphasic response suggests that stimulation may be mediated by a high-affinity, low-K_m receptor, and inhibition is mediated by a low-affinity, high-K_m H_2 receptor.[59]

This observation has been reported in both normal and duodenal ulcer subjects,[60] with low doses of histamine causing an increase in pepsin secretion whereas higher doses produced inhibition. A possible explanation for apparent stimulation of pepsin secretion by histamine in these human studies may be the fact that conventional H_1 antagonists given concurrently to block histamine side effects possess additional inherent cholinergic actions. Using the H_2 receptor specific agonist impromidine[19] in humans, in the absence of H_1 receptor blockade, inhibition of pepsin secretion has been demonstrated.[61] However, the effect of impromidine in dogs is similar to that of histamine in that low doses stimulate and high doses inhibit pepsin secretion.[62] These observations have in the past been attributed to the "washout" phenomenon, in which there is a large discharge of preformed pepsinogen granules from the chief cell, giving rise to an *apparent* stimulation followed by diminution of pepsin secretion as the granule supply becomes exhausted.

In clinical studies, cimetidine competitively inhibits histamine-stimulated acid secretion but changes the biphasic pepsin dose–response curve (in which low doses of histamine stimulate and higher doses inhibit) to one that parallels the acid output curve.[63] A similar phenomenon has been observed overnight in duodenal ulcer patients free of exogenous stimulation, although endogenous stimulation by excessive vagal drive remains one possible explanation.

The control of pepsin secretion in humans has yet to be finally determined, and in the majority of clinical situations suppression of acid secretion is sufficient to render this potent proteolytic enzyme inactive. However, without pepsin, ulceration does not occur[31–33] thus warranting an improved understanding of the control mechanisms and the potential for the development of a truly antipeptic agent.

3. DEFENSIVE FACTORS

The property of the gastric mucosa to protect itself against acid and pepsin digestion, termed the "mucosal barrier," was developed as a concept by Davenport[64] in 1964. Since that time considerable interest has been focused on the factors that alter mucosal integrity. This review will focus on gastric mucosal blood flow, mucosal integrity, mucus, and bicarbonate secretion (Fig. 2).

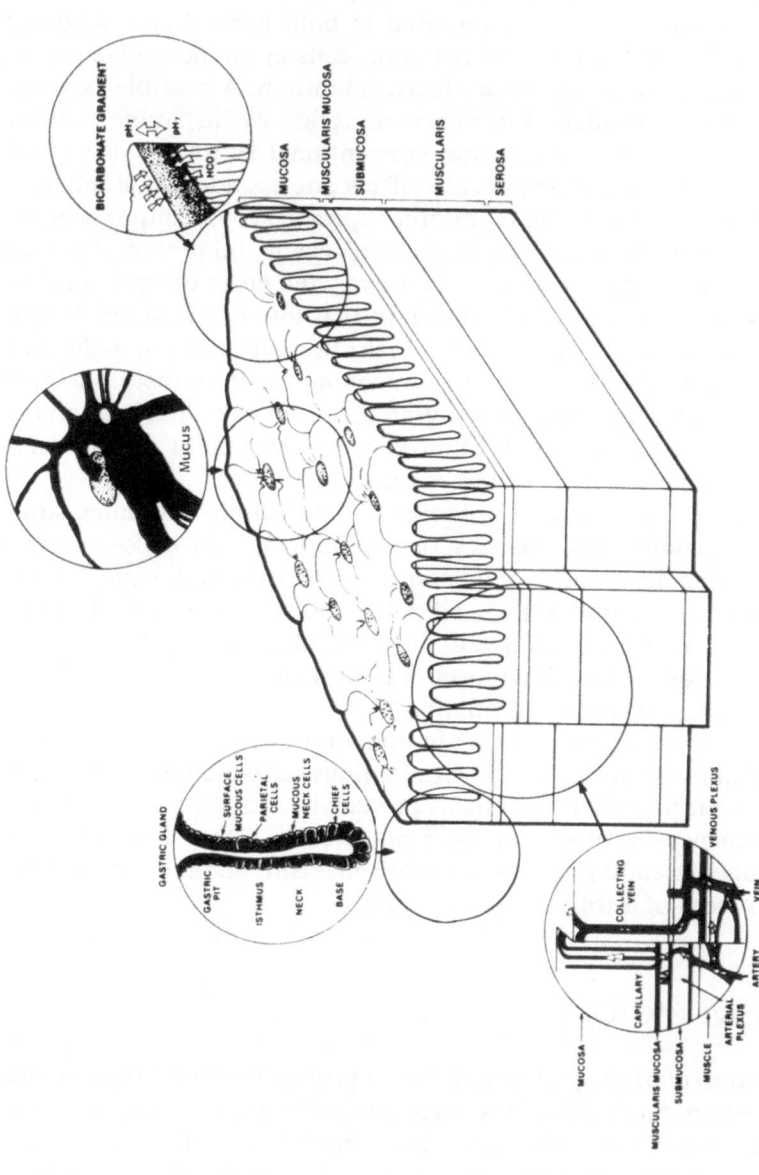

Figure 2. Schematic model of the functional morphology of the gastric mucosa showing the sites of secretion of acid, pepsin, and mucus in the gastric gland, together with a representation of the primary means of achieving mucosal integrity—mucosal blood flow, mucus, and bicarbonate.

3.1. Mucosal Blood Flow

The gastric mucosa receives approximately 70% of the total gastric blood flow. A variety of techniques for the study of mucosal blood flow have been described including [¹⁴C]aminopyrine clearance,[65] indicator-dilution with ^{42}K[66] or ^{86}Rb,[67] heat clearance,[68] and inert gas indicator washout technique using ^{85}Kr,[69] ^{133}Xe,[70] or hydrogen clearance. The control of mucosal blood flow involves an interplay between the central and autonomic nervous systems, the peptidergic system, and tissue amines. Studies on anterior and posterior hypothalamic stimulation and left gastric artery blood flow[71] revealed an increased flow and acid output with anterior stimulation and had the opposite effect with posterior stimulation. Electrical stimulation of the lateral hypothalamic area[72] showed an increase in blood flow and acid secretion in rats which was reversed by instillation of norepinephrine into the lateral ventricle. A noradrenergic inhibitory mechanism may therefore be involved in the regulation of mucosal blood flow. Stimulation of sympathetic fibers to the stomach decreases both total and mucosal blood flow, through reduction in submucosal arteriolar blood flow. Parasympathetic supply, via the vagus, when stimulated, increases blood flow, an effect that can be reversed by atropine[73] and vagotomy.[74] An interaction between the sympathetic and parasympathetic systems has been demonstrated in the dog[75] such that activation of muscarinic receptors on adrenergic nerve endings mediate inhibition of adrenergic neurotransmission.

Histamine has been shown to increase gastric blood flow through both H_1 and H_2 receptors on the submucosal arterioles.[76] The H_2 receptor antagonists metiamide and cimetidine have no effect on resting mucosal blood flow, but, in some species studied, reduce the ischemia produced by experimental hemorrhagic shock.[77] Many of the gastrointestinal hormones including VIP,[78] secretin, vasopressin,[79] and somatostatin[80] while inhibiting stimulated gastric acid secretion also produce a reduction in gastric blood flow. The ratio of blood flow to acid secretion remained unchanged, indicating that the reduction was secondary to the inhibition of acid secretion.

Studies into the effects of prostaglandins (PGs) on the gastric mucosal vasculature have to be interpreted with caution since many have potent antisecretory properties. PGI_2 in the rat, for example, increases resting gastric blood flow, inhibits pentagastrin-stimulated acid secretion, and causes an increase in the mucosal blood flow–acid output ratio.[81] Similarly, PGs A and E inhibit acid secretion and vasodilate rat gastric mucosa.[82] Drugs such as indomethacin and aspirin which inhibit the synthesis of prostaglandins have been shown to decrease both resting and pentagastrin-stimulated mucosal blood flow.[83]

The importance of mucosal blood flow in the maintenance of mucosal integrity has been demonstrated in animal studies with induced mucosal ischemia where high concentrations of acid produced no injury in normotensive rats, but erosions occurred even with very low acid concentrations in hypotensive animals.[84] Furthermore, agents that tend to increase mucosal blood flow, such as prostaglandins, have a protective effect against substances known to produce mucosal injury such as bile salts.

3.2. Mucosal Integrity

The gastric mucosa behaves as a semipermeable barrier, and luminal acid has the ability to back-diffuse from lumen into the mucosa. A variety of agents have been shown to increase mucosal permeability to H^+ by both *in vitro* and *in vivo* methods. *In vivo* methods of study include isolated gastric pouches,[63] a mucosal flap with an intact blood supply,[85] or the ligated stomach with continuous perfusion.[86] These studies involve placing a solution of known composition into the pouch, flap, or stomach and analyzing the changes in ionic flux over a given time period. The Ussing chamber[87] provides an *in vitro* perfusion system divided into a luminal and serosal half by the mucosa. With electrodes connnected to a voltmeter any changes of potential difference (PD) may be recorded. PD has been suggested as a sensitive index of mucosal integrity in such a system[88] since PD routinely falls when there is increased mucosal permeability.

Exposure to damaging agents produces a rapid change in mucosal ultrastructure, with intracellular changes in mucus cells occurring prior to cell membrane changes. Intracellular changes in parietal cells are more apparent in the midupper regions of the gastric pits.[89] Ito[90,104] has termed the reparative changes that occur as gastric mucosal restitution. He has demonstrated that this restitution is rapid, i.e., 30 min, if damage is mild. Cells adjacent to a damaged area throw out lamelapodia, with surface mucous cells migrating over the basal lamina, leading to the formation of new tight junctions and the re-establishment of normal electrophysiology and secretory properties.

Bile and bile salts frequently reflux from the duodenum into the stomach in patients with gastritis and gastric ulcer, and their effect on mucosal permeability is both pH and concentration dependent.[91] The actions are related to their detergent or lipid-disrupting properties which cause dissolution of mucosal phospholipid and leakage of acid hydrolases.[92] Pancreatic juice alone does not alter mucosal permeability,[93] but lysolecithin, which is formed in the presence of bile salts and pancreatic enzymes, causes changes in a concentration-dependent, pH independent manner.[94]

The damaging effects of alcohol are pH independent, but are dependent on carbon chain length, lipid solubility, and concentration; ethyl alcohol, at a concentration of 10% or less, does not alter mucosal permeability,[95] whereas increasing concentrations do. Salicylates are a potent cause of mucosal damage, and do so by a variety of mechanisms. Actions include a nonspecific increase in mucosal permeability,[96] decrease in cellular ATP,[97] dose-dependent decrease in protein synthesis,[98] and interference with oxidative phosphorylation.[99] Of importance is the exposed carboxyl group common to salicylates and many of the nonsteroidal anti-inflammatory agents, which has been implicated in increasing mucosal permeability and the inhibitory effects on active ion transport.[100] Although direct contact of the gastric mucosa with steroids[101] or long-term parenterally administered steroids does not alter mucosal permeability, prednisolone does potentiate the effects of acetylsalicylic acid.[102]

The ability of low-dose, non-antisecretory doses of prostaglandins to protect mucosal integrity produced by ethanol and boiling water has been termed "cytoprotection."[103] This concept has recently been challenged by Lacy and Ito,[104] who have shown histologically that rat gastric mucosa was not protected from the damaging effects of absolute ethanol by 16,16-dimethyl prostaglandin E_2 in 77% of animals although no macroscopic lesion was evident. Various amino acids have been claimed to have protective effects, but may in fact represent the alkaline pH of amino acids in solution or their weak buffering action.[105] The mechanisms by which prostaglandins maintain the mucosal integrity are complex including inhibition of H^+ secretion, increase of cyclic AMP activity, active Na^+ transport, HCO_3^- secretion, blood flow, and mucus secretion, and stabilization of lysosomal membranes.[106] Whether H_2 receptor antagonists prevent mucosal damage or act solely by acid inhibition is controversial; in some studies the effect appears to be H^+ related,[107] and in others the protective effect appears independent of acid inhibition.[108] The most recent theory of cellular defense has been proposed by Hills, Butler, and Lichtenberger[109] whereby surface-active phospholipids in gastric mucosa form a hydrophobic protective lining, which can be disrupted by aspirin or bile salts.

3.3. Mucus

Mucus forms a thin continuous layer of water-insoluble viscoelastic gel adherent to the epithelium, Gel formation is due to high-molecular-weight (2×10^6) glycoproteins, which consist of polymers of four sub-units (mol. wt. 5×10^5) joined covalently by disulfide bridges and containing short carbohydrate side chains.[110] Free gastric juice mucus is made up largely of pepsin-degraded mucus subunits. Adherent epithelial mucus is 0.5 mm thick[111] and contains 5% glycoprotein at a concentration of 30–50 mg/ml and 90% water.[112]

A variety of methods have been described for the study of mucus including carbohydrate composition by colorimetry or gas liquid chromatography, radiolabeling of glycoprotein precursors, histochemical staining, radioimmunoassay, viscosity measurements, and precipitation and turbidity studies.[110]

Mucus is produced by specific glands throughout the gastrointestinal tract including Brunner's glands. Secretion is by continuous exocytosis of granules or by explosive release by apical expulsion of older cells in the interfoveolar area and, rarely, by cell exfoliation. The synthesis of mucus is complex, involving multiple steps in the biosynthetic pathway.[113] The protein core is made by translation of mRNA with attachment of N-acetylgalactosamine to serine and threonine residues; then carbohydrate side-chain biosynthesis begins in the rough endoplasmic reticulum (ER). In the smooth ER and Golgi apparatus, stepwise addition of sugars to the precursor glycoprotein occurs. The glycoprotein is packed into secretory vesicles and secreted as new mucus from these vesicles by plasma membrane fusion. The degradation involves proteolysis of the glycoprotein with solubilization of the gel and subsequent breakdown of the soluble glycoprotein into low-molecular-weight sugars and amino acids that can be reutilized by the body or enteric flora.

A variety of neural and humoral factors can increase luminal mucus. Splanchnic or vagal nerve stimulation or topical acetylcholine produces copious mucus,[114] although glycoprotein synthesis is not increased.[115] Secretin has been shown to increase the sugar content of glycoprotein in humans[116] and increase mucus viscosity in cats. Prostaglandins increase the amount of soluble mucus in rats without changing the glycoprotein content of surface mucus.[117] Cholecystokinin, gastrin, histamine,[118] serotonin, and carbachol (reversible by atropine)[119] also increase gastrointestinal mucus. The ulcer healing drug *carbenoxolone* increases the life-span of mucus-producing cells and the amount of stable mucus.[120] On the other hand, salicylates[121] and steroids decrease stainable mucus in the mucosa and the glycoprotein sugars in gastric juice.[122]

The glycoprotein content of mucus has been shown to be increased in patients with gastric ulcer compared to normal controls and those with duodenal ulcer.[123] Increased luminal glycoprotein sugars have been found in human stress erosions,[124] and duodenal ulcer patients have been found to have increased viscosity.[125] There is also histochemical and biochemical evidence that the nature of mucus is altered in malignant disease.[126]

Although considerable data have accumulated regarding the nature of gastric mucus, the physiological control mechanisms and the *in vivo* dynamic changes of pepsin-degraded soluble mucus versus mucosal surface have yet to be determined. Of considerable interest is the process by which not only ions such as H^+, but also large molecules, for example, pepsin, pass through the mucus layer from the mucosa into the lumen.

3.4. Bicarbonate Secretion

Secretion of bicarbonate by the stomach was first proposed by Schierbeck[127] in 1892, and Pavlov, 6 years later, suggested that an "alkaline mucus" lined the gastric mucosa and neutralized luminal acid.[128] In 1959 Heatley[129] presented evidence for a zone of low turbulence produced by mucus adherent to the mucosa, which allowed for gradients of bicarbonate secreted by the epithelium and H^+ ions diffusing from the lumen. The bicarbonate would protect the epithelium against acid by neutralizing the H^+ ions diffusing through the mucus layer to the mucosa. The study of bicarbonate secretion is hampered by the fact that stimuli for bicarbonate lead to a much greater simultaneous stimulation of acid secretion.

The human stomach secretes bicarbonate at basal rates varying between 0.4 and 2.6 mmol/hr.[129] Prostaglandin E_2 and its methyl derivatives in high intraluminal concentrations stimulate gastric alkali secretion.[130] This fact may contribute to its theoretical usefulness in peptic ulcer disease. Lower doses do not appear to produce stimulation, and this may represent a dose-related phenomenon. Aspirin and taurocholate, which produce mucosal damage, have been shown to inhibit alkali secretion,[131] and it has been suggested that mucosal injury may be due to a diminished neutralizing capacity, thus permitting greater H^+ ion back-diffusion. Urecholine, a cholinomimetic, increases bicarbonate secretion whereas histamine and gastrin have no effect.[132]

Recent work has revealed that gastric and duodenal epithelia secrete bicarbonate by an energy-dependent process at a maximum rate that is about 10% of that for acid.[133] The use of microelectrodes has demonstrated experimentally the existence of pH gradients, with neutralization of H^+ by secreted bicarbonate within the unstirred layers of mucus adherent to the mucosa,[134] the pH at the cell surface being much higher than in the luminal bulk solution.

Although it appears that a variety of agents can stimulate or inhibit gastric and duodenal bicarbonate secretion, interpretation of results remains difficult. The mucosa of the fundus or antrum contains tight junctions which have a low permeability for the passive transfer of ions.[135] Many agents, including aspirin and ethanol, described earlier, change mucosal permeability by their actions on tight junctions or by destruction of epithelium which leads to a marked increase in the passive migration of ions including bicarbonate from tissue and blood to the gastric lumen. This effect then gives rise to an apparent increased secretion of bicarbonate but merely represents a leaky gastric mucosa. To overcome this possible artifact, concurrent measurement of the electrical characteristics of the mucosa may help to differentiate true increases in secretion from luminal bicarbonate accumulation due to passive transfer since a leaky mucosa has a low potential difference and resistance.

Insights into mucosal defense mechanisms are only now beginning to answer the question proposed by Archibald Pitcairn (1652–1713): " . . . why, upon the Digestion of Food in the Stomach, which is as easily digestible as the Food, yet, the stomach itself should not be dissolved."[136]

4. A PHYSIOLOGICAL BASIS FOR THE CHOICE OF ULCER THERAPY

Epidemiological, clinical, and pathophysiological evidence indicates that the etiology of peptic ulceration is heterogeneous if unknown. On a background of genetic predisposition and certain environmental conditions, such as alcohol, analgesics, or indigestion, peptic ulcer may be due to an increase in gastric acidity and/or pepsin release, or a defect in mucosal resistance (Fig. 3). Thus, methods used to treat ulcers and thereby achieve the goals of medical therapy may be divided into two major categories: (1) drugs that reduce gastric acidity and peptic activity, and (2) drugs that enhance mucosal resistance (Table 1). This provides a working formula for drug prescription in peptic ulcer disease, although some agents, such as H_2-receptor antagonists, sucralfate, and the antacids, may have more than one effect.

4.1. Acid- and Pepsin-Inhibiting Drugs

This group includes H_2-receptor antagonists, proton pump inhibitors, anticholinergic agents and antacids. The mechanism of action differs but the end result is nevertheless elevation of intragastric pH. Contrary to original concepts, recent evidence suggests that acid suppression need

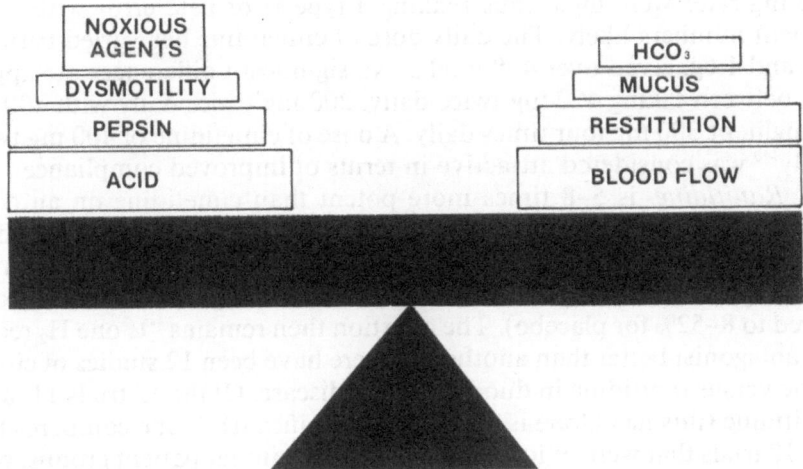

Figure 3. The occurrence of peptic ulceration may be viewed as a result of an imbalance between aggressive factors (left) and defensive factors (right). Therapy is aimed at restoration of this balance.

Table 1. Drugs Used in Peptic Ulcer Disease Divided into Those Which Reduce Acid and Peptic Activity and Those Which Enhance Mucosal Resistance

Controlling acid/pepsin	Enhancing defense
H_2-receptor antagonists	Prostaglandins
Prostaglandins	Carbenoxolone
Antacids	?Sucralfate
Anticholinergics	?Antacids
Benzimidazoles	?Bismuth
Trimipramine	

only be at night rather than for the whole 24 hr to obtain comparable 4-week healing rates.[137,138] The precise amount of acid inhibition required to promote ulcer healing has yet to be determined.

4.1.1. H_2-Receptor Antagonists

Since its release on the British market in 1976, *cimetidine* has been used in 30 million patients in 123 countries.[139] There have been over 35 trials of cimetidine versus placebo in duodenal ulcer healing. In all studies, cimetidine was superior to placebo, with 16 of the 23 studies showing significant improvement with cimetidine (61–90%) over placebo (14–59%). In the seven studies not showing a significant difference, placebo healing rates were high, thus making a type II or beta error with small patient numbers likely. The daily dose of cimetidine has varied between 0.8 and 1.6g, given over 4–8 weeks. No significant differences are apparent between taking 400 mg twice daily, 200 mg thrice daily with 400 mg at night, or 300 mg four times daily. A dose of cimetidine of 400 mg twice daily[140] was considered attractive in terms of improved compliance.

Ranitidine, is 5–8 times more potent than cimetidine on an equimolar basis, allowing a twice-daily dose of 150 mg to be used. Ranitidine is consistently better than placebo in duodenal ulcer healing, all 20 trials showing a significant advantage (54–100% healing for ranitidine compared to 8–52% for placebo). The question then remains "Is one H_2 receptor antagonist better than another?" There have been 12 studies of cimetidine versus ranitidine in duodenal ulcer disease. Of the 12 trials 11 favor ranitidine (this fact alone is statistically significant). If one compares 8 of the 12 trials that were of identical design with similar patient groups, with about 700 patients in each group (approximately the number calculated by Peterson and Elashoff[141] required to show a 10% significant difference when the less effective therapy is successful in 70% of patients), ranitidine's healing rate of 74% becomes statistically significantly superior to cimetidine's rate of 64% ($p < 0.05$).

A recent clinical pharmacological study of ranitidine, 300 mg at night,[137] showing a superior reduction in nocturnal acid secretion to conventional twice-daily administration has led to a five-center therapeutic trial conducted in the United Kingdom and Canada of ranitidine, 300 mg at night versus 150 mg twice daily in duodenal ulcer healing.[142] Ranitidine given as a nighttime dose gave a healing rate of 95% compared to 84% for twice-daily treatment, although this difference was not significant. The deleterious effect of smoking on ulcer healing was reaffirmed in this study, and could be overcome by the large evening dose of ranitidine.

The different efficacies of H_2 receptor antagonists in ulcer healing probably represent the effect of different potencies to inhibit gastric acid secretion at any given dose. Equipotency can be achieved if molar equivalent doses are administered.[143] This may account for the fact that the 4-week healing rate can be increased to 95% or better with most H_2 receptor antagonists continued for 6–8 weeks.

4.1.2. Proton Pump Inhibitors

The only clinically available example of this new and exciting group of compounds is the substituted benzimidazole *omeprazole*. One study[144] has shown dramatic healing rates in duodenal ulcer patients of 63% and 100% at 2 weeks with 20 mg and 60 mg respectively. At 4 weeks, healing rates reach 93% and 100%, respectively. The healing rate with omeprazole is dose dependent, since Prichard et al.[145] have shown healing rates of 50% and 78% at 2 weeks with 10 mg and 30 mg, increasing to 83% and 94%, respectively, at 4 weeks. This striking healing rate suggests that clinical benefit can be gained by stronger and longer-lasting inhibition of acid secretion.

At the time of writing, phase III clinical studies of this drug have been suspended because of the development of enterochromaffinlike cell hyperlasia in the 2-year rat toxicology studies. It has been proposed that these lesions have developed as a consequence of prolonged anacidity causing a sustained hypergastrinaemia, rather than as a direct toxicological effect. Further studies are awaited.

4.1.3. Antacids

Antacids have been renowned as effective agents in dyspepsia for two thousand years. Whereas the primary goal in antacid therapy has been to neutralize gastric acid, aluminium hydroxide gels, for example, are capable of inactivating pepsin independently of their pH effect. Additionally, antacids are potent binders of bile acids, and this property is of potential therapeutic value in gastric ulceration where duodenogastric reflux may be a contributing factor. A recent study has suggested that an additional property of antacids may be that of cytoprotection.[146] This could explain why healing rates for antacids, which essentially only buffer daytime acidity, are similar to single nocturnal H_2 receptor antagonist therapy.

Although antacids are principally used for pain relief, there have been seven studies of antacids in duodenal ulcer healing. In the original study by Peterson et al.,[147] antacids with a buffering capacity in excess of 1000 mmol/day healed 78% of ulcers, in 4 weeks, compared with 45% on placebo. Three other studies, using antacid doses of as little as 175 mmol/day, have also shown significant healing compared with placebo. Comparisons with cimetidine, however, have shown no significant differences.

There is some evidence that smaller doses of antacids can be used if combined with anticholinergics. In one study[148] 100% healing rates were achieved with antacid and l-hyoscyamine compared with 39% on placebo, with a significant reduction in anticholinergic side effects normally encountered with anticholinergics alone.

4.1.4. Anticholinergic Agents

Despite the fact that anticholinergics have been in use for several decades, only recently has there been a resurgence of interest in their use in peptic ulcer healing. Previous dissatisfaction with anticholinergic agents had arisen because of the unpleasant side effects associated with atropine. The isolation of gastric-specific muscarinic receptors and the development of a specific antagonist, pirenzepine, has resulted in a large number of endoscopically controlled studies; 12 studies have examined pirenzepine versus placebo, eight versus cimetidine, and five versus both cimetidine or placebo. According to earlier published results, pirenzepine probably fails to exhibit healing efficacy in duodenal ulcer when administered in a daily dose of 75 mg or less. Healing rates after 4–6 weeks of therapy with a dose of 100 mg or more range from 62 to 90%. Not all of the placebo-controlled studies reached significance, and in all of the comparisons with cimetidine, no significantly different healing rates were found.

4.1.5. Trimipramine

Trimipramine—a combination of the tricyclic antidepressant imipramine and levomepromazine—slightly inhibits basal and pentagastrin-stimulated acid and pepsin secretion. The precise mechanism of action in peptic ulcer disease is unknown since it is neither H_2-receptor blocker nor anticholinergic. An ulcer healing effect through a central antidepressive action has been suggested.[149]

The healing efficacy of trimipramine in duodenal ulcer has been compared in four trials each of placebo and cimetidine. Healing rates after 4–6 weeks' therapy were 46–100% with trimipramine compared with 15–48% for placebo (significant at 4 weeks in all four trials). When compared with cimetidine, healing rates with trimipramine were inferior.

4.2. Drugs That Enhance Mucosal Resistance

As outlined previously, mucosal resistance is dependent on a number of factors, including mucosal blood flow, stimulation of mucus and bicarbonate secretion, and mucosal cell turnover. Agents that may promote any of these factors, or allow regeneration of mucosa by physical exclusion of acid, pepsin, and bile salts, may then have a place in the therapy of peptic ulcer disease. These agents include carbenoxolone, tripotassium dicitratobismuthate, sucralfate, and prostaglandins.

4.2.1. Carbenoxolone

Carbenoxolone was first shown to promote ulcer healing 20 years ago. In both gastric and duodenal ulcer there is an average of a twofold improvement in ulcer healing over placebo in 11 studies. Comparison with cimetidine show a marginal superiority toward the H_2 antagonist in the treatment of gastric ulceration.[150,151]

Carbenoxolone, although effective in promoting gastric ulcer healing in particular, has the serious side effect of mineralocorticoid and aldosteronelike actions thus limiting its use in those patients most prone to develop gastric ulceration—the elderly.

The mode of action in ulcer healing is not well defined. Although it has weak antipeptic activity, other properties may be of more importance. Carbenoxolone increases glycoprotein synthesis, which is necessary for mucus formation and also reduces the activity of prostaglandin-inactivating enzymes in the mucosa.[152] Since spironolactone is known to nullify its healing action, interference with intracellular aldosterone receptor, or some dependence on maintenance of sodium–potassium fluxes, may be related to ulcer healing.

4.2.2. Tripotassium Dicitratobismuthate (TDB)

Colloidal bismuth (TDB) is a complex bismuth salt which forms insoluble complexes at acid pH. TDB selectively chelates with the proteinaceous material of the ulcer base forming a protective coating against acid, pepsin, and bile. There have been 21 trials of TDB in duodenal ulcer healing, 12 versus placebo and nine versus cimetidine. All of the placebo-controlled studies showed a significant healing rate (50–89%) over placebo. None of the cimetidine comparisons reached a statistically significant difference, with no trend in either direction.

An intriguing finding has been the suggestion that the relapse rate of duodenal ulcers after prior treatment with cimetidine is faster than after TDB,[153,154] although one particular study disagrees.[155] Whether ulcer healing with TDB really protects against relapse requires further study.

4.2.3. Sucralfate

Sucralfate is the basic aluminium salt of sucrose, substituted with eight sulfate groups. At acid pH, polymerization of sucrose octasulfate occurs leading to the deposition of a viscous paste which adheres to the gastric and duodenal mucosa. Sucralfate has a 6–7 times greater affinity for the ulcer base than for normal mucosa, thus providing a barrier to injurious agents. Additionally, the negatively charged sulfated macroanions of sucralfate bind to positively charged protein substrates and inhibit the formation of a pepsin–substrate complex, which suggests a specific antipeptic action of sucralfate.[156]

Of the 15 trials of sucralfate for duodenal ulcers, 10 have been against placebo and five versus cimetidine. Sucralfate, in a dose of 4 g/day, results in a healing rate of 60–100%. Placebo studies show high healing rates up to 64%. Therefore, 5 of the 10 studies did not show a statistically significant improvement on sucralfate, although a trend in favor of sucralfate is seen in all studies suggesting a type II error. The five comparative studies with cimetidine show no significant difference between sucralfate and cimetidine, with duodenal ulcer healing in both groups of the order of 70–80%.

4.2.4. Prostaglandins

Prostaglandin E_2 (PGE_2) and certain methyl analogs of PGE_2 inhibit gastric secretion in animals and humans, and they prevent the formation of experimental gastric and duodenal ulcers. 15 [R]-15-methyl PGE_2 (Arboprostil) improves healing in gastric ulcers, and more recently, a multicenter study of 173 patients has demonstrated that 67% of patients with duodenal ulcers were healed at 4 weeks compared with 39% receiving placebo.[157] Diarrhea is a common side effect of prostaglandin therapy, which may be less of a problem with newer analogs.

At the present time it is too early to determine the precise role of prostaglandins in peptic ulcer therapy, and true cytoprotective effects can be difficult to evaluate owing to the dose-dependent antisecretory property of the PGE_2 analogs.

5. CONCLUSION

The pathogenesis of peptic ulcer disease is believed to be multifactorial. However, a conceptual subdivision of the mechanisms into hyperacidity states and/or defective mucosal resistance allows a rational approach to the treatment of peptic ulceration. Healing rates on the standard therapies (Fig. 4) continue to improve with more logical timing of dose administration. However, significant failure and relapse rates still occur, which represents imperfect disease understanding accompanied by an inability to tailor therapy to the individual resistant patient. The advent of new, highly potent antisecretory drugs coupled with research into synthetic prostaglandins may provide a dual approach to the management of the patient with peptic ulcer disease and hopefully an improved understanding of disease etiology.

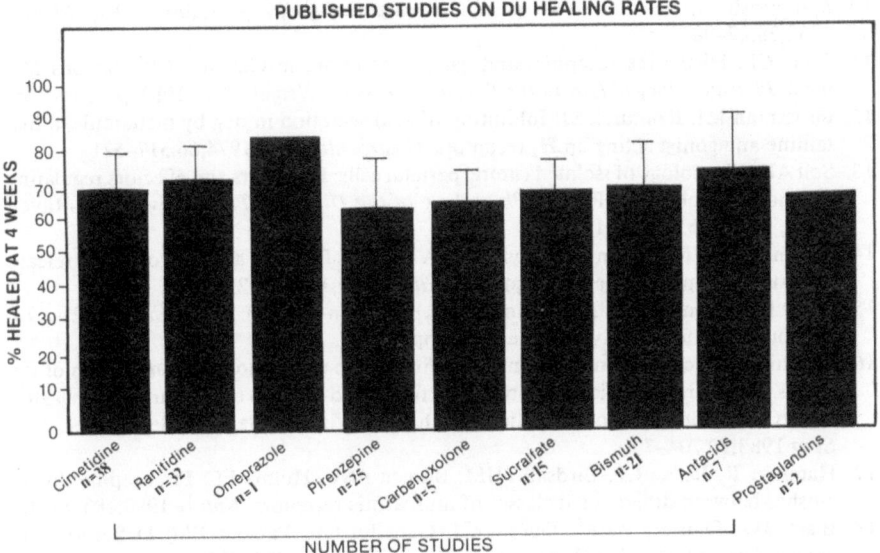

Figure 4. Mean (± SEM) healing rates after 4 weeks' treatment of duodenal ulcers for various agents.

REFERENCES

1. Cox AJ: Stomach size and its relation to chronic peptic ulcer. *Arch Pathol* 1952;54:407–422.
2. Card WI, Marks IN: The relationship between the acid output of the stomach following "maximal" histamine stimulation and the parietal cell mass. *Clin Sci* 1960;19:147–163.
3. Schwarz K: Ueber Penetrierende Magen-Und Jejunal Geschwure. *Beitr Z Klin Chir Tubing* 1910;67:96–128.
4. Feldman M: Comparison of acid secretion rates measured by gastric aspiration and by *in vivo* intragastric titration in healthy human subjects. *Gastroenterology* 1979;76:954–957.
5. Malagelada JR, Longstreth, GF, Summerskill WHJ, Go VJW: Measurement of gastric functions during digestion of ordinary solid meals in man. *Gastroenterology* 1976;70:203–210.
6. Forte JG, Forte TM, Machen TE: Histamine stimulated hydrogen ion secretion by *in vitro* piglet gastric mucosa. *J Physiol* 1975;244:15–31.
7. Berglindh T, Obrink KJ: A method for preparing isolated glands from the rabbit gastric mucosa. *Acta Physiol Scand* 1976;96:150–159.
8. Soll AH: The actions of secretagogues on oxygen uptake by isolated mammalian parietal cells. *J Clin Invest* 1978;61:370–380.
9. Grossman MI: Chemical messengers: A view from the gut. *Fed Proc* 1979;38:2341–2343.

10. MacIntosh FC: Histamine as normal stimulant of gastric secretion. *J Exp Physiol* 1938;28:87–98.
11. Code CF: Histamine receptors and gastric secretion, in Ganellin CR, Parsons ME (eds): *Pharmacology of Histamine Receptors*. Bristol: Wright, PSG, 1982, pp. 217–235.
12. Grossman MI, Konturek SJ: Inhibition of acid secretion in dog by metiamide, a histamine antagonist acting on H_2 receptors. *Gastroenterology* 1974;66:517–521.
13. Soll AH, Physiology of isolated canine parietal cells: Receptors and effectors regulating function, in Johnson LR (ed): *Physiology of the Digestive Tract*. New York: Raven Press, 1981, pp. 673–691.
14. Feldman M, Richardson CT, Taylor IL, Walsh JH, Effect of atropine on vagal release of gastrin and pancreatic polypeptide. *J Clin Invest* 1979;63:294–298.
15. Hunt RH: Non-responders to cimetidine, in Baron JII (ed): *Cimetidine in the 80's*. Edinburgh: Churchill Livingstone, 1981, pp. 34–41.
16. Gledhill T, Buck M, Paul A, Hunt RH: Cimetidine or vagotomy? Comparison of the effects of proximal gastric vagotomy, cimetidine and placebo on nocturnal intragastric acidity and acid secretion in patients with cimetidine resistant duodenal ulcer. *Br J Surg* 1983;70:704–706.
17. Hammer R, Berrie CP, Birdsall NJM, Burgen ASV, Hulme EC: Pirenzepine distinguishes between different subclasses of muscarinic receptors. *Nature* 1980;283:90–92.
18. Black JW, Duncan WAM, Durant CJ, Ganellin CR, Parsons EM: Definition and antagonism of histamine H_2-receptors. *Nature* 1972;236:385–390.
19. Hunt RH, Mills JG, Beresford J, Billings JA, Burland WL, Milton-Thompson GJ: Gastric secretory studies in humans with impromidine (SKF92676) a specific histamine H_2-receptor agonist. *Gastroenterology* 1980;78:505–512.
20. Berglindh T, Sachs G, Takeguchi N: Ca^{++}-dependent secretagogue stimulation in isolated rabbit gastric glands. *Am J Physiol* 1980;239:G90–G94.
21. Machen TE, Rutten MJ, Ekblad EBM: Histamine, cAMP, and activation of piglet gastric mucosa. *Am J Physiol* 1982;242:G79–G84.
22. Berglindh T, Dibona DK, Ito S, Sachs G: Probes of parietal cell function. *Am J Physiol* 1980;238:G165–G176.
23. Soll AH, Grossman MI: The interaction of stimulants on the function of the isolated canine parietal cells. *Philos Trans R Soc, London (Biol)* 1981;296:5–15.
24. Shaltz LJ, Bools C, Reimann EM: Phosphorylation of membranes from the rat gastric mucosa. *Biochim Biophys Acta* 1981;673:539–551.
25. Knight DE, Baker PF: Calcium dependence of catecholamine release from bovine adrenal medullary cells after exposure to intense electric fields. *J Membrane Biol* 1982;68:107–140.
26. Sachs G, Chang HH, Rabon E, Schackman R, Lewin M, Saccomani G: A nonelectrogenic H^+ pump in plasma membranes of hog stomach. *J Biol Chem* 1976;251:7690–7698.
27. Fellenius E, Elander B, Wallmark B, Helander HF, Berglindh T: Inhibition of acid secretion in isolated gastric glands by substrated benzimidazoles. *Am J Physiol* 1982;243:G505–G510.
28. Lind T, Cederberg C, Ekenved G, Haglund U, Olbe L: Effect of omeprazole—A gastric proton pump inhibitor on pentagastrin stimulated acid secretion in man. *Gut* 1983;24:270–276.
29. Muller P, Dammann HG, Seitz H, Simon B: Effect of repeated once daily oral omeprazole on gastric secretion. *Lancet* 1983;1:66 (letter).

30. Schwann T: Ueber das Wesen des Verdauungsprocesses. *Mullers Arch J Anat Physiol* 1836;90–138
31. Schiffrin MJ, Warren AA: Some factors concerned in the production of experimental ulceration in the GI tract in cats. *Am J Dig Dis* 1942;9:205–209.
32. Driver RL, Chappell RH, Carmichael EB: Effect of concentration of pepsin and the differential susceptibility of jejunal segments in experimental jejunal ulcers in the dog. *Am J Dig Dis* 1945;12:166–167.
33. Alphin RS, Vokac VA, Gregory RL, Bolton PM, Tawes JW III: Role of intragastric pressure, pH and pepsin in gastric ulceration in the rat. *Gastroenterology* 1977;73:495–500.
34. Northrop, JH: Crystalline pepsin: Isolation and tests of purity. *J Gen Physiol* 1933;16:615–623.
35. Herriott RM, Northrop JH: Isolation of crystalline pepsinogen from swine gastric mucosae and its autocatalytic conversion to pepsin. *Science* 1936;83:469–470.
36. Janowitz HD, Hollander F: The exocrine–endocrine partition of enzymes in the digestive tract. *Gastroenterology* 1951;17:591–592.
37. Ellis A, McConnell RB: Duodenal ulcer and urinary pepsinogen phenotypes. *Gastroenterology* 1982;83:1261–1263.
38. Rotter JI, Sones JQ, Samloff IM, et al: Duodenal ulcer disease associated with elevated serum pepsinogen I: An inherited autosomal dominant disorder. *N Engl J Med* 1979;300:63–66.
39. Samloff IM, Townes PL: Electrophoretic heterogeneity and relationships of pepsinogens in human urine, serum and gastric mucosa. *Gastroenterology* 1970;58:462–469.
40. Burhol PG, Hirschowitz BI: Dose responses with subcutaneous infusion of histamine in gastric fistula chickens. *Am J Physiol* 1972;222:308–313.
41. Hirschowitz BI: Secretion of pepsinogen, in Code CF (ed): *Handbook of Physiology.* Section 6. Washington, DC: American Physiology Society, 1967,pp.889–918.
42. Bynum TE, Johnson LR: Stimulation of human pepsin output by topical hydrochloric acid. *Am J Dig Dis* 1975;20:7:607–612.
43. Johnson LR: Regulation of pepsin secretion by topical acid in the stomach. *Am J Physiol* 1972;223:4:847–850.
44. Berstad A, Petersen H, Roland M, Liavag I: The effect of secretin on pentagastrin-stimulated gastric acid and pepsin secretion after vagotomy in man. *Scand J Gastroenterol* 1973;8:119–122.
45. Hirschowitz BI, London J: Studies of the secretion of acid, water and pepsinogen by the human stomach. *J Lab Clin Med* 1955;46:826–827.
46. Hirschowitz BI, Hutchinson GA: Evidence for a histamine H_2 receptor that inhibits pepsin secretion in the dog. *Am J Physiol* 1977;233:E225–228.
47. Brooks AM, Isenberg J, Grossman MI: The effect of secretin, glucagon and duodenal acidification on pepsin secretion in man. *Gastroenterology* 1969;57:159–162.
48. Gibson, R, Hirschowitz BI, Hutchinson G: Actions of metiamide, an H_2-histamine receptor antagonist, on gastric H^+ and pepsin secretion in dogs. *Gastroenterology* 1974;67:93–99.
49. Hirschowitz BI, Molina E: Effects of four H_2 histamine antagonists on bethanechol-stimulated acid and pepsin secretion in the dog. *J Pharm Exp Ther* 1983;224(2):341–345.
50. Fritsh WP, Scholten T, Muller J, Hengew KJ, in Holtermuller, Malagelada (eds): *Advances in Ulcer Diseases.* Munich: JR Excerpta Medica, 1980, pp.427–449.

51. Johnston D, Wilkinson AR: Highly selective vagotomy without a drainage procedure in the treatment of duodenal ulcer. *Br J Surg* 1970;57:289–296.
52. Gledhill T, Buck M, McEwan J, Hunt H: The effect of cimetidine 1g/day and cimetidine 2g/day on 24 hr intragastric acidity and nocturnal acid secretion in cimetidine nonresponders. *Gut* 1982;23:A456.
53. Berstad A, Petersen H: Comparison of histamine and pentagastrin in stimulation of pepsin secretion in man. *Scand J Gastroenterol* 1971;6(3):209–216.
54. Aagaard P, Christiansen J: Dose–response studies of gastric pepsin secretion in man after stimulation with pentagastrin. *Digestion* 1970;3:279–284.
55. Waldum HL, Burhol PG, Straume BK: Serum group I pepsinogens during prolonged infusion of pentagastrin and secretin in man. *Scand J Gastroenterol* 1979;14(6):761–768.
56. Limbosch JM, de Graef J: Comparative effects of gastrin, pentagastrin and insulin on acid and pepsin secretion in man. *Acta Hepatogastroenterol (Stuttg)* 1972;19(1):19–24.
57. Hirschowitz BI: The control of pepsinogen secretion. *Ann NY Acad Sci* 1967;140(2):709–723.
58. Linde S: Studies on stimulation mechanism of gastric secretion. *Acta Physiol Scand* 1950;21(Suppl 74):1–92.
59. Hirschowitz BI, Hutchinson GA: Evidence for a histamine H_2 receptor that inhibits pepsin secretion in the dog. *Am J Physiol* 1977;233(3):E225–8.
60. Desai HG, Zaveri MP, Antia FP: Minimal dose of a stimulus for maximal pepsin secretion. *Postgrad Med J* 1973;49:258–260.
61. de Gara CJ, Gledhill T, Silletti C, Sivakumaran T, Hunt RH: Impromidine and Pentagastrin: a dose response inhibition of pepsin output. *Gastroenterology* 1984;86(Part 2):1059.
62. Hirschowitz, BI, Rentz J, Molina E: Histamine H_2 receptor stimulation and inhibition of pepsin secretion in the dog. *J Pharmacol Exp Ther* 1981;218(3):676–680.
63. Hirschowitz BI, Gibson RG: Effect of cimetidine on stimulated gastric secretion and serum gastrin in the dog. *Am J Gastroenterol* 1978;70(5):437–447.
64. Davenport HW: Gastric mucosal injury by fatty and acetylsalicylic acids. *Gastroenterology* 1964;46:245–253.
65. Jacobson ED, Linford RH, Grossman MI: Gastric secretion in relation to mucosal blood flow studied by a clearance technic. *J Clin Invest* 1966;45:1–13.
66. Delaney JP, Grim E: Canine gastric blood flow and its distribution. *Am J Physiol* 1964;207:1195–1202.
67. Steiner SH, Muller GCE: Distribution of blood flow in the digestive tract of the rat. *Circ Res* 1961;9:99–102.
68. Bell PRF, Shelley T: Gastric mucosal blood flow and acid secretion in conscious animals measured by heat clearance. *Am J Dig Dis* 1968;13:685–696.
69. Bell PRF, Battersby C: Effect of vagotomy on gastric mucosal blood flow. *Gastroenterology* 1968;54:1032–1037.
70. Levitt MD, Levitt DG: Use of inert gases to study the interaction of blood flow and diffusion during passive absorption from the gastrointestinal tract of the rat. *J Clin Invest* 1973;52:1852–1862.
71. Leonard AS, Long D, French LA, Peter ET, Wangensteen OH: Pendular pattern in gastric secretion and blood flow following hypothalamic stimulation—origin of stress ulcer? *Surgery* 1964;56:109–120.
72. Osumi Y, Aibara S, Sakae K, Fujiwara M: Central noradrenergic inhibition of gastric mucosal blood flow and acid secretion in rats. *Life Sci* 1977;20:1407–1416.

73. Martinson J: Studies on the efferent vagal control of the stomach. *Acta Physiol Scand* 1965;65(Suppl 255):1-24.

74. Nakamuray K, Ishi K, Kusano M, Hayashi S: Acute and longterm effects of vagotomy on gastric mucosal blood flow, in Halle F, Andersson S (eds): *Vagotomy: Latest Advances with Special Reference to Gastric and Duodenal Ulcer.* New York: Springer-Verlag, 1974, pp. 109-111.

75. Van Hee RH, Vanhoutte PM: Cholinergic inhibition of adrenergic neuro transmission in the canine gastric artery. *Gastroenterology* 1978;74:1266-1270.

76. Guth PH, Smith E: Histamine receptors in the gastric microcirculation. *Gut* 1978;19:1059-1063.

77. Levine BA, Schwesinger WH, Sirinek KR, Jones D, Pruitt BA: Cimetidine prevents reduction in gastric mucosal blood flow during shock. *Surgery* 1978;84:113-119.

78. Konturek SJ, Dembinski A, Thor P, Krol R: Comparison of vasoactive intestinal peptide (VIP) and secretin in gastric secretion and mucosal blood flow. *Pfluegers Arch* 1976;361:175-181.

79. Skarstein A: Effect of vasopressin on blood flow distribution in the stomach of cats with gastric ulcer. *Scand J Gastroenterol* 1978;13:783-788.

80. Konturek SJ, Tasler J, Cieszkowski M, Coy DH, Schally AV: Effect of growth hormone release inhibiting hormone on gastric secretion, mucosal blood flow, and serum gastrin. *Gastroenterology* 1976;70:737-741.

81. Whittle BJR, Boughton-Smith NK, Moncada S, Vane JR: Actions of prostacyclin (PGI$_2$) and its product 6-oxo-PGF$_1$ alpha on the rat gastric mucosa *in vivo* and *in vitro.* *Prostaglandins* 1978;15:955-967.

82. Main IHM, Whittle BJR: The effects E and A prostaglandins on gastric mucosal blood flow and acid secretion in the rat. *Br J Pharmacol* 1973;49:428-436.

83. Gerkens JF, Shand DG, Flexner C, Nies AS, Oates JA, Data JL: Effect of indomethacin and aspirin on gastric blood flow and acid secretion *J Pharmacol Exp Ther* 1977;203:646-652.

84. Whittle BJR: Mechanisms underlying gastric mucosal damage induced by indomethacin and bile salts and the actions of prostaglandins. *Br J Pharmacol* 1977;60:455-460.

85. Moody FG, Durbin RP: Effects of glycine and other instillates on concentration of gastric acid. *Am J Physiol* 1965;209:122-126.

86. Smith P, O'Brien P, Fromm D, Silen W: Secretory state of gastric mucosa and resistance to injury by exogenous acid. *Am J Surg* 1977;133:81-85.

87. Ussing HH, Zerahn K: Active transport of sodium as the source of electric current in the short-circuited isolated frogskin. *Acta Physiol Scand* 1951;23:110-127.

88. Geall MG, Phillips SF, Summerskill DM: Profile of gastric potential difference in man. *Gastroenterology* 1970;58:437-443.

89. Rainsford KD, Whitehouse MW: Gastric irritancy of aspirin and its congeners: antiinflammatory activity without this side effect. *J Pharmacol* 1976;28:599-601.

90. Hingson DJ, Ito S: Effect of aspirin and related compounds on the fine structure of mouse gastric mucosa. *Gastroenterology* 1971;61:156-177.

91. Black RB, Hole D, Rhodes J: Bile damage to gastric mucosal barrier: the influence of pH and bile acid concentration. *Gastroenterology* 1971;61:178-184.

92. Wassef MK, Lin YN, Horowitz MI: Phospholipid-deacylating enzymes of rat stomach mucosa. *Biochim Biophys Acta* 1978;528:318-330.

93. Davenport HW: Protein losing gastropathy produced by sulfhydryl reagents. *Gastroenterology* 1971;60:870-879.

94. Kivilaakso E, Fromm D, Silen W: Effects of lysolecithin on isolated gastric mucosa. *Surgery* 1978;84:616-621.

95. Cooke AR, Kienzle MG: Studies of anti-inflammatory drugs and aliphatic alcohols on antral mucoa. *Gastroenterology* 1974;66:56–62.

96. Fromm D: Ion selective effects of salicylate on antral mucosa. *Gastroenterology* 1976;71:743–749.

97. Kuo YJ, Shanbour LL: Inhibition of ion transport by bile salts in canine gastric mucosa. *Am J Physiol* 1976;231:1433–1437.

98. Mitznegg P, Estler CJ, Loew FW, van Seil J: Effects of salicylates on cyclic AMP in isolated rat gastric mucosa. *Acta Hepatogastroenterol (Stuttg)* 1977;24:372–376.

99. Tompkins L, Lee KH: Studies on the mechanism of action of salicylates IV: Effect of salicylate on oxidative phosphorylation. *J Pharm Sci* 1969;58:102–105.

100. Fuhro R, Fromm D: Effects of compounds chemically related to salicylate on isolated antral mucosa of rabbits. *Gastroenterology* 75;661–667.

101. Chvasta TE, Cooke AR: The effect of several ulcerogenic drugs on the canine gastric mucosal barrier. *J Lab Clin Med* 1972;79:302–315.

102. Chung RSK, Field M, Silen W: Effects of methylprednisolone on hydrogen ion absorption in the canine stomach. *J Clin Invest* 1978;62:262–270.

103. Robert A: Anti-secretory, anti-ulcer, cytoprotective and diarrheogenic properties of prostaglandins, in Samuelsson B, Paoletti R (eds): *Advances in Prostaglandin and Thromboxane Research,* Vol. 2. New York: Raven Press, 1976, pp. 507–521.

104. Lacy ER, Ito S: Microscopic analysis of ethanol damage to rat gastric mucosa after treatment with a prostaglandin. *Gastroenterology* 1982;83:619–625.

105. O'Kabe S, Takeuchi K, Honda K, Takagi K: Effects of various amino acids on gastric lesions induced by acetylsalicylic acid (ASA) and gastric secretion in pylorus ligated rats. *Drug Res* 1976;26:534–537.

106. Miller TA, Jacobson ED: Gastrointestinal cytoprotection by prostaglandins. *Gut* 1979;20:75–87.

107. Carmichael HA, Nelson LM, Russell RI: Cimetidine and prostaglandin: Evidence for different modes on action of the rat gastric mucosa. *Gastroenterology* 1978;74:1229–1232.

108. Bommelaer G, Guth PH: Protection by histamine receptor antagonists and prostaglandin against gastric mucosal barrier disruption in the rat. *Gastroenterology* 1979;77:303–308.

109. Hills BA, Butler BD, Lichtenberger LM: Gastric mucosal barrier: Hydrophobic lining to the lumen of the stomach. *Am J Physiol* 1983;244:G561–G568.

110. Pearson J, Allen A, Venables C: Gastric mucus: Isolation and polymeric structure of the undegraded glycoprotein: its breakdown by pepsin. *Gastroenterology* 1980;78:709–715.

111. Bickel M, Kauffman GL: Gastric gel mucus thickness: Effect of distension 16, 16-dimethyl prostaglandin E_2 and carbenoxolone. *Gastroenterology* 1981;80:770–775.

112. Schacter H: Glycoprotein synthesis, in Horowitz, Pigman (eds): *Colon v Glycocongugates,* Vol II. New York: Academic Press, 1978, pp. 87–181.

113. MacDermott RP, Donaldson RM, Trier JS: Glycoprotein synthesis and secretion by mucosal biopsies of rabbit colon and human rectum. *J Clin Invest* 1974;54:545–554.

114. Horowitz MI, Hollander F: Evidence regarding the chemical complexity of acetylcholine-stimulated gastric mucus. *Gastroenterology* 1961;40:785–793.

115. Andre C, Lambert R, Descos F: Stimulation of gastric mucous secretions in man by secretion. *Digestion* 1972;7:284–293.

116. Kaura R, Allen A, Hirst BH: Mucus in the gastric juice of cats during pentagastrin and secretin infusions: The viscosity in relation to glycoprotein structure and concentration. *Biochem Soc Trans* 1980;8:52–53.

117. Bolton JP, Palmer D, Cohen MM: Stimulation of mucus and nonparietal cells secretion by the E_2 prostaglandins. *Am J Dig Dis* 1978;23:359–367.
118. Vagne M, Perret G: Regulation of gastric mucus secretion. *Scand J Gastroenterol* 1976;11(Suppl 42):63–74.
119. Black JW, Bradbury AE, Wyllie JH: Stimulation of colonic mucus output in the rat. *Br J Pharmacol* 1979;66:456P–457P.
120. Steer HW, Colin-Jones DG: Mucosal changes in gastric ulceration and their response to carbenoxolone sodium. *Gut* 1975;16:590–597.
121. Menguy R, Masters YF: Effects of aspirin on gastric mucous secretion. *Surg Gynecol Obstet* 1965;120:92–98.
122. Desbaillets L, Menguy R: Inhibition of gastric mucous secretion by ACTH. *Am J Dig Dis* 1967;12:582–588.
123. Roberts-Thompson IC, Clarke AE, Maritz VM, Denborough MA: Gastric glycoproteins in chronic peptic ulcer. *Aust NZ J Med* 1975;5:507–514.
124. Glass GBJ, Slomiany BL: Derangements in gastrointestinal injury and disease, in Elstein M, Parke DV (eds): *Mucus in Health and Disease*. New York: Plenum Press, 1977, pp. 227–238.
125. Pringle R: Gastric mucus viscosity and peptic ulcer, in Elstein M, Parke DV (eds): *Mucus in Health and Disease*. New York: Plenum Press, 1977, pp. 227–238.
126. Kimoto E, Kuranari T, Masuda H, Takeughi M: Isolation and characterization of a glycopeptide from mucinous carcinoma of human stomach. *J Biochem* 1968;63:542–549.
127. Schierbeck NP: Ueber Kohlensaure im Ventrikel. *Skand Arch Physiol* 1892;3:437–474.
128. Pavlov JP: *Die Arbeit der Verdauu In Gsdrusen*. Wiesbaden: JF Bergman Verlag, 1898.
129. Heatley NG: Mucosubstance as a barrier to diffusion. *Gastroenterology* 1959;37:313–317.
130. Flemstrom G, Heylings JR, Garner A: Gastric and duodenal HCO_3^- transport *in vitro:* Effects of hormones and local transmitters. *Am J Physiol* 1982;242:G100–G110.
131. Rees WDW, Gibbons LC, Warhurst G, Turnberg LA: Studies of bicarbonate secretion by the normal human stomach *in vivo*—Effect of aspirin, sodium taurocholate and prostaglansin E_2, in: Allan A, Flemstrom G, Garner A (eds): *Mechanisms of Mucosal Production in the Upper Gastrointestinal Tract*. New York: Raven Press, 1983, pp. 119–123.
132. Feldman M, Barnett CC: Gastric bicarbonate secretion in humans. Effects of pentagastrin, bethanechol and 11, 16, 16-trimethyl prostaglandin E_2. *J Clin Invest* 1983;72:295–303.
133. Johansson C, Aly A, Nilsson E, Flemstrom G: Stimulation of gastric bicarbonate secretion by E_2 prostaglandins in man, in Samuelsson B, Paoletti R, Ramwell D (eds): *Advances in Prostaglandin, Thromboxane and Leukotriene Research*, Vol. 12. New York: Raven Press, 1983, pp. 395–401.
134. Rees WDW, Botham D, Turnberg LA: A demonstration of bicarbonate production by the normal human stomach *in vivo*. *Dig Dis Sci* 1982;27:961–966.
135. Spenney JG, Shoemaker RL, Sachs G: Microelectrode studies of fundic gastric mucosa: Cellular coupling and shunt conductance. *J Membrane Biol* 1974;19:105–128.
136. Pitcairn A: The dissertation upon the motion which reduces the aliment in the stomach to a form proper for the supply of blood, in *The Whole Works*, 2 ed (Sewell G,) transl. London: JT Desaguliers, 1727, pp. 106–38.
137. Gledhill T, Howard OM, Buck M, Paul A, Hunt RH: Single nocturnal dose of an H_2 receptor antagonist for the treatment of duodenal ulcer. *Gut* 1983;24:904–908.

138. de Gara CJ, Burget D, Siletti C, Hunt RH: Is the daytime control of acid secretion really necessary? *Scand J Gastroenterol* 1984;19:(Suppl 98):7.

139. McGuigan JE: Safety of cimetidine: An overview, in Cohen S (ed): *Update: H₂-Receptor Antagonists.* New York: Biomedical Information, 1984, pp. 179–184.

140. Kerr GD: Cimetidine. Twice daily administration in duodenal ulcer—Results of the UK and Ireland multicentre study, in Baron JH (ed): *Cimetidine in the 80's.* Edinburgh: Churchill Livingstone, 1981, pp. 9/13.

141. Peterson WL, Elashoff J: Placebo in clinical trials of duodenal ulcer: The end of an era? *Gastroenterology* 1980;79:585–588.

142. Ireland A, Colin-Jones DG, Gear P, et al: Ranitidine 150 mg twice daily versus 300 mg nightly in treatment of duodenal ulcers. *Lancet* 1984;2(8397):274–276.

143. Milton-Thompson GJ: Comparative clinical pharmacology of the H₂ receptor antagonists, in Cohen S (ed): *Update: H₂ Receptor Antagonists.* New York: Biomedical Information, 1984, pp. 3–8.

144. Gustavsson S, Adami HO, Loof A, Nyberg A, Nyren O: Rapid healing of duodenal ulcers with omeprazole: Double-blind dose-comparative trial. *Lancet* 1983;2(8342):124–125.

145. Prichard PJ, Rubenstein D, Jones DB, et al: Omeprazole: Double-blind comparison of 10mg versus 30mg for healing duodenal ulcers. *Gastroenterology* 1984;86:1213.

146. Hollander D, Tarnawski A, Cummings D, Krause WJ, Gergely H, Zipser RD: Cytoprotective action of antacids against alcohol induced gastric mucosal injury. Morphologic, ultrastructural and functional time sequence analysis. *Gastroenterology* 1984;86:1114.

147. Peterson WL, Sturdevant RAL, Frankl HD, et al: Healing of duodenal ulcer with an antacid regimen. *N Engl J Med* 1977;297:341–345.

148. Strom M, Gotthard R, Bodemar G, Walan A: Antacid/anticholinergic, cimetidine and placebo in treatment of active peptic ulcers. *Scand J Gastroenterol* 1981;16:593–602.

149. Siurala M: The possible significance of the central action of trimipramine in the treatment of functional "non-ulcer" dyspepsia and peptic ulcer with masked depression. *Scand J Gastroenterol* 1979;15(Suppl 58):57–58.

150. Colin-Jones DG, Misiewicz JJ, Milton-Thompson GJ, Hunt RH, Golding PI: Cimetidine and carbonoxolone in gastric ulcer, in Wastell C, Lance P (eds): *Cimetidine: The Westminster Hospital Symposium.* Edinburgh: Churchill Livingstone, 1978, pp. 289–291.

151. Petrillo M, Bianchi Porro G, Valantini M, Dobrilla G: Cimetidine and carbonoxolone sodium in the treatment of gastric ulcer: An open pilot study. *Curr Ther Res* 1979;26:990–994.

152. Domschke W, Domschke S, Hagel J, Demling L, Croft DN: Gastric epithelial cell turnover, mucus production and healing of gastric ulcers with carbenoxolone. *Gut* 1979;18:817–820.

153. Martin DF, Hollanders D, May SJ, Ravenscroft MM, Tweedle DE, Miller JP: Difference in relapse rates of duodenal ulcer after healing with cimetidine or tripotassium dicitratobismuthate. *Lancet* 1981;1:7–10.

154. Bianchi Porro G, Lazzaroni M, Petrillo M, de Nicola C: Relapse rates in duodenal ulcer patients formerly treated with bismuth subcitrate or maintained with cimetidine. *Lancet* 1984;2:698 (letter).

155. Kang JY, Piper DW: Cimetidine and colloidal bismuth in the treatment of chronic duodenal ulcer: Comparison of initial healing and recurrence after healing. *Digestion* 1982;23:73–79.

156. Samloff IM: Inhibition of peptic aggression by sucralfate. A view from the ulcer creator. *Scand J Gastroenterol* 1983;18(Suppl 83):7–11.
157. Vantrappen G, Janssens J, Popiela T, et al: Effect of 15 (R)-15-methyl prostaglandin E₂ (arbaprostil) on the healing of duodenal ulcer: A double-blind multicentre study. *Gastroenterology* 1982;83:357–363.

2

Peptic Ulcer Disease
Is There a Need to Be Selective or Superselective?

David Fromm

1. INTRODUCTION

As technical details and acid secretory consequences of the various operative procedures for peptic ulcer disease became better understood in the 1950s and 1960s, greater emphasis was placed on determining the incidence of dumping and other long-term sequelae of peptic ulcer surgery. The frequency of various syndromes occurring after gastrectomy and/or vagotomy ranged from practically none to uniform occurrence. These figures were used to support employment of one operation over others, but agreement was far from uniform. However, it remained for the Leeds/York prospective study, published in 1968, to put the problem in proper perspective.[1] As the incidence of sequelae related to removal or destruction or bypass of the pylorus and vagotomy became better appreciated, interest in the 1970s gravitated toward proximal gastric (or highly selective) vagotomy. This acid-reducing operation could safely permit leaving the pylorus intact.

The 1970s were also marked by closer scrutiny of the incidence of recurrent ulcer after operation. Previous reports were confusing because of inclusion of both proven and "suspected" recurrences in the data. Furthermore, medication-induced ulceration in patients who had undergone gastric surgery was not readily appreciated or even well understood. With

David Fromm ● Department of Surgery, State University of New York–Upstate Medical Center, Syracuse, New York 13210.

the introduction of proximal gastric vagotomy and the ready availability of a more acceptable and reliable method for upper gastrointestinal endoscopy, there was increasing enthusiasm for prospective studies. Studies appeared in increasing numbers, but none had long-term endoscopic follow-up. Answers to a number of difficult questions relating to operative treatment were eagerly awaited, but suddenly the reports of prospective studies became few indeed. In fact, a large cooperative study in the United States was disbanded because of the dearth of patients.

Just as enthusiasm for proximal gastric vagotomy was increasing in the United States, cimetidine became clinically available. Although the incidence of peptic ulcer surgery had been progressively declining since 1973, this became more noticeable in 1978, the year after the introduction of a practical H_2 receptor antagonist.[2] The decline continued thereafter on its previous straight-line course. Reasons for the continuing decline in peptic ulcer disease requiring operation are speculative even though they are undoubtedly related to the decreasing incidence of ulcer. In the United States, the incidence of peptic ulcer disease as a whole has decreased from 1968 to 1975. Along with this trend there has been a decline in hospitalization rates for uncomplicated peptic ulcer disease. This is, at least in part, due to changes in the criteria for hospital admission, coding practices, and diagnostic procedures. Yet, there has been little or no change in hospitalization rates for perforated duodenal ulcer and only a slight decrease in admissions for hemorrhage. Deaths from peptic ulcer, both as an underlying and as a contributing cause, also have been declining since 1962. Thus, the impact of newer modes of nonoperative treatment on the necessity for operation is unclear and even difficult to determine.

Now that the presence of peptic ulcer can be established with precision, now that the etiology of certain types of ulcers is known, and now that the side effects of various operations are fairly well appreciated, the question of the degree of selectivity can be applied to many areas of surgery for peptic ulcer disease. However, this discussion will be confined to certain preoperative considerations that dictate a highly selective approach and the results of various operations done electively for peptic ulcer that should dictate a selective approach.

2. INTRACTABILITY AS AN INDICATION FOR OPERATION

In addition to the H_2 receptor antagonists, newer classes of medications for the treatment of peptic ulcer disease have been introduced recently. Present-day nonantacid medications taken for relatively short periods can be very effective, but there are concerns about the unknown long-term side effects of such medications. Even if it can be shown that these medications are safe when taken for the prolonged periods necessitated by the natural history of peptic ulcer disease, it appears unlikely that they will have a significant long-term impact on the indications for operation.

An important benefit of effective medications more readily taken than frequent antacids is that failure of compliance as an indication for operation has become much less common. Peptic ulcer disease appears to be a lifelong phenomenon, marked by periodic healing and recurrence. The majority of recurrences respond to repeated courses of medications. Prolonged liquid antacid use is impractical for many patients, but the long-term effects of H_2 receptor antagonists and other more easily taken medications are unclear.

Frequently, it is helpful to make a distinction between asymptomatic and symptomatic recurrence, since symptomatic patients are more likely to opt for operation, especially when these symptoms interfere with their daily activities. However, asymptomatic ulcers also present a threat, as illustrated by the patient who perforates or bleeds as the first recognized manifestation of the disease. Although many such patients will on careful inquiry have premonitory symptoms, they are often mild enough that patient and physician pay little attention.

Certain types of ulcers are notorious in terms of failing to heal or of recurring. Examples include giant duodenal, pyloric channel, and post-bulbar ulcers. Whereas in the past, patients with these types of ulcers were advised to have an early operation, the situation is less clear today because such ulcers may heal with cimetidine treatment. Although the data are not yet entirely clear, one of the advantages of readily acceptable medication such as an H_2 receptor antagonist may be that it more readily helps to select out those patients who are prone to frequent, threatening recurrences despite adequate nonoperative treatment.

Although intractability as an indication for operation is becoming easier to define as more patients comply with their treatment, there still is a wide range of disagreement about when nonoperative treatment has indeed failed, particularly in the absence of obstruction, perforation, or bleeding.

3. OTHER PREOPERATIVE CONSIDERATIONS

It is helpful to have certain information about the serum gastrin, the location of the ulcer, perhaps the level of gastric secretion, and, in the case of gastric ulcer, whether or not malignancy is present prior to operation. This facilitates proper planning of surgery and thus minimizes morbidity.

3.1. Serum Gastrin

With the ready availability of immunoassay for serum gastrin, there is little reason why this measurement should not be done preoperatively. Although it may be argued that the incidence of gastrinoma or antral G-cell hyperfunction (a term preferable to antral G-cell hyperplasia because not all agree that there is an increased number of G cells) is rare relative to ordinary peptic ulcer disease, significant morbidity can occur as a result of incorrect operative treatment. Less than the complete removal of the antral mucosa (anatomic antrectomy) is insufficient for the treatment of antral G-cell hyperfunction, though the approach to patients with gastrinoma is controversial; not knowing the diagnosis usually leads to inaccurate exploration and operation. The majority of patients with gastrinoma seen today have ulcer disease that is difficult to distinguish on the basis of history or location from the garden-variety disease.

Serum gastrin measurements are frequently neglected in patients who present with an acute complication of peptic ulcer disease such as obstruction, bleeding, or perforation. While waiting for the result of this measurement will unnecessarily delay an urgent or emergent operation until the result of the preoperative gastrin level is known, full treatment with an H_2 receptor antagonist can be continued postoperatively. An abnormally elevated serum gastrin measurement demands further study using the secretin and perhaps calcium as well as protein stimulation tests. Gastric analysis is not a substitute for serum gastrin measurement, as the analysis often is inaccurate, and overlap of secretory values between gastrinoma and ordinary duodenal ulcer disease is not unusual.

3.2. Location of the Ulcer

It is generally accepted that different operative concepts apply to gastric as opposed to duodenal ulcer. Yet, controversy continues about the correct approach to the treatment of ulcers in certain specific locations. A prepyloric ulcer, although anatomically in the stomach, is believed to be physiologically and clinically more akin to a duodenal ulcer than to an ordinary gastric ulcer. Data regarding this point are unclear, primarily because of the overlap of acid secretory values between gastric and duodenal ulcers, the location of the prepyloric ulcer with respect to the antral and parietal cell-bearing mucosa, and the variable definition of what represents a prepyloric ulcer.[3] The definition of "prepyloric" by site has ranged from those presenting to the right of the gastric anulus to those within 2–3 cm of the pylorus. Accepted operative treatment is to deal with a prepyloric ulcer as a duodenal ulcer, even though the adequacy of proximal gastric vagotomy for such an ulcer has been questioned by at least one report.[4] However, the issues are compounded by the lack of precise definition, by the lack of acceptable control patients, and by adequate prospective study.

Those patients with ulcers of both the stomach and duodenum are believed to generally belong to a hypersecretory group that behaves primarily as duodenal ulcer disease. The majority of such patients are believed to have an element of pyloric stenosis and large, deep gastric ulcers. Epidemiological data, however, indirectly suggest that the gastric ulcer precedes the duodenal ulcer more frequently than does the reverse situation.[5]

Until data further clarify whether or not prepyloric ulcers behave like gastric or duodenal ulcers, it is best to continue to treat these as if they were duodenal lesions. In the case of combined ulcers, elements of treatment of both (antrectomy for the gastric ulcer and vagotomy for the duodenal ulcer) should be incorporated into the operative procedure.

3.3. Gastric Analysis

It is tempting to think that an operative procedure for duodenal ulcer can be tailored to the individual patient based on preoperative acid secretory studies. The premise of this type of selective surgery is that an operation associated with a greater, or perhaps more lasting, reduction in acid secretion (for example, vagotomy with antrectomy) is necessary for those with high acid secretory rates, whereas a less radical procedure (for example, vagotomy without resection) will suffice for those with normal or low acid secretory rates. Although there are data to support this view, the bulk of clinical experience does not support the approach. The concept of selective surgery based on acid levels implies that there is a secretory threshold necessary for ulceration, but this threshold must vary in order to accommodate a large amount of data. Furthermore, the selective operative approach based on acid secretory levels does not encompass certain features about the pathophysiology of ulcers, such as the extent of mucosal permeability to acid, the degree of bicarbonate and mucus secretion, and the ability of the mucosa to buffer acid diffusing back from the lumen to the gastric epithelium. Presumably, these and perhaps other factors may explain why some patients with acid hypersection do not ulcerate and why others with normal secretory rates do.

3.4. Malignancy

Even though the incidence of carcinoma of the stomach is decreasing, the possibility of malignancy should not be neglected in a patient with a gastric ulcer. It is generally agreed that the best method for obtaining tissue diagnosis preoperatively is by simultaneous endoscopic biopsy and brush ctyology. This combination has a reported diagnostic accuracy of 97%. Preoperative knowledge of the presnce or absence of malignancy is of value in planning an operation, especially for ulcers situated in the proximal body of the stomach. It must be stressed that some infiltrative cancers can be difficult to diagnose by endoscopic biopsy. Thus, one should not ignore very suggestive radiographic criteria or the failure of complete healing of the ulcer after 3 months of acceptable medical therapy.

4. CHOICE OF OPERATION FOR DUODENAL ULCER

Before undertaking operation and considering the question of a selective operative approach, it is helpful to know the advantages and disadvantages of the currently accepted surgical procedures.

4.1. Truncal Vagotomy, Vagotomy with Antrectomy, Subtotal Gastrectomy

Truncal vagotomy with drainage, truncal vagotomy with antrectomy, and subtotal gastrectomy are the three generally accepted operative procedures for peptic ulcer disease of the duodenum. For the purposes of the discussion that follows, it makes no difference whether the drainage is a pyloroplasty or a gastrojejunostomy, or whether the reconstruction after resection involves a gastroduodenostomy (Billroth I) or gastrojejunostomy (Billroth II). Unless stated otherwise, the term antrectomy as used here (in contrast to anatomic antrectomy) refers to what some surgeons consider to be a hemigastrectomy, but reference to antrectomy is frequently made in the literature. This loose definition does not imply all of the antral mucosa is removed. Subtotal gastrectomy refers to excision of 70–75% of the distal stomach.

Prospective studies indicate that there are no significant differences in operative mortality between the three operative procedures.[1,6–8] This is in contrast to suggested differences reported by retrospective studies. In fact, two studies reported no mortality.[1,6] The reason for this is that the prospective studies were not only performed under elective circumstances, but the protocols contained an escape clause which permitted rejection of a specific operative procedure if it was not technically safe to perform in a given patient. This selective feature is of prime importance in minimizing operative mortality and morbidity. In one prospective study, the operative complications related to the specific procedure were not significantly different,[6] but in another the incidence of complications was significantly lower following vagotomy with drainage.[7]

Prospective studies[1,6-8] comparing the three standard operative procedures indicate that although the majority of patients are pleased with the results of their operations, new symptoms can occur as a consequence of the surgery (Table 1). Such new symptoms include epigastric fullness, heartburn, abdominal pain, nausea, regurgitation, bile vomiting, food vomiting, dumping syndrome, flatulence, diarrhea, and hypoglycemia (sometimes referred to as late dumping). The incidence of these side

Table 1. Combined Results of Three Prospective Trials of Standard Ulcer Operations[1,6-8a]

	Percent V and D	Percent V and A	Percent STG
Fullness	14–40	29–36	16–37
Heartburn	20	16	8
Abdominal pain	19–30	20–29	19–24
Nausea	13–20	17–24	23–31
Reflux	4	7	4
Regurgitation	3	12	4
Bile emesis	15	14	13
Food emesis	4	10	6
Dumping	9–27	9–33	22–42
Flatulence	18	23	20
Diarrhea	14–26	21–23	7–17
Hypoglycemia	6–12	4–16	1–12
Operative death	0–2	0–3	0–2
Operative complications	6	6–12	8–9
Recurrence	6–10	1–4	2–5
Overall result			
Excellent–good	70–83	78–91	77–90
Fair	12–19	7–14	7–17
Poor	5–11	2–8	3–6

[a]V and D, vagotomy with drainage; V and A, vagotomy with antrectomy; STG, subtotal gastrectomy.

effects of operation varies from series to series, in part owing to definition. A number of claims have been made suggesting that the incidence
of certain symptoms is more or less after one of three standard operative
procedures, but by and large these claims are not substantiated by prospective studies.

The most common long-term symptom of gastric surgery is the sensation of epigastric fullness. This is not usually incapacitating, and its
etiology is speculative. It is probably related to the loss of receptive relaxation of the fundus following vagotomy. In the case of subtotal gastrectomy without vagotomy, the reduced size of the gastric pouch may contribute to the sensation of fullness. The incidence of fullness is not
significantly different between the three standard operative procedures.[1]

The most frequent troublesome sequela of gastric surgery is the
dumping syndrome. The incidence of the dumping symptoms is confusing because of the variability of its definition. For example, in the Minnesota study[6] the incidence of dumping was significantly less after vagotomy with drainage than for other procedures. There was a significant
increase in severity of dumping as the amount of stomach excised
increased in the VA study.[7,8] In contrast, the incidence of dumping was
significantly less after vagotomy with antrectomy in the Leeds/York
study in the 5 to 8-year period of follow-up[1]; this difference was no longer
significant with further follow-up 10–16 years postoperative.[9]

A major difficulty in determining the true incidence of dumping is
that the diagnosis is usually based on history rather than on the oral
administration of a standard osmotic load. Thus, other postgastrectomy
disorders may be erroneously labeled as part of the dumping syndrome.
A hypertonic glucose load given orally provokes dumping symptoms in
20% of duodenal ulcer patients prior to operation, in 73% of patients with
truncal vagotomy with pyloplasty, in 80% of patients with selective
vagotomy with pyloroplasty, and in 47% of patients with proximal gastric
vagotomy.[10] Since these figures are higher than those generally encountered clinically, it is likely that patients do not ordinarily ingest a similar
hypertonic load to that used for the test meal. It is also possible that in
time the patients consciously or subconsciously adjust their diets to prevent symptoms of dumping.

Many physicians still believe that diarrhea is not a significant problem following operation. The Minnesota and VA data suggest that the
occurrence of postvagotomy diarrhea has been overemphasized, because
the incidence following vagotomy was not significantly different from
that occurring after subtotal gastrectomy.[6,7] Others argue that little attention is usually paid to preservation of the vagal divisions during subtotal
gastrectomy.[11] The incidence of diarrhea was significantly less after sub-

gastrectomy.[11] The incidence of diarrhea was significantly less after subtotal gastrectomy in only one study.[1] However, prospective data for selective vagotomy leave little doubt that there is an increased incidence of diarrhea after truncal vagotomy.[12,13] For reasons that are unclear, the differing incidence of diarrhea following vagotomy with gastric resection and vagotomy without resection disappeared with longer follow-up in the Leeds/York study.[9]

The etiology of postvagotomy diarrhea is poorly understood. However, it appears that the incidence is much greater in patients who have undergone or who will undergo cholecystectomy. It has been suggested that preservation of the hepatic division of the left anterior vagus nerve minimizes the incidence of diarrhea.[11] Diarrhea tends to be ignored postoperatively because it is usually not a severe problem in the majority of patients. However, as many as 5–10% of patients with diarrhea find it troublesome, and in less than 1% the diarrhea is disabling.

Prospective studies indicate that the major difference between vagotomy with drainage, vagotomy with antrectomy, and subtotal gastrectomy relates to the incidence of recurrent ulceration. In four prospective studies,[3] the incidence of recurrent ulcer ranged from 7 to 10% after vagotomy with drainage. This is in contrast to a 1–4% incidence after vagotomy with antrectomy and a 2–5% incidence after subtotal gastrectomy.[3] Although some data suggest otherwise,[9] it is generally accepted that the incidence of recurrent ulcer is least after vagotomy with antrectomy. This is most likely due to the dual protective nature of the operation: antrectomy compensates for an incomplete vagotomy, and vagotomy compensates for an incomplete antrectomy.[14]

Although it is clear that residual antral mucosa in the duodenal stump of a Billroth II reconstruction places the patient at great risk for the recurrent ulcer, the role of residual antrum in the gastric stump is not clear. It cannot be assumed that the operation of hemigastrectomy always removes the antrum, since the proximal extent of the antrum varies from patient to patient on both the greater and lesser curvature aspects of the stomach.[15] Conceptually, it appears that if gastric resection is done, an anatomic antrectomy (which removes all of the antral mucosa) should be done.[3] That this is accomplished can be verified by histological examination of both greater and lesser curves of the proximal aspect as well as the distal most aspect of the specimen.

The most important observation emerging from the prospective studies of the three standard operations for duodenal ulcer is that there is no significant difference between them in terms of long-term sequelae. However, the incidence of recurrent ulcer is least with vagotomy and antrectomy but still within an acceptable range following vagotomy with

one of the three standard operations can be done with minimal immediate postoperative morbidity and mortality. Thus, if one plans a vagotomy with antrectomy preoperatively and the duodenum is found to be
markedly scarred or edematous intraoperatively, one need not undertake
a potentially hazardous resection. Furthermore, there are no substantive
data indicating any long-term differences between the various types of
drainage procedures accompanying vagotomy. Thus, if the duodenum is
scarred or edematous, a gastroenterosomy as a drainage procedure can be
done without hesitation.

My preference is to generally avoid subtotal gastrectomy because of
my impression that although the incidence of symptoms is not greater
compared to the other standard procedures, the severity of symptoms is
greater. Subtotal gastrectomy, however, can be a useful procedure in the
presence of severe portal hypertension, a situation where one may want
to avoid dissection around the esophagus. Some surgeons continue to do
truncal vagotomy along with subtotal gastrectomy, but this combination
usually is unnecessary and may place the patient at additional risk for
diarrhea.

4.2. Selective Vagotomy with Drainage

The incidence of diarrhea can be minimized by doing a selective
vagotomy. The only major difference between truncal and selective
vagotomy in two prospective studies was a significantly lower incidence
of diarrhea with the selective technique.[12,13] Selective vagotomy has not
caught on as a standard operative procedure for duodenal ulcer disease
because the overall results of the technically more difficult selective
vagotomy are not different from those of the less difficult truncal vagotomy. Yet, there is a role for selective vagotomy in patients who are prone
to diarrhea. For example, patients with prior cholecystectomy or patients
who require gastroenterostomy as a result of Crohn's disease may benefit
from selective as opposed to truncal vagotomy.

4.3. Drainage Procedure

Truncal vagotomy classically involves division of the vagal trunks
proximal to the celiac and hepatic divisions and thus also interrupts vagal
flow to the nerves of Latarjet innervating the parietal cell-bearing and
antral mucosa. Selective vagotomy, on the other hand, involves division
of the nerves of Latarjet at their origins, thereby preserving the hepatic
and celiac divisions. Since both types of vagotomy interrupt the parasympathetic flow to the antrum, there is impairment of the emptying of solids

from the stomach. However, it appears that only about 20% of patients will have clinically significant impaired gastric emptying if truncal or selective vagotomy is done without an accompanying drainage procedure. Although this figure invites the tempting possibility of doing a truncal vagotomy without an accompanying drainage procedure, insufficient information is available for the group of patients absolutely requiring drainage. It is doubtful that scarring from the ulcer alone is the sole determinant of the necessity for drainage, because at least 20% of patients can be shown to have impaired gastric emptying following esophagoproximal gastrectomy without a drainage procedure.

The drainage procedure is in itself a cause of morbidity, especially dumping, bilious vomiting, and hypoglycemia. The majority of patients either do not have the symptoms to a significant degree or are able to cope with them. Nevertheless, there remains a group of patients with long-term operative sequela that are difficult to treat, and this has led to enthusiasm for proximal gastric vagotomy.

4.4. Proximal Gastric Vagotomy without Drainage

Proximal gastric vagotomy differs from the other types of vagotomy in that the nerves of Latarjet innervating the antrum remain intact whereas branches of these nerves innervating the parietal cell mass are severed. Thus, the celiac and hepatic divisions also remain intact. Because the antral mill is preserved, it is unnecessary to do a drainage procedure with proximal gastric vagotomy. It is generally agreed that all symptoms, with the exception of epigastric fullness, are decreased in incidence following proximal gastric vagotomy. However, prospective studies indicate that the major difference between proximal gastric vagotomy and selective vagotomy relates to the dumping syndrome,[16-20] the incidence of which is lower after proximal gastric vagotomy, both by history and after a standard osmotic load given orally. The incidence of dumping reported by prospective studies comparing selective to proximal gastric vagotomy ranges from 28 to 59% for the former and 4 to 17% for the latter. Even though the pylorus is intact with this procedure, dumping may occur because of the faster emptying of liquids as a result of the loss of receptive relaxation of the fundus.

The operative mortality of proximal gastric vagotomy is not significantly different from that of other procedures. On a retrospective basis, however, proximal gastric vagotomy is associated with a lower operative mortality, 0.3% in over 5500 operations.[21] This figure for mortality is less than that reported by other retrospective series involving gastric resection or vagotomy with drainage.

The major question concerning proximal gastric vagotomy is its durability in terms of recurrent ulceration. Although the mean numerical incidence of recurrence tends to be higher in the relatively short follow-up available from most prospective studies, the statistical incidence of recurrence in most reports is not significantly different from that following other forms of vagotomy. However, it is clear that lack of attention to technical details of the procedure will result in unacceptably high recurrence rates.[3] Now that greater emphasis has been placed on the periesophageal dissection of the vagal branches, the incidence of postoperative dysphagia appears to have increased, but this is usually mild and is rarely permanent.

Proximal gastric vagotomy usually is begun 7 cm proximal to the pylorus. This landmark generally corresponds to being just proximal to the so-called "crow's feet" of the nerves of Latarjet. The results using the 7-cm landmark do not differ from the antral mapping technique, which is perhaps a more physiological approach. However, a potential problem with proximal gastric vagotomy is that the extent of antral mucosa may differ from the external landmark(s) of the antrum. It has been suggested that as many as 20% of patients may not have complete denervation of the distal fundic mucosa.[22] This consideration has not yet been shown to be clinically significant, but it may account for some of the recurrences after a technically well-performed operation. It is of interest that many surgeons believe that the incidence of incomplete truncal vagotomy also is about 20%.

5. CHOICE OF OPERATION FOR GASTRIC ULCER

Fewer operative options are available for the treatment of gastric ulcer. Although there are claims that vagotomy is an effective operative procedure for gastric ulcer, this is not supported by prospective[23,24] and several retrospective studies. Relatively short-term follow-up in prospective studies report a 10–13% incidence of recurrence following vagotomy with drainage, and some retrospective studies with longer follow-up report an incidence of at least 30%.

Since the overwhelming majority of gastric ulcers occur within the 2-cm transitional zone between the antral and parietal cell-bearing mucosa,[15] complete removal of the antral mucosa (anatomical antrectomy) is the treatment of choice. If this is done, recurrence rates of 1% or less can be expected, simply because the peptic ulcer-bearing area is removed. It should be appreciated that ulcers occuring in locations proximal to the transitional zone are not peptic in origin.

The importance of complete removal of all antral mucosa for gastric ulcer is emphasized by the results of another operative procedure, pylorus-preserving gastrectomy. Since anatomical antrectomy necessitates removal of the pylorus, pylorus-preserving antrectomy was proposed in order to minimize long-term postoperative sequelae. The operation involves removal of all but the distal 1.5–2 cm of antrum and anastomosis of the residual stomach to the cuff of antrum. In addition to delayed gastric emptying, vomiting, and epigastric pain, there is a 13% incidence of recurrent gastric ulcer in the retained *antral cuff* (even in the absence of obstruction) following relatively short follow-up.

6. IS THERE A NEED TO BE SELECTIVE OR SUPERSELECTIVE?

The need to be selective or superselective cannot be answered in a dogmatic fashion, as the goals of therapy must be matched to the individual patient. Thus, the degree of selectivity should depend on some of the following considerations:

1. The decision as to when medical therapy has failed should take into account the effect of symptoms and the treatment itself on the patient's daily activities, as well as the short- and long-term side effects of medical treatment. Time of declaration of failure of nonoperative treatment (in the absence of obstruction, bleeding, or perforation) should take into account the magnitude of interference of symptoms and treatment itself with daily activities of the patient as well as the short- and long-term side effects of medicinal treatment.
2. The serum gastrin, location of the ulcer, and question of malignancy will influence the type of operative procedure that is done, just as will the anatomical circumstances found at operation and the surgeon's technical experience.
3. The incidence and potential severity of symptoms resulting from destruction or bypass or excision of the pylorus must be weighed against the incidence of recurrent ulcer following proximal gastric vagotomy. If the incidence of recurrent ulcer remains the same for proximal gastric vagotomy and the other types of vagotomy, then there is every reason to do the former operation, provided the ulcer is duodenal and there is no element of obstruction. On the other hand, if proximal gastric vagotomy is not done for duo-

denal ulcer and anatomical circumstances permitting, anatomical antrectomy with vagotomy will result in a lower incidence of recurrent ulcer. The incidence of diarrhea can be lessened if selective rather than truncal vagotomy is done.

Although data are not yet available, it is probable that proximal gastric vagotomy will generally lessen the risk of subsequent operation. All patients who have had their pylorus altered, bypassed, or excised are at potential risk for requiring subsequent operation for incapacitating sequela.

REFERENCES

1. Goligher JC, Pulvertaft CN, de Dombal FT, et al: Five- to eight-year results of Leeds/York controlled trial of elective surgery for duodenal ulcer. *Br Med J* 1968;2:781.
2. Fineberg HV, Pearlman LA: Surgical treatment of peptic ulcer in the United States. *Lancet* 1981;1:1305.
3. Fromm D: Peptic Ulcer, in Fromm D (ed): *Gastrointestinal Surgery*. New York: Churchill-Livingstone, 1985, pp. 233–323.
4. Andersen D, Amdrup E, Hostrup H, et al: The Aarhus County vagotomy trial. *World J Surg* 1982;6:86.
5. Bonnevie O: Gastric and duodenal ulcers in the same patient. *Scand J Gastroenterol* 1975;10:657.
6. Howard RJ, Murphy WR, Humphrey EW: A prospective randomized study of the elective surgical treatment for duodenal ulcer: Two- to ten-year followup study. *Surgery* 1973;73:256.
7. Postlethwait RW: Five year follow-up results of operations for duodenal ulcer. *Surg Gynecol Obstet* 1973;137:387.
8. Price WE, Grizzle JE, Postlethwait RW, et al: Results of operation for duodenal ulcer. *Surg Gynecol Obstet* 1970;131:233.
9. Goligher JC, Feather DB, Hall R, et al: Several standard elective operations for duodenal ulcer. Ten to 16 year clinical results. *Ann Surg* 1979;189:18.
10. Humphrey CS, Johnston D, Walker BE, et al: Incidence of dumping after truncal and selective vagotomy with pyloroplasty and highly selective vagotomy with drainage procedure. *Br Med J* 1972;3:785.
11. Fromm D: *Complications of Gastric Surgery*. New York: John Wiley & Sons, 1977.
12. Kennedy T, Connell AM, Love AHG, et al: Selective or truncal vagotomy? Five-year results of a double-blind randomized, controlled trial. *Br J Surg* 1973;60:944.
13. Kronborg O, Malmstrom J, Christiansen PM: A comparison between the results of truncal and selective vagotomy in patients with duodenal ulcer. *Scand J Gastroenterol* 1970;5:519.
14. Stempien SJ, Lee ER, Dagradi AE: The role of distal gastrectomy, with and without vagotomy, in the control of cephalic secretion and peptic ulcer disease. *Surgery* 1972;71:110.
15. Oi M, Oshida K, Sugimura S: The location of gastric ulcer. *Gastroenterology* 1959;36:45.

16. Amdrup E, Andersen D, Hostrup H: The Aarhus County vagotomy trial. I. An interim report on primary results and incidence of sequelae following parietal cell vagotomy and selective gastric vagotomy in 748 patients. *World J Surg* 1978;2:85.
17. Andersen D, Hostrup H, Amdrup E: The Aarhus County vagotomy trial. II. An interim report on reduction in acid secretion and ulcer recurrence rate following parietal cell vagotomy and selective gastric vagotomy. *World J Surg* 1978;2:91.
18. Faxen A, Kewenter J, Stockbrugger R: Clinical results of parietal cell vagotomy and selective vagotomy with pyloroplasty in the treatment of duodenal ulcer. *Scand J Gastroenterol* 1978;13:741.
19. Jordan PH Jr: A prospective study of parietal cell vagotomy–antrectomy for treatment of duodenal ulcer. *Ann Surg* 1976;183:619.
20. Kennedy T, Johnston GW, Macrae KD, et al: Proximal gastric vagotomy: Interim results of a randomized controlled trial. *Br Med J* 1975;2:301.
21. Johnston D: Operative mortality and postoperative morbidity of highly selective vagotomy. *Br Med J* 1975;4:545.
22. Nielsen HO, Monoz JD, Kronborg O, et al: The antrum in duodenal ulcer patients. *Scand J Gastroenterol* 1981;16:491.
23. Duthie HL, Kwong NK: Vagotomy or gastrectomy for gastric ulcer. *Br Med J* 1973;4:79.
24. Madsen P, Kronborg O, Hart-Hansen O: Billroth I gastric resection versus truncal vagotomy and pyloroplasty in the treatment of gastric ulcer. *Acta Chir Scand* 1976;142:151.

3

Disordered Gastrointestinal Motility Syndromes
Is the Gastrointestinal Tract Inflamed or Irritable?

Walter J. Hogan

1. INTRODUCTION

Certain disordered gastrointestinal (GI) motility syndromes are caused by demonstrable primary alterations in structure. Cases in point are achalasia of esophagus, Hirschsprung disease, and certain types of pseudointestinal obstruction. Although the definitive pathophysiology is not completely known, a cause for the motor disturbance is apparent. This discussion will concern motor disorders of the GI tract which, to our current state of knowledge, are *not* associated with recognizable morphological alteration. Disordered GI motility disturbances of this genre are often observed in association with "functional GI disorders." Are these syndromes closely related? Are they cause and effect? Or are these motility disorders simply an epiphenomenon—a chance relationship with little meaningful clinical correlation?

This type of disordered GI motility may be far more relevant clinically but much more difficult to bring into meaningful focus in a discussion of the "scientific basis for therapeutic decision."

Walter J. Hogan ● Froedtert Memorial Lutheran Hospital, Milwaukee, Wisconsin 53226.

2. DEFINITION

Disordered GI motility syndromes that occur in a structurally intact GI tract, in the absence of a biochemical or infective cause, are often associated with a complex of symptoms. Apparently, the symptoms can occur anywhere along the length of the GI tract. They can be intermittent, chronic, or recurrent. There is almost always a setting or undercurrent of stress on the individual—albeit acute or chronic. Motor abnormalities may sometimes be characteristic or specific and associated with clinical symptoms. More frequently, motor abnormalities may be inconsistent or lacking in symptom correlation. How, then, do we approach the relationship of functional GI tract disease to disordered motility syndromes and expect to make any sensible deductions for enhanced clinical recognition and effective treatment choices?

3. INCIDENCE

The prevalence of functional GI disorders in the general population is unknown. Functional disorders comprise approximately half of the gastrointestinal complaints encountered by physicians.[1] The symptoms of at least 20% of the patients who consult a gastroenterologist remain unexplained.[2] Despite the fact that only a small proportion of patients with functional GI disorders become hospitalized patients, they comprise a significant number of a hospital's population and take a good share of the health dollar. Although difficulties with identifiable terminology and coding exist, nonetheless, there were 37,000 patients discharged from U.S. hospitals with a diagnosis of "psychogenic GI disorder" in 1976. At the same time, 181,000 patients were discharged from a hospital with a primary or secondary diagnosis of "irritable bowel syndrome."[3]

4. FUNCTIONAL DISEASE

The concept of "functional" GI tract disorders is assuming an increasingly important "organic" meaning as a result of recent research investigations. Newer knowledge concerning the relationships of the central nervous system and the gut has been obtained. Peptide-containing cells have been identified in both the brain and the GI tract. Increasing information concerning the innervation, myoelectrical activity, and humoral and hormonal function of the digestive tract has resulted from advanced methodology and study techniques by GI investigators.

Despite this informational explosion about the human GI tract and its function, research to date has yielded very little new, practical information to help improve our diagnosis and treatment of functional GI tract disorders.

At the outset, therefore, our focus will be directed to the most important clinical aspects of functional GI disorders, i.e., pain symptomatology, stress, and psychoneurotic factors.

4. CLINICAL APPRAISAL

4.1. Pain

Functional GI disorders may present with a specific complaint, i.e., "lump in the throat," or a multiplicity of symptoms, such as bowel dysfunction, nausea, vomiting, and abdominal pain. However, at least 30% of patients with GI symptomatology have pain as a predominant complaint.[4] In an English population sample, one-fifth of the subjects indicated they had experienced abdominal pain more than six times in the preceding year.[5] One study of functional GI patients with abdominal pain demonstrated four features that were more common to that group than to a comparable group with organic diseases: loose or frequent stools (or both) at pain onset, pain relief upon defecation, and abdominal distention.[6] Significant discrimination of patient groups was obtained using a combination of these symptoms; e.g., half of the patients with organic disease did not have any of these complaints, whereas two-thirds of functional GI patients had three or four of these symptoms. Pain is often the keystone in the functional GI symptom complex and a major determinant to patient–physician interaction and subsequent clinical decision making. For example, functional GI disease types appear predicated by location of pain symptoms, e.g., right epigastric pain is "biliary," noncardiac chest pain is "esophageal," and right-lower-quadrant pain is "chronic appendicitis." Since the pain symptoms can be so important, can we say anything more specific about it?

Patients with functional GI tract disorders appear to have an over-responsiveness or hypersensitivity to GI tract luminal distention. For example, during progressive distention of the rectosigmoid area, patients with functional bowel symptoms experienced pain sooner than control subjects.[7] Often when the gastrointestinal tract is distended with air during endoscopy or at the time of barium enema x ray, pain is experienced. Routine visceral stimulation appears to be magnified beyond acceptable boundaries of comfort in these patients.

A recent study demonstrated that the distribution of pain in control subjects caused by colonic balloon distention at several sites was felt predominantly in the central, lower, and left abdomen. Pain was felt in any part of the abdomen in 48 patients with painful functional bowel syndrome, however, and in distant referral sites such as the back, shoulders, thigh, and perineum. Furthermore, the original pain was reproduced by such distention in approximately half of the patients.[8] Balloon distention of the esophagus, stomach, biliary tree, and colon has been used to induce pain. In one such study, unexplained pain was reproduced in two-thirds of the patient group, including some who possessed two widely separate trigger zones within the GI tract.[9] Perhaps this information helps to explain why some patients with functional GI disease seem to have an abdominal "tenderness" on physical examination or, possibly, why "chest pain" may not arise exclusively from thoracic organs!

In addition to balloon distention of the GI tract, other provocative methods have been tried to "reproduce" the patient's pain. For example, a host of drugs ranging from intravenous ergonovine to edrophonium have been used to reproduce distress in patients with suspected noncardiac, esophageal chest pain.[10] Cholecystokinin (CCK) i.v. has caused spasm and pain of the colon[11] and sphincter of Oddi.[12] The induction of a specific pain may be helpful in focusing the patients' attention on the fact that the "source of the symptoms has been found, even though no abnormality of structure is demonstrable."[13] A caveat must be raised about the "reproduction" or "provocation" of pain in a patient with functional GI disease. First this observation may not necessarily be cause-effect related. We have seen as many "normal" patients complain of biliary tract pain with initial ERCP contrast injection into the common bile duct as those patients with suspected biliary dyskinesia. The occurrence of pain, therefore, does not imply sphincter of Oddi (SO) dysfunction per se. The prostigmine–morphine test is not discriminatory. It can elicit pain and enzyme elevations in normal subjects as well as patients with suspected SO dysfunction.[14] Additionally, does right-upper-quadrant pain after intravenous CCK imply biliary dyskinesia, irritable bowel syndrome—or both? In the postcholecystectomy syndrome, the problem has always been to determine how much of the right-upper-quadrant distress before and after the operation is due to biliary tract disorder and how much to the failure to recognize an irritable bowel syndrome in the same patient. "The interactions of local functional disorders make their rigid categorization, to some extent, a distortion of nature."[15] It is not uncommon to observe an overlap of functional syndromes in the same patient with expressive symptomatology oscillating back and forth over periods of time.

4.2. Psychological Factors

The role of stress and psychoneurosis in functional GI tract distress is not completely defined but appears significant. The gut is well known as a sensitive organ of emotional expression. Spastic contractions, induced reflexly or by stress, characterize both functional esophageal[16] and colonic disorders.[17] Startling noises have been demonstrated to trigger esophageal contractions in humans,[18] distal nonpropulsive contractions can be induced by stressful interviews in normal subjects,[19] and cold pressor stress testing significantly alters esophageal contractions in a high percentage of normals causing a marked increase in peristaltic amplitude.[20] "There is abundant evidence that many, if not all, of the underlying physiological changes in the more common functional disorders are normal bodily accompaniments of emotional tension."[15] Whether stress induces increased sensitivity to somatic symptoms or certain individuals have a personality type characterized by hypersensitivity to stressful events is uncertain. In either situation, the link between stress and disease suggests a far clearer relationship to treatment-seeking behavior than to onset of illness.

The relationship between functional GI symptoms and psychopathology is suggested by the high incidence of somatic complaints in patients with psychiatric disorders such as depression, anxiety disorders, and hysteria. A striking prevalence of psychiatric illness has been reported in patients with irritable bowel syndrome when systematic psychiatric diagnostic criteria were used.[21] In a study of 29 patients with irritable bowel syndrome and a control group of 33 patients, only six patients in the control group (18%) had an identifiable psychiatric disorder as compared with 21 (72%) of the patients with irritable bowel syndrome. Among this latter group, depression, hysteria, and anxiety neurosis were detected. These psychiatric symptoms presented simultaneously or preceded those of irritable bowel syndrome in the majority of patients. No definite association could be made between the chronicity or episodic nature of the psychiatric disorder and the type of GI complaints. Interestingly, the diagnosis of a psychiatric disorder was missed in the majority of these patients by their private medical physicians.

There are inconsistencies, however, in the theory that psychopathology plays the major role in functional GI disorders. The association between psychiatric illness and esophageal motility disorders was evaluated in a group of 50 patients referred for esophageal manometry.[16] There was a markedly high incidence of psychiatric illness in 21 (84%) of the 25 patients with contraction abnormalities in the esophageal body, suggesting a relationship between emotional and GI motility disturbances. However, a study of psychoneurotic patients with no bowel complaints and irritable bowel patients with pain demonstrated no significant differences in colonic motor or myoelectrical abnormalities, despite the fact that both groups had similar psychometric test indices.[22] Finally, most individuals who have functional GI complaints apparently do not consult a physician[5]; additional motivating factors appear necessary for treatment-seeking behavior. It remains to be determined whether the role of psychoneurosis in functional GI disorders is one of cause, effect, or coincidence.

5. DISORDERED GI MOTILITY SYNDROME: THE SPECTRUM OF PRIMARY ESOPHAGEAL MOTOR DISORDERS

Motility disorders have been linked to a number of functional GI disturbances. Esophageal dysmotility is described frequently in "noncardiac chest pain" patients. Gastric dysrhythmia seemingly characterizes a group of patients with pernicious nausea and vomiting. SO dyskinesia often is implicated in the symptom complex of postcholecystectomy distress, and colonic motor abnormality is reported in some patients with irritable bowel syndrome. Although evidence of the association of motility disorders with GI functional syndromes continues to accumulate, a cause-and-effect relationship has yet to be established.

In the past, the variety of primary motor disorders of the esophagus encountered by the clinician was limited. Achalasia was the most frequently recognized motor disturbance. The condition is associated with denervation of the smooth muscle segment of the gullet; manometric criteria are quite specific and serve as the "gold standard" for all other primary esophageal motor disorders (Table 1). Diffuse esophageal spasm (DES), on the other hand, is a more nebulous, less frequently encountered esophageal motor disturbance.

Table 1. Achalasia: Manometric Criteria[a]

Modality	Finding	Criteria
Primary peristalsis	Absent	Major
LES relax	Impaired	Major
LESP	Elevated	Minor
Pharmacologic test	Positive	Minor

[a]The manometric diagnosis of achalasia requires the presence of two major criteria and at least one minor criterion.

DES is considered by many to be part of the spectrum of esophageal motility dysfunction, which includes achalasia. The evidence for associated denervation or smooth muscle alteration of the esophagus in DES patients is skimpy, at best. Although the patient with suspected DES complains of frequent intermittent chest pain and dysphagia for both liquids and solids, esophageal manometric study is often normal. On other occasions, positive manometric findings suggesting esophageal "spasm" may be noted in the absence of patient complaints.

The manometric criteria for DES remain variable and confusing. Unlike the achalasia patient, however, the esophagus in DES syndrome retains its ability to propagate primary peristaltic waves the majority of the time. The manometric "criteria" for DES have recently been reported from two centers. In the first report,[23] DES patients demonstrate at least 30% of swallow-induced wave contractions that occur simultaneously. Both the amplitude and duration of these esophageal contractions are prolonged (i.e., >100 mm Hg and >7.5 sec mean duration, respectively). Multiple pressure peaks following swallows are described in the majority of patients, and "spontaneous" contractions occur in more than half the patients with DES. In the second report,[24] manometric criteria for DES included the "requirement" that simultaneous wave contractions occur in >10% of swallowing sequences after a liquid bolus, in the presence of intermittent primary peristalsis. Repetitive, prolonged, spontaneous, high-amplitude wave contractions were "associated findings." The lower esophageal sphincter may show incomplete relaxation and/or high resting pressure—or it may behave normally! Figure 1 illustrates the manometric trace of a patient with symptomatic DES.

The spectrum of primary esophageal motor disorder types has expanded dramatically in recent years. This is due, in large part, to the fact that esophageal manometric technology has evolved from a qualitative to a quantitative method for evaluating esophageal pressure dynamics.[25] A variety of esophageal motor abnormalities may be seen which do not fulfill the manometric criteria for either achalasia or DES and which may or may not be associated with clinical symptoms.

The esophagus, like other organ systems, has a limited mode of expression to reflect a variety of disorders. The esophageal body displays various combinations of dysrhythmic wave forms, and the lower esophageal sphincter exhibits a variable range of resting pressures and "completeness" of relaxation with swallows. Combinations of these motor abnormalities are present with all primary swallowing disorders, but few patterns are sufficiently repetitive or unique to be diagnostic. Categorization of these "motility variants" or "combinations" has been discouraged,[26] and the generic term of "nonspecific esophageal motility disorder"

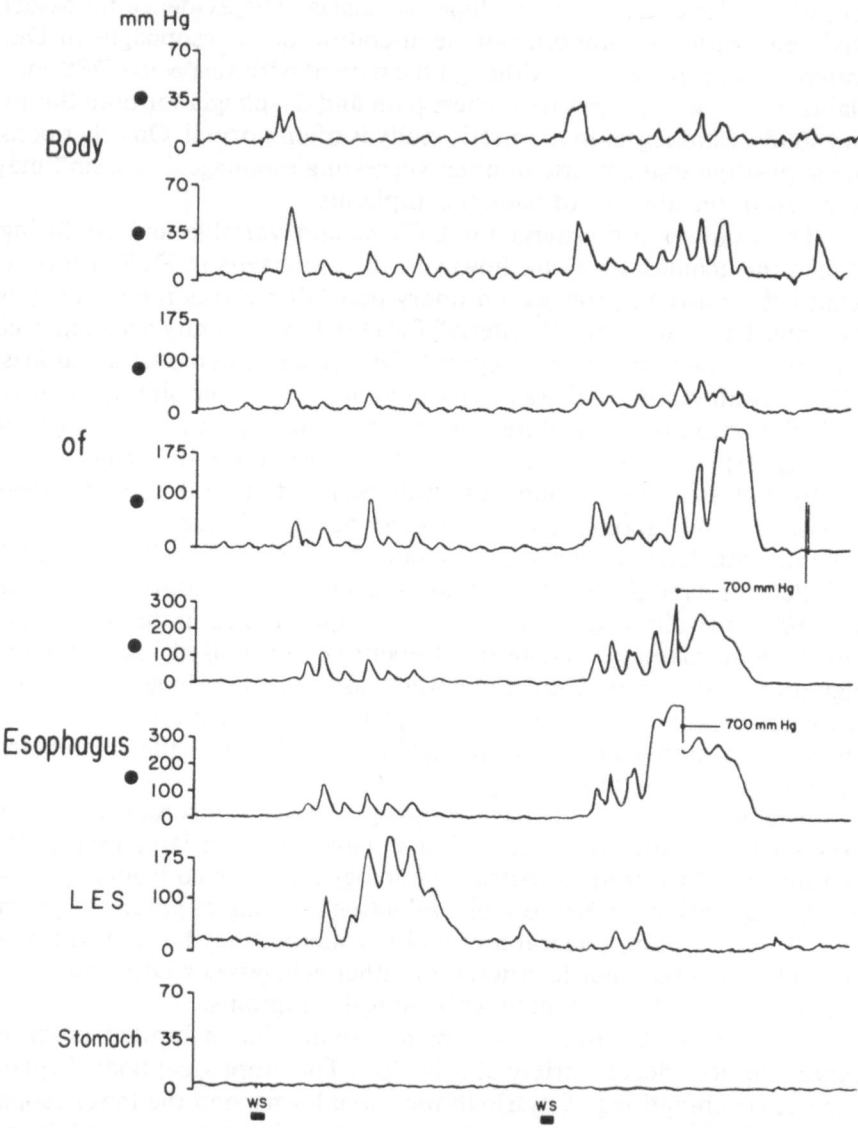

Figure 1. During manometric pressure recording in a patient with DES, esophageal wave contractions following deglutition demonstrate extremely elevated amplitudes. Attenuation of the recording scale to the 700-mm Hg range was necessary to accurately trace the amplitude of wave height in the two distal esophageal recording tips.

seems most applicable presently. Manometric study of the esophagus in these conditions remains, for the most part, a descriptive art requiring close correlation and sensitive interpretation based on the clinical situation.

The problem of noncardiac chest pain has enlivened the controversy regarding the relationship of motility disorders to pain syndromes. According to a recent report, chest pain has now surpassed all other causes of patient referral for esophageal manometric study in the United States.[27] It is estimated that 45% of chest pain patients without coronary artery disease have some form of esophageal dysmotility.[28] Theoretically, 25,000–75,000 patients per year meet this criterion! This intense interest in the noncardiac chest pain patient has resulted in reports of a number of "new" esophageal manometric motor disorders, e.g., the "tender esophagus,"[29] the hypertensive lower esophageal sphincter (LES),[30] and the "nutcracker esophagus."[31] Odynophagia is experienced during swallows by patients with a tender esophagus. The hypertensive LES is characterized by a markedly elevated sphincteric resting pressure (>50 mm Hg) with normal relaxation and normal peristalsis in the esophageal body.

The nutcracker esophagus is touted to be the most common esophageal motor disturbance responsible for chest pain. The nutcracker esophagus is characterized by high-amplitude, peristaltic contractions (>180 mm Hg) in the distal esophagus and, frequently, prolonged duration of

Table 2. Noncardiac Chest Pain: Provocative Tests during Esophageal Manometry[a]

Authors[a]	Patients	Drug	Dose	Motor abnormal/pain
Siegel and Tucker	25	Tensilon	10 mg i.v.	40%
Nostrant et al.	87	Urecholine	50 μg/kg s.c. × 2	77%
Lee et al.	120	Tensilon	10 mg i.v.	34%
Jobin et al.	21	Ergonovine	0.025–0.4 mg i.v.	40%
Ippoliti	36	Tensilon	100 μg/kg i.v.	66%

[a]Abstracts:

Siegel D, Tucker H: Comparison of provocative tests to identify an esophageal origin of chest pain. *Gastroenterology* 1985;86:1251.

Nostrant TT, Huber TP, Sams JS, Goldstein NG: Urecholine enhances diagnostic yield of esophageal manometry in evaluating patients with chest pain. *Gastroenterology* 1985;86:1196.

Lee CA, Reynolds JC, Ouyang A, Baker L, Cohen S: Esophageal chest pain: Diagnostic value of high-dose tensilon provocative testing. *Gastroenterology* 1985;86:1156.

Jobin G, Bouchard A, Aumais G, Miller DD, Waters DD: Ergonovine-induced esophageal spasm and angina-like chest pain: Prevalence, diagnosis and response to treatment with nifedipine. *Gastroenterology* 1985;86:1126.

Ippoliti A: Tensilon stimulation for the manometric diagnosis of diffuse esophageal spasm. *Gastroenterology* 1985;86:1121.

wave contraction (>6 sec). Similar to this entire spectrum of motility disorders, the nutcracker esophagus may have intermittent clinical and motor expression. Patients are often asymptomatic when studied, or they may have an esophageal motor disorder without associated symptoms. Because of this problem with diagnosis, provocative tests, using drug administration or noxious stimuli, have been used to "reproduce" esophageal manometric abnormalities and chest pain. A proliferation of provocative tests (Table 2) have been described with positive results ranging

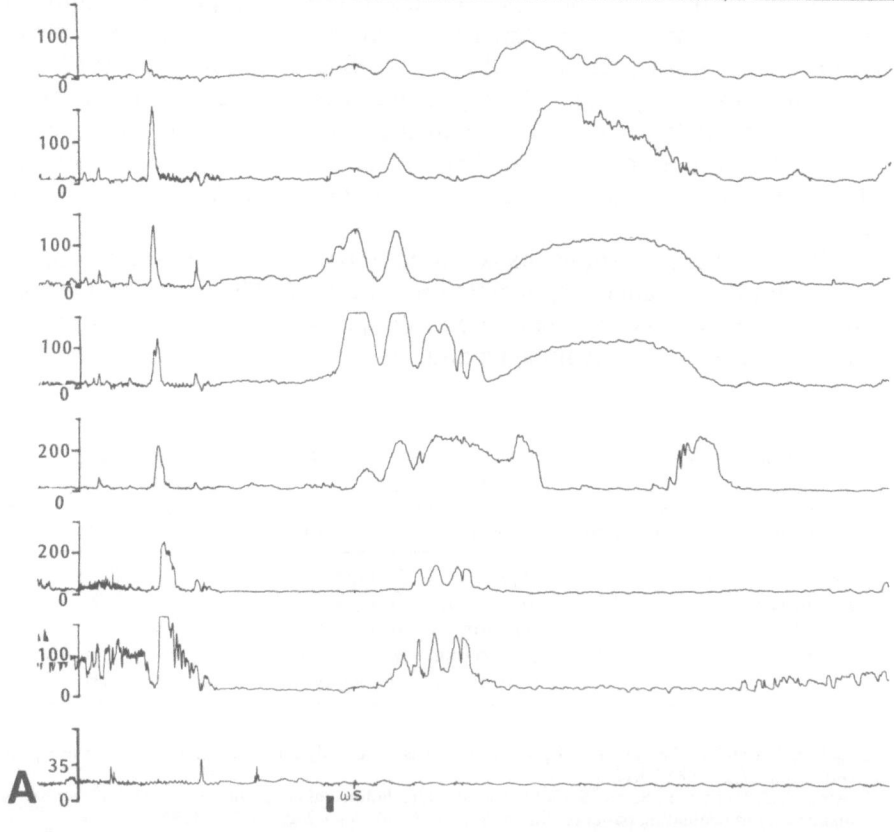

Figure 2. (A) Marked esophageal motor disturbance immediately following tensilon administration (80 μg/kg i.v.) in a patient with "nutcracker esophagus." The simultaneous, prolonged spasm complexes are noted only in the top four recording tips because of esophageal shortening and subsequent intragastric placement of the lower four tips. This motor response was associated with chest pain which reproduced the patient's symptoms. (B) Two

from 40 to 80%. If the provocative test brings on the esophageal manometric abnormality and the chest pain closely resembles the pain from which the patient originally sought relief, the esophagus is felt to be the cause of the clinical problem.[32] A positive esophageal manometric and symptomatic response to edrophonium chloride (80 µg/kg i.v.) by a noncardiac chest pain patient is shown in Fig. 2A and B.

There are problems with "provocative tests," however. Normal patients can respond to edrophonium provocative challenge with abnormal esophageal wave contraction amplitude and duration, albeit the degree of response in patients who do experience pain appears quantita-

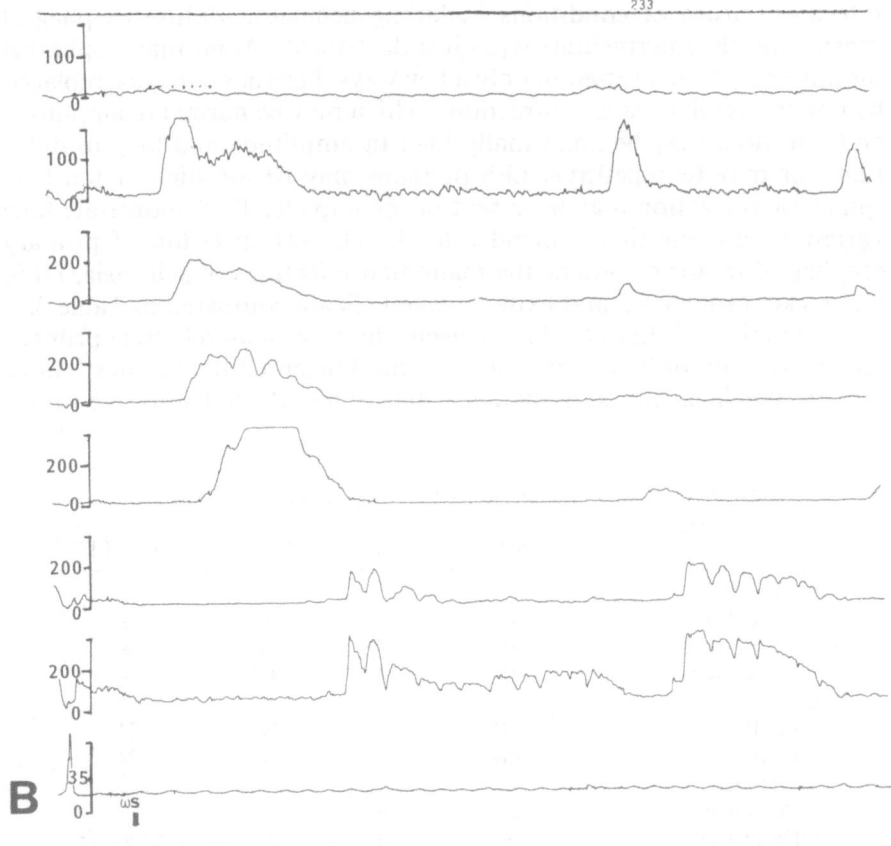

minutes after tensilon, the patient still demonstrates high-amplitude, prolonged-duration wave contractions in the esophageal body after swallows. Note the marked postdeglutition contractile pressures in the distal esophagus and lower esophageal sphincter zone (second recording tip from bottom).

tively greater.[33] Finally, to bring this subject into appropriate perspective, Clouse et al.[34] studied nine patients with intermittent chest pain thought clinically to be secondary to esophageal "spasms." The patients developed typical pain while being studied during esophageal manometry, but exhibited no evidence of unusual motor activity at that time. It was concluded that "patients clinically suspected of having esophageal 'spasms' as the source of chest pain frequently do not, regardless of the presence or absence of motility abnormalities." Additionally, psychological profiling of a group of patients with esophageal motility disorders was very similar to that of patients with irritable bowel syndrome.[35] Perhaps the irritable bowel syndrome is really the irritable gut syndrome, after all!

There is evidence that primary esophageal motility disorders constitute a spectrum of conditions including achalasia, diffuse esophageal spasm, and the intermediate types just described.[36] Abnormal esophageal motility may be expressed in only a few ways. Peristalsis may be replaced by nonprogressive wave contractions, which may be normal in amplitude and duration, may be abnormally high in amplitude and long in duration—or may be repetitive. LES pressure may be too high or too low; spincteric relaxation may be absent or incomplete. To demonstrate how variations on this theme blend into the clinical spectrum of primary esophageal motor disorders, the manometric features of achalasia, DES, nutcracker esophagus, and hypertensive LES are compared in Table 3.

A number of pharmacological agents have been used to treat primary esophageal motor disorders. Short- and longer-acting nitrates[37] have proven beneficial for some patients, but others do not improve or are

Table 3. Spectrum of Primary Esophageal Motor Disorders[a]

	Achalasia	DES	Nutc.	Hyper LES
Body				
Peristalsis	0	+	+	+
Amplitude	0	↑	↑↑	+
Duration	0	↑	N/↑	+
LES				
LESP	N/↑	N	N	↑↑
LESR	0/inc	N	N	N
Symptoms				
Chest pain	±	+	±	±
Dysphagia	+	+	±	±

[a]O, none; ↑, elevated; inc, incomplete; ±, present/absent; LESP, lower esophageal sphincter. Comparison of manometric features characteristic for achalasia, diffuse esophageal spasm (DES), nutcracker esophagus (Nutc.) and hypertensive lower esophageal sphincter (LES).

intolerant of side effects. The calcium channel-blocking drugs[38] have shown promise and can be very effective in controlling symptoms in patients with chest pain of esophageal origin. Their use may be limited also by disturbing side effects. Hydralazine[39] has been evaluated in patients with chest pain and may be effective at the same dosage used for treating hypertensive patients. For patients with underlying psychiatric problems, formal psychiatric counselling and the use of psychotrophic drugs may be of considerable help.

The esophagus, the portal to the gastrointestinal tract, is accessible to research investigations directed to smooth muscle motor dysfunction and its correlation to clinical symptomatology. Perhaps the key necessary to unlock this paradox may reside in the upper recesses of the GI tract. The search is far from over, however.

REFERENCES

1. Alpers DH: Functional gastrointestinal disorders. *Hosp Pract,* April 1983, pp. 139–153.
2. Switz DM: What the gastroenterologist does all day: A survey of a state society's practice. *Gastroenterology* 1976;70:1048–1050.
3. Mendeloff AL: Epidemiology of functional gastrointestinal disorders, in Chey WY (ed): *Functional Disorders of the Gastrointestinal Tract.* New York: Raven Press, 1983, pp. 13–19.
4. Chaudray NA, Truelove SC: The irritable colon syndrome. *Q J Med* 1962;31:307–322.
5. Thompson WG, Heaton KW: Functional bowel disorders in apparently healthy people. *Gastroenterology* 1980;79:283–288.
6. Manning AP, Thompson WG, Heaton KW, Morris AF: Towards positive diagnosis of the irritable bowel. *Br Med J* 1978;2:653–654.
7. Ritchie J: Pain from distension of the pelvic colon by inflating a balloon in the irritable colon syndrome. *Gut* 1973;14:25–32.
8. Swarbrick ET, But L, Hogarty JE, Williams CB, Dawson AM: Site of pain from irritable bowel. *Lancet* 1980;2:443–446.
9. Moriarty KJ, Dawson AM: Functional abdominal pain: Further evidence that the whole gut is affected. *Br Med J* 1982;284:1670–1672.
10. Blackwell JN, Castell DO: Oesophageal chest pain: A point of view. *Gut* 1984;25:1–6.
11. Harvey RF, Read AE: Effect of cholecystokinin on colonic motility and symptoms in patients with irritable bowel syndrome. *Lancet* 1973;1:1–3.
12. Hogan WJ, Geenen JE, Dodds WJ, Toouli J, Venu R, Helm JF: Paradoxical motor response to cholecystokinin (CCK-OP) in patients with suspected sphincter of Oddi dysfunction. *Gastroenterology* 1982;82:1085.
13. Lennard-Jones JE: Functional gastrointestinal disorders. *N Engl J Med* 1983;308:431–435.
14. LoGiudice JA, Geenen JE, Hogan WJ, Dodds WJ: Evaluation of the morphine-prostigmine test in patients with suspected papillary stenosis. *Gastrointest Endosc* 1978;24:204.
15. Almy TP: Clinical features and diagnosis of functional GI disorders, in Chey WY (ed): *Functional Disorders of the Digestive Tract.* New York: Raven Press, 1983, pp. 7–11.

16. Clouse RE, Lustman PJ: Psychiatric illness and contraction abnormalities of the esophagus. *N Engl J Med* 1983;309:1337–1342.
17. Whitehead WE, Engel BT, Schuster MM: Irritable bowel syndrome: Physiological and psychological differences between diarrhea-prominent and constipation-prominent patients. *Dig Dis Sci* 1980;25:404–413.
18. Stacher G, Steinringer H, Blau A, Landgraf M: Acoustically evoked esophageal contractions and defense reaction. *Psychophysiology* 1979;16:234–241.
19. Rubin J, Nagler R, Spiro HM, Pilot ML: Measuring the effect of emotions on esophageal motility. *Psychosom Med* 1962;24:170–176.
20. Obrecht WF, Richter JE, Katz PO, et al: Stress in the healthy esophagus. *Dig Dis Sci,* 1984;29:568.
21. Young SJ, Alpers DH, Norland CC, Woodruff RA: Psychiatric illness and the irritable bowel syndrome. *Gastroenterology* 1976;70:162–166.
22. Latimer P, Sarna S, Campbell D, Latimer M, Waterfall W, Daniel EE: Colonic motor and myoelectrical activity: A comparative study of normal subjects, psychoneurotic patients and patients with irritable bowel syndrome. *Gastroenterology* 1981;80:893–901.
23. VanTrappen G, Hellemans J: Esophageal motility disorders, in Chey WY (ed): *Functional Disorders of the Digestive Tract.* New York: Raven Press, 1983, pp. 117–124.
24. Richter JE, Castell DO: Diffuse esophageal spasm. A reappraisal. *Ann Intern Med* 1984;100:242–245.
25. Arndorfer RC, Stef JJ, Dodds WJ, Linehan JH, Hogan WJ: Improved infusion system for intraluminal esophageal manometry. *Gastroenterology* 1977;73:23–27.
26. Cohen S: The classification of the esophageal motility disorders (editorial). *Gastroenterology* 1983;84:1050–1051.
27. Blackwell JN, Castell DO: Oesophageal chest pain: A point of view. *Gut* 1984;25:1–6.
28. Meyer GW, Castell DO: Human esophageal response during chest pain induced by swallowing cold liquids. *JAMA* 1981;246:2057–2059.
29. Edwards DAW: "Tender esophagus": A new syndrome (abstract). *Gut* 1982;23:A919.
30. Berger K, McCallum RW: The hypertensive lower esophageal sphincter. *Gastroenterology* 1981;80:1109.
31. Benjamin SB, Gerhardt DC, Castell DO: High amplitude peristaltic esophageal contractions associated with chest pain and/or dysphagia. *Gastroenterology* 1979;77:478–483.
32. Benjamin SB, Richter JE, Cordova CM, Knuff TE, Castell DO: Prospective manometric evaluation with pharmacological provocation of patients with suspected esophageal motility dysfunction. *Gastroenterology* 1983;84:893–901.
33. Richter JE, Wu WC, Blackwell JN, Johns DN, Hackshaw BT, Castell DO: The edrophonium response: Use in diagnosis and possible understanding of mechanism of esophageal chest pain (abstract). *Gastroenterology* 1983;84:1285.
34. Clouse RE, Staiano A, Landau DW, Schlachter JL: Manometric findings during spontaneous chest pain in patients with presumed esophageal "spasms." *Gastroenterology* 1983;85:395–402.
35. Obrecht WF, Richter JE, Castell DO, Bradley LA, Young LD, Anderson KO: Is the nutcracker esophagus part of the spectrum of irritable bowel syndrome? *Dig Dis Sci* 1984;29:568.
36. VanTrappen G, Janssens J: Diffuse muscle spasm of the esophagus and the hypertensive lower esophageal sphincter. *Clin Gastroenterol* 1976;5:59–72.
37. Swamy N: Esophageal spasm: Clinical and manometric response to nitroglycerin and long-acting nitrites. *Gastroenterology* 1977;72:23–27.

38. Richter JE, Spurling TJ, Cordova CM, Castell DO: Effects of oral calcium blocker, Diltiazem, on esophageal contractions: Studies in volunteers and patients with nutcracker esophagus. *Dig Dis Sci* 1984;7:649–656.
39. Mellow MH: Effect of isosorbide and hydralazine in painful primary esophageal motility disorders. *Gastroenterology* 1982;82:364–370.

4

Medical Dissolution of Gallstones
When Is Cholecystectomy Indicated?

Roy M. Preshaw

1. INTRODUCTION

Oral agents capable of slow dissolution of cholesterol gallstones are currently prescribed in Western Europe and the United States and will soon be widely available in Canada. The initial enthusiasm for this novel therapy has dimmed slightly following publication of the results of controlled trials, such that at least some authorities have been able to forecast that "cholecystectomy continues to be the treatment of choice for a great majority of patients with cholelithiasis"[28]; "no more than 10% of gallstone patients can be successfully treated (with dissolution therapy)"[47]; and "(surgical) treatment, although threatened, is not yet outmoded."[41]

Perhaps it is appropriate on the eve of the introduction of these agents to Canada to reconsider the place of routine elective cholecystectomy in Canada, where there is evidence that we volunteer our patients for this operation more than in any other nation. In 1971 in Windsor or Kapuskasing, Ontario the crude rate of cholecystectomy was 7 times higher than in Luton, England and 5 times higher than the rate in Rennes, France, communities of similar size.[33] In 1976 the annual rate of cholecystectomy in Canada was 1.4 times the rate in the United States and 4 times the rate in England and Wales.[44] In 1978 in Canada there were 131

Roy M. Preshaw ● Department of Surgery and Gastrointestinal Research Unit, University of Calgary Medical School, Calgary, Alberta, Canada T2N 4N1.

cholecystectomies per 100,000 males and 357/100,000 females, almost double the rate for appendectomy.[40]

2. EPIDEMIOLOGY OF GALLSTONES

Examination of the indications for gallstone therapy is incomplete without consideration of estimates of prevalence of calculi in the general population. For example, a simple explanation of the high rate of cholecystectomy in Canada would be that asymptomatic gallstones are much commoner north of the 49th parallel. Unfortunately, estimates of gallstone prevalence in this country are also incomplete. Seventy-five years ago in Toronto the number of subjects with gallstones at the time of autopsy was 4%[36]; in more recent studies, 16% of males and 33% of females over the age of 10 years and coming to autopsy in North Bay, Ontario either had gallstones or had a previous cholecystectomy.[17] Canadians do not appear to differ substantially from other races, where current estimates of gallstone prevalence vary from 3% in Portuguese males to 57% in Swedish females (Table 1).

The diagnosis of gallstones during life depends on screening with oral cholecystography or ultrasound. Clearly these techniques are dependent on subject cooperation, and screening has therefore been restricted to specific groups within larger populations. In Wales, Bainton et al.[4] found 6% of males and 12% of females below the age of 70 to have gallstones. In Canada, surveys of Nova Scotian women between the ages of 15 and 50 years showed a 17% prevalence of gallstones in Caucasians and 21% in Micmac Indians.[49] In the southwestern United States even higher rates of gallstone disease have been described in Mexican Americans[9] and in local Indian tribes.[37]

Table 1. Prevalence of Gallstones

	Method	Males %	Females %	Comments
Wales[4]	X-ray	6.2	12.1	
Portugal[11]	Autopsy	3.3	7.3	
Germany[13]	Autopsy	17	34	
Germany[27]	Autopsy	26	55	
Sweden[20]	Autopsy	30	57.	
Canada				
Toronto[36]	Autopsy		4	
Ontario[17]	Autopsy	16	33	Including cholecystectomy
Nova Scotia[49]	X-ray	—	21	MicMac 15–50 years
Nova Scotia[48]	X-ray	—	17	Caucasian 15–50 years

Many of these quoted studies confirm a tendency for gallstone disease to be more prevalent with increasing age. In groups of elderly persons in selected populations (most notably southwestern American Indians), the proportion of individuals having gallstones greatly exceeds 50%. This raises the interesting problem of definition of a disease state and suggests that, at least for some populations, the presence of gallstones in the elderly has become the norm.

Current prevalence rates for gallstones suggest that many cause little or no symptoms. The proportion of symptomatic gallstones in a population is even more difficult to define, because of the general nature of the complaints presently assigned to gallbladder disease. Two studies from Britain that identified gallstones by screening techniques were unable to separate subjects with and without calculi on the basis of nonspecific dyspeptic symptoms (e.g., abdominal pain or discomfort, belching, flatus, postprandial discomfort). The authors concluded that such complaints were surprisingly common and could not routinely be ascribed to gallstones.[4,34] The definition of minimally symptomatic gallstones becomes blurred when it is reported that 50% of a sample of over 1 million North Americans will list periodic gastrointestinal symptoms of this nonspecific nature.[16]

3. INDICATIONS FOR CHOLECYSTECTOMY

Sharply defined indications for biliary surgery have appeared by consensus in the literature, contrasting with the vagueness of other studies on gallstone prevalence and symptomatology. Acute inflammation associated with gallstone disease (cholecystitis, cholangitis, pancreatitis) is best treated by surgical intervention, with controversy restricted to whether the operation should be performed immediately or after the acute process has resolved. Obstructive jaundice secondary to choledocholithiasis in the presence of an intact gallbladder may be relieved by endoscopic papillotomy, but most opinion favors subsequent cholecystectomy if there are no other clear contraindications to this surgery.

There is also little doubt that subjects experiencing intermittent attacks of severe upper abdominal or chest wall pain associated with nausea and vomiting (biliary colic), in whom gallstones can be demonstrated radiologically, are best subjected to elective cholecystectomy.

Perhaps most of current elective cholecystectomies are, however, performed when gallstones are demonstrated radiologically as part of the investigation of ill-defined abdominal complaints. In the absence of strong reasons to avoid anesthesia or surgery, current surgical opinion has tended toward defining the presence of gallstones per se as an indication for cholecystectomy. One notable American authority suggested that "patients with cholelithiasis who are carefully evaluated and who have no contraindication to operation should be treated surgically. . . . such an approach will reduce the sequelae and complications in later life when the morbidity and mortality are highest."[12] In Canada the statement has been made that " . . . most surgeons would opt for cholecystectomy in a healthy subject with radiologically demonstrated gallstones and equivocal or absent symptoms. . . ."[6]

4. EFFICACY AND COMPLICATIONS OF CHOLECYSTECTOMY

Numerous series by individual surgeons or institutions demonstrate mortality rates for elective cholecystectomy which approach that for general anesthesia alone.[24,28] Although such publications bear witness to the skill and dedication of individuals, of more interest are estimates of the overall mortality following this procedure. Table 2 shows the mortality rates for cholecystectomy recorded in the National Halothane Study in the United States, which confirms the low risk in subjects below the age of 50 years. However, the mortality rate from cholecystectomy alone rises alarmingly in poor-risk patients, especially those above the age of 70.[5] Similar high mortality rates in elderly patients undergoing cholecystectomy have been recorded in Canada.[31]

Extension of the operative procedure appears to increase the morbidity and mortality. In a prominent U.S. institution, addition of common bile duct exploration to simple cholecystectomy raised the mortality rate from 0.5 to 3.2%.[29]

Biliary calculi may still form after cholecystectomy, but there is evidence suggesting that removal of the gallbladder in man may decrease cholesterol saturation in the bile,[32] thus diminishing the chances of forming further cholesterol stones. Cholecystectomy does not diminish intraluminal micellar lipid concentrations during digestion,[39] and there is no demonstrable change in the ability to absorb lipid.[10]

Table 2. Mortality Rate for Cholecystectomy (Percent)[5]

Age	Good risk		Poor risk	
	Males	Females	Males	Females
<50	0.10	0.05	2.40	1.26
50–69	0.54	0.28	3.26	1.71
>70	2.49	1.32	9.51	5.16

Thus, long-term effects of cholecystectomy, once the operative procedure is safely passed, appear to be negligible. Studies suggesting an association between cholecystectomy and cancer, especially of the colon,[21,45] have been interpreted by others as an expression of cholesterol disease, since the same slight association may be present before cholecystectomy.[22]

5. INDICATIONS FOR AGENTS PROMOTING GALLSTONE DISSOLUTION

Most gallstones in North America are primarily due to precipitation of cholesterol in bile contained in the gallbladder. It is not the purpose of this chapter to consider current theories of the pathogenesis of cholesterol gallstones. It is sufficient to note that bile which is supersaturated with cholesterol will interact with abnormalities promoting cholesterol crystal formation to cause the formation of calculi.[15] The supersaturation theory is supported by evidence that cholesterol gallstones are more common in obesity, especially with recent weight loss; in subjects on high-fat diets; in patients with disease of the ileum; in diabetes mellitus; with hyperlipidemias; with total parenteral nutrition; with primary biliary cirrhosis; and during therapy with serveral pharmacological agents, including estrogens and clofibrate.[18]

Expansion of the bile acid pool to avoid cholesterol saturation is an elegant theoretical technique for cholesterol gallstone dissolution. By 1972 it was possible to demonstrate that prolonged therapy with oral chenodeoxycholic acid caused radiological dissolution of cholesterol gallstones.[8] Surprisingly, detailed study of this effect in the ensuing decade showed that dissolution of gallstones was not due to a simple expansion of the bile acid pool, but to a reduction in the biliary secretion of cholesterol relative to total bile acids and phospholipids.[1,19]

Controversy over the mechanism of action of chenodeoxycholic acid has only been exceeded by arguments over its efficacy. In subjects with radiolucent gallstones (i.e., probably cholesterol stones) and a functioning gallbladder, complete dissolution occurred in perhaps 25% of subjects when a substantial number of studies are pooled: the range is from 0 to 53%. The largest and probably best controlled trial has been the National Cooperative Gallstone Study (NCGS) in the United States: using a relatively low dose of chenodeoxycholic acid, gallstone dissolution was achieved in a disappointing 14% of subjects.[38]

The most important side effect of treatment with chenodeoxycholic acid has been diarrhea: sufficient oral bile acid may directly damage colonic mucosa and certainly induces net colonic secretion of fluid.[30]

Diarrhea occurred in 41% of subjects receiving 750 mg/day in the NCGS. The diarrhea may be sufficiently severe to cause some subjects to drop out of a trial of prolonged therapy, and in others it may be necessary to reduce the dose of chenodeoxycholic acid and therefore reduce the efficiency of gallstone dissolution.

Of perhaps more concern are elevated levels of serum aminotransferase which occur in about 50% of subjects, associated with minor changes on liver biopsy. These biochemical and ultrastructural changes also appear to be dose-related and tend to regress when therapy is discontinued.[50] Chenodeoxycholic acid therapy also reduces serum triglyceride levels significantly, yet causes about a 10% rise in serum cholesterol, located in the low-density-lipoprotein fraction.[2] This raises the possibility of increased atherogenesis, especially with prolonged therapy.

Selection of patients for oral chenodeoxocholic acid therapy instead of surgery is therefore difficult. Absolute requirements are radiolucent stones in a gallbladder which visualizes on oral cholecystography. It is not known what proportion of the current gallstone population meets this definition, but estimates range from 10% to over 70%. It should be noted that about half of pigment gallstones are also radiolucent, and these are not likely to respond to oral chenodeoxycholic acid.[42] Perhaps up to 30% of calculi removed at cholecystectomy in the United States are predominantly pigment.[43]

Features that improve the chances of successful stone dissolution include a normal body weight (i.e., nonobese) and the presence of small, rather than large, stones. Absolute contraindications include complications of gallstone disease which are life threatening, such as acute cholangitis, cholecystitis, or pancreatitis. Chenodeoxycholic acid should not be used in the presence of certain other gastrointestinal diseases, including peptic ulcer, cirrhosis, or other significant liver disease, or Crohn's disease or ulcerative colitis, because of its effects of gastric mucosal permeability to ions, the propensity to diarrhea, and the observed ultrastructural changes in hepatic morphology. Its safety in pregnancy has not been established, and perhaps its efficacy will be reduced in women of childbearing age who are on oral contraceptives.

Zak and co-workers[50] suggested that chenodeoxycholic acid is the therapy of choice in subjects with significant pulmonary or cardiac disease who meet the other qualifications, and perhaps also in severe diabetics, who would be expected to have a higher incidence of infection and other complications after surgery. Of course, dissolution therapy would be appropriate in subjects who cannot accept anesthesia or elective surgery. These authors favor cholecystectomy in patients in presenting with episodic, severe biliary colic. The recommended dose of chenodeoxycholic acid is greater than 10 mg/kg per day and is probably optimal at 12–15 mg/kg per day, given in two divided doses with meals. Higher doses and the administration of the total daily amount as a single dose may cause increased problems with diarrhea. It is possible that a slow build of chenodeoxycholic acid up to a final ideal dose level over several weeks may increase tolerance to diarrhea.

Experience in the NCGS suggests monitoring of serum aminotransferase levels at monthly intervals for 3 months and then every 3–6 months, with serum cholesterol measurements performed at 6-month intervals. Oral cholecystography or ultrasound should be used after 1 year to evaluate the progress of gallstone dissolution; partial dissolution indicates successful therapy which should be reviewed after another 12 months. No change after 1 year should result in a decision either to attempt an increase in dose or to discontinue the therapy. It is recommended that chenodeoxycholic acid be continued for a final 3 months after successful dissolution.

Subjects who will have their stones after therapy for 2 years should probably give up if there has been no change in gallstone size as assessed radiologically. There will be, however, a certain number who will exhibit a definite decrease in stone size at this stage: if therapy is continued for another year or two, complete dissolution will probably be achieved in some such subjects. In the NCGS, further therapy for 2 years with 750 mg/day increased the total number with complete dissolution from 14% to about 20%. The exact number reaching complete dissolution is not clear because of failure to examine all subjects radiologically.[25]

Other bile acids that are effective in causing dissolution of cholesterol gallstones have been studied. Ursodeoxycholic acid has been subjected to considerable investigation, but adequate long-term clinical trials comparing this agent with chenodeoxycholic acid are not yet available. It appears at this point that ursodeoxycholic acid is at least as effective as chenodeoxycholic acid and may have fewer side effects: less diarrhea, less transaminase changes, and no changes in serum lipids. The optimal dose of ursodeoxycholic acid is probably between 10 and 15 mg/kg per day.[3] It is also likely to become available shortly for prescription use in Canada.

6. THE GALLSTONES ARE DISSOLVED—WHAT NOW?

After successful cholecystectomy, further formation of biliary calculi will only occur in the main biliary duct system. After successful dissolution therapy, the subject is left with an intact and presumably functioning gallbladder. In the absence of further intervention, the patient is subject to the same conditions that generated the gallstones in the first place. Thus, the recurrence of gallstones is not surprising. Follow-up of subjects whose gallstones have been successfully dissolved show that a substantial number develop recurrence in the subsequent years. In a follow-up to the NCGS, 27% of such subjects had proven recurrence within 3.5 years,[26] and similar rates of recurrence have been recorded by other workers. In Marks' study, a group randomized to a low maintenance dose of cheno-deoxycholic acid (375 mg/day) demonstrated similar rates of recurrence. It is not known whether a higher maintenance dose or added dietary manipulation such as a low-cholesterol and/or high-fiber diet might be more effective in the prevention of recurrence. Conversely, it appears likely that recurrent stones, after initial dissolution, will also respond to a further course of chenodeoxycholic acid.

7. COMPARISON OF ORAL BILE ACID THERAPY WITH CHOLECYSTECTOMY

The spectrum of biliary tract disease is wide, and different opinions on the value or otherwise of the specific therapies are also widely pro-moted. There appears to be general agreement between proponents of oral dissolution and surgical authorities that severe acute episodes of bil-iary tract disease, especially if life threatening, are best treated by surgical intervention. Surgeons will also not dispute the argument that severe con-comitant disease in other organ systems, which greatly increases the risk of cholecystectomy,[5] should be an indication for selection of oral bile acid therapy as an initial treatment.

Probably more than 50% of Canadians with gallstones, however, do not meet the definitions above. Many if not most will have gallstones which are asymptomatic or are, at best, associated with mild, nonspecific symptoms. It is of interest to this author that both surgeons and bile acid enthusiasts claim priority in their approach to this group of patients with minimally symptomatic gallstones. Some surgical authorities have even suggested that even completely asymptomatic gallstones are best removed while the subject is relatively young and healthy.[12] On the other hand, Zak and co-workers[50] have suggested that chenodeoxycholic acid is the treatment of choice for patients with mild or absent biliary symp-toms. These authors even promote this therapy for trials in subjects with normal gallbladders but who are at high risk for gallstone formation, such as American Indians or obese persons.

In view of this aggressive approach by both surgeons and internists to the innocent (or nearly innocent) gallstone, it is worth searching for evidence that such calculi threaten to cause future pain and suffering and perhaps life-threatening events. The surgical opinion appears based on studies in which gallstones were identified, either by radiology or at the time of laparotomy for other reasons, and when the patient was not subjected to cholecystectomy. Four such series (Table 3) are available, and all are in agreement that between 30 and 50% of such subjects will have further symptoms, and perhaps 20% will develop significant complications.[7,23,38,46] Unfortunately, there is one problem with these four series: the subjects all must have had some symptoms that led initially either to oral cholecystography or, in some, to laparotomy. Therefore, these series are correctly labeled as dealing with minimally symptomatic gallstones.

Only one study has examined the fate of gallstones discovered in subjects without even minimal symptoms. For several years at the University of Michigan, faculty members were required to take an initial medical examination on appointment, which included an oral cholecystogram. One hundred and twenty-three subjects, mostly men, were identified to have gallstones and were followed for up to 24 years.[14] As would be expected, some elected to have cholecystectomy, but of the remainder who did not have cholecystectomy, only 18% developed significant symptoms probably associated with their gallstones: two patients had acute cholecystitis and one had pancreatitis. None died from biliary tract disease, and the three men with complications had uneventful cholecystectomies. This important study badly needs replication in populations other than faculty at the University of Michigan and, of course, in women. As noted earlier, in 1978 73% of cholecystectomies in Canada were in women.

This study by Gracie and Ransohoff[14] has encouraged the calculation of the effects of surgical intervention in large populations with asymptomatic gallstones.[35] Elective cholecystectomy will result in some deaths, with the chance of dying increasing with age: older subjects unfortunately appear to have the highest prevalence of gallstones. In Canada, it appears

Table 3. Minimally Symptomatic Gallstones

	Number	Follow-up (years)	Symptoms %	Complications %
Comfort et al.[7]	112	24	45	Not stated
Lund[23]	34	5–20	33	20
Wenckert and Robertson[46]	781	1–11	51	18
Schoenfeld et al.[38]	305	2	45	4

probable that the percentage of the population having gallstones is between 4 and 24%[17,36]: this calculates to between 1 and 6 million subjects. Using the smallest death rates for elective cholecystectomy in the National Halothane Study[5] of 0.10% in males and 0.05% in females below the age of 50 years, elective surgery in this large number of subjects would result in between 750 and 4500 deaths. It has been effectively argued that the University of Michigan study indicates that surgical intervention in asymptomatic subjects cannot be justified, but that one should wait for the few who will develop symptoms or complications. Perhaps this approach is also useful in subjects with minimally symptomatic gallstones.

These calculations also point out that, despite aggressive surgical pronouncements on the advisability of cholecystectomy in all gallstone subjects, even the high rate of cholecystectomy in Canada barely dents the surface of the gallstone population. In 1978 there were 57,333 cholecystectomies in Canada[40]: using the estimate above of a total gallstone population of between 4 and 24%, this represents surgical cure in that 1 year of only between 1 and 6% of the total numbers at risk.

This process can also be used to calculate costs of aggressive versus expectant oral dissolution therapy for asymptomatic gallstones. Here the limiting factor is not operative mortality, but costs of the treatment plus rather nebulous long-term effects, which may include increased atherogenesis. Treatment with cheno- or ursodeoxycholic acid is not cheap: costs in Canada will depend on final marketing decisions for each agent, but experience elsewhere suggests the daily cost will be between $1.50 and $2.00 a day for a dose between 10 and 15 mg/kg per day. Most subjects will require a minimum of 2 year's therapy, at a cost of between $1100 and $1500 for the drug alone. The worst case scenario—treating every gallstone subject in Canada with these agents for 2 years and using the estimate of 24% for the total gallstone population—results in the absurd estimate of 9 billion dollars for drug costs alone. This amount is exceeded only by the costs of cholecystectomy in the same population.

8. SUMMARY

The evidence available now suggests that if you are discovered to have gallstones, further action should depend on assessment of your symptomatology. If the gallstones are truly asymptomatic, there is good evidence that you have an 80% change of *not* having either significant symptoms or complications in the next 10–20 years, and that if you do develop problems, they can be safely dealt with at that time. If the gallstones are causing significant problems, such as acute complications or repeated bouts of pain requiring narcotics for relief, with return visits to hospital emergency departments, all authorities agree that elective cholecystectomy is justified. If, however, you fall between these two extremes, as undoubtedly most subjects demonstrated to have gallstones do, further treatment should be left up to you. If you choose to have no therapy, the indications are that you have a 30–50% chance of further symptoms in the next 1–25 years (Table 3) and a less than 20% chance of significant complications in the same period. You should know that the mortality rate from these complications and the attendant surgery increases with increasing age. These facts have led surgical authorities to suggest intervention when your gallstones have been discovered, and medical authorities to offer you oral dissolution therapy, particularly as you grow older.

Despite the side effects of oral bile acids and the patience required to maintain the therapy, I suspect that many Canadians will elect for this treatment in the next decade. Given the choice, most people will probably choose pharmacology over surgery, knowing that eager and willing surgeons are always available if the therapy is unsuccessful. Perhaps they also realize that improved agents for oral dissolution are likely to be developed, and innocuous programs to prevent gallstone recurrence may be discovered. The only certain forecast is that gallstone disease will continue to appropriate a substantial portion of the Canadian health dollar.

REFERENCES

1. Adler RD, Bennion LJ, Duane WC, et al: Effects of low dose chenodeoxycholic acid feeding on biliary lipid metabolism. *Gastroenterology* 1975;68:326–334.
2. Albers JJ, Grundy SM, Cleary PA, et al: National Cooperative Gallstone Study. The effect of chenodeoxycholic acid on lipoproteins and apolipoproteins. *Gastroenterology* 1982;82:638–646.
3. Bachrach WH, Hofmann AF: Ursodeoxycholic acid in the treatment of cholesterol cholelithiasis: A review. *Dig Dis Sci* 1982;27:737–761, 833–856.
4. Bainton D, Davies GT, Evans KT, et al: Gallbladder disease. Prevalence in a South Wales industrial town. *N Engl J Med* 1976;294:1147–1149.
5. Bishop YMM, Mosteller F: Smoothed contingency table analysis, in: Bunker JP, Forrest WP (eds): *The National Halothane Study*. Bethesda, MD: National Institute of General Medical Sciences, 1969, pp. 238–272.
6. Carroll SE: Indications for cholecystectomy. *Can J Surg* 1974;17:1–2.
7. Comfort MW, Gray HK, Wilson JM: The silent gallstone: A ten to twenty year follow up study of 112 cases. *Ann Surg* 1948;128:931–937.
8. Danziger RG, Hofmann AF, Schoenfield LJ, et al: Dissolution of cholesterol gallstones by chenodesoxycholic acid. *N Engl J Med* 1972;286:1–8.

9. Diehl AK, Stern MP, Ostrower VS, et al: Prevalence of clinical gallbladder disease in Mexican-American, Anglo and Black women. *South Med J* 1980;73:438–443.
10. Fedor EJ, Fisher B: The use of radioactive iodine labelled triolein in the evaluation of fat absorption following cholecystectomy. *Surg Gynecol Obstet* 1960;111:206–210.
11. Galvao H, Menezes ML, Correia JP: The prevalence of gallstones in the Portuguese population: A necropsy study. *Ital J Gastroenterol* 1981;13:100–104.
12. Glenn F: Biliary tract disease. *Surg Gynecol Obstet* 1981;153:401–402.
13. Goebell VH, Rudolph HD, Breuer N, et al: The frequency of gallstones in liver cirrhosis. *Z Gastroenterol* 1981;19:345–355.
14. Gracie WA, Ransohoff DF: The natural history of the silent gallstone: The innocent gallstone is not a myth. *N Engl J Med* 1982;307:798–800.
15. Grundy SM: Mechanism of cholesterol gallstone formation. *Semin Liver Dis* 1983;3:97–111.
16. Hammond EC: Some preliminary findings on physical complaints from a prospective study of 1,064,004 men and women. *Am J Public Health* 1964;54:11–12.
17. Karnauchow PN, Mylne GE: Whither cholecystectomy? *Can J Surg* 1974;17:25–29.
18. Kern F: Epidemiology and natural history of gallstones. *Semin Liver Dis* 1983;3:87–96.
19. LaRusso NF, Hoffman NE, Hofmann AF, et al: Effect of primary bile acid ingestion on bile acid metabolism and biliary lipid secretion in gallstone patients. *Gastroenterology* 1975;69:1301–1314.
20. Lindstrom CG: Frequency of gallstone disease in a well-defined Swedish population. *Scand J Gastroenterol* 1977;12:341–346.
21. Linos D, O'Fallon WM, Beard CM, et al: Cholecystectomy and carcinoma of the colon. *Lancet* 1981;2:379–381.
22. Lowenfels AB, Domellof L, Lindstrom CG, et al: Cholelithiasis, cholecystectomy and cancer: A case-control study in Sweden. *Gastroenterology* 1982;83:672–676.
23. Lund J: Surgical indications for cholelithiasis: Prophylactic cholecystectomy elucidated on the basis of long-term follow-up in 526 nonoperated cases. *Ann Surg* 1960;151:153–162.
24. MacLean LD, Goldstein M, MacDonald JE, et al: Results of cholecystectomy in 1000 consecutive patients. *Can J Surg* 1975;18:459–465.
25. Marks JW, Baum RA, Hanson RF, et al: Additional chenodiol therapy after partial dissolution of gallstones with two years of treatment. *Ann Intern Med* 1984;100:382–384.
26. Marks JW, Lan SP, Baum RA, et al: Low-dose chenodiol to prevent gallstone recurrence after dissolution therapy. *Ann Intern Med* 1984;100:376–381.
27. Massarrat VS, Klingemann HG, Kappert J, et al: Incidence of gallstone disease in autopsy material and outpatients from West Germany. *Z Gastroenterol* 1982;20:341–345.
28. McSherry CK: The National Cooperative Gallstone Study report: A surgeon's perspective. *Ann Intern Med* 1981;95:379–380.
29. McSherry CK, Glenn F: The incidence and causes of death following surgery for nonmalignant biliary tract disease. *Ann Surg* 1980;191:271–275.
30. Mekhjian HS, Phillips SF, Hofmann AF: Colonic secretion of water and electrolytes induced by bile acids. Perfusion studies in man. *J Clin Invest* 1971;50:1569–1577.
31. Mylne GE, Karnauchow PN: Cholecystectomy and related procedures in two community hospitals. *Can J Surg* 1974;17:20–24.
32. Palmer RH: The gallbladder and bile composition. *Am J Dig Dis* 1976;21:795–796.
33. Plant JCD, Percy I, Bates T, et al: Incidence of gallbladder disease in Canada, England and France. *Lancet* 1973;2:249–251.

34. Price WH: Gall-bladder dyspepsia. *Br Med J* 1963;2:138–141.
35. Ransohoff DF, Gracie WA, Wolfenson LB, et al: Prophylactic cholecystectomy or expectant management for silent gallstones: A decision analysis to assess survival. *Ann Intern Med* 1983;99:199–204.
36. Ryerson E: Aetiology of cholelithiasis with special reference to the age-incidence. *Can Med Assoc J* 1911;1:832–841.
37. Sampliner RE, Bennett PH, Comess LJ, et al: Gallbladder disease in Pima Indians. Demonstration of high prevalence and early onset by cholecystography. *N Engl J Med* 1970;283:1358–1364.
38. Schoenfield LJ, Lachlin JM: Chenodiol (chenodeoxycholic acid) for dissolution of gall-stones: The National Cooperative Gallstone Study. A controlled trial of efficacy and safety. *Ann Intern Med* 1981;92:257–282.
39. Simmons F, Bouchier IAD: Intraluminal bile salt concentrations and fat digestion after cholecystectomy. *S Afr Med J* 1972;46:2089–2092.
40. Statistics Canada: Surgical procedures and treatments, 1978. Cat. 82.208. Minister of Supply and Services, Ottawa, Ontario: 1982.
41. Sutherland LR: Medical dissolution of gallstones: An illusion? *Can Med Assoc J* 1983;129:232.
42. Trotman BW: Pigment gallstone disease. *Semin Liver Dis* 1983;3:112–119.
43. Trotman BW, Soloway RD: Pigment v. cholesterol cholelithiasis: Clinical and epidemiological aspects. *Am J Dig Dis* 1975;20:735–740.
44. Vayda E, Mindell WR, Rutkow IM, et al: A decade of surgery in Canada, England and Wales, and the United States. *Arch Surg* 1982;117:846–853.
45. Vernick LJ, Kuller LH, Lohsoonthorn P, et al: Relationship between cholecystectomy and ascending colon cancer. *Cancer* 1980;45:392–395.
46. Wenckert A, Robertson B: The natural history of gallstone disease: Eleven-year review of 781 non-operated cases. *Gastroenterology* 1966;50:376–381.
47. Whiting MJ, Bradley BM, Watts JM, et al: Chemical and physical properties of gall-stones in South Australia: Implications for dissolution treatment. *Gut* 1983;24:11–15.
48. Williams CN, Johnston JL: Prevalence of gallstones and risk factors in Caucasian women in a rural Canadian community. *Can Med Assoc J* 1980;122:664–668.
49. Williams CN, Johnston JL, Weldon KLM: Prevalence of gallstones and gallbladder disease in Canadian MicMac Indian women. *Can Med Assoc J* 1977;117:758–760.
50. Zak RA, Marks JW, Schoenfield LJ: Current status of chenodeoxycholic acid (chenodiol) therapy of cholesterol gallstones. *Semin Liver Dis* 1983;3:132–145.

5

Interventional Endoscopy
Sclerotherapy, Sphincterotomy, and Laser Coagulation

Bryce R. Taylor

1. INTRODUCTION

Upper gastrointestinal endoscopy was originally developed as a diagnostic procedure. Technological advances have gradually led to the use of sophisticated flexible fiberoptic instruments, which can now be employed therapeutically as well as diagnostically. Three such modalities are the subject of this chapter: injection sclerotherapy, endoscopic sphincterotomy, and laser photocoagulation.

2. ENDOSCOPIC INJECTION SCLEROTHERAPY

Endoscopic injection sclerotherapy represents the latest example of a fascinating series of management regimens for bleeding esophageal varices. The problem of bleeding varices, especially in the alcoholic, accounts for approximately 75% of cases in North America. Bleeding varices remain a difficult and frustrating problem to manage. The patient's outcome may well be determined more by the type, extent, and activity of his liver disease than by the efficacy of one particular method of control and prevention of hemorrhage. In addition, the alcoholic patients are

---

Bryce R. Taylor • Toronto General Hospital, Toronto, Ontario, Canada M5KG 1L7.

often noncompliant and difficult to follow and may have active alcoholic hepatitis related to recent ethanol abuse. All these factors make even the most carefully planned randomized trial extremely difficult to control. The solution in the last 40 years, therefore, has apparently been one of enthusiastic support of the current popular regimen. At the moment, after a patient with bleeding varices is stabilized, usually with blood transfusions, intravenous Pitressin, and/or balloon tamponade, the management options or combinations of options are legion. To stop and protect against hemorrhage, the physician or surgeon can reduce portal pressure or attempt to devascularize the gastroesophageal junction. It is this one area of portasystemic collateralization that is producing a life-threatening situation. The reduction in portal pressure can be accomplished medically with β blockers or surgically with either total or selective shunts. Devascularization can be attempted endoscopically with endoscopic injection sclerotherapy, angiographically with percutaneous transhepatic obliteration of the coronary vein, and surgically with a variety of devascularization procedures. The most extensive devascularization procedure is the "Sugiura" procedure. At present, all these options have their enthusiastic supporters.

Endoscopic injection sclerotherapy is undoubtedly the most popular interventional therapy at the moment, and it the purpose of this chapter to assess what has been learned about the procedure in the last 5 years and to reach a conclusion as to what its role might be in the next 5. There has been a veritable explosion of literature regarding the selection of patients, timing of therapy, sclerosants used, type of injection employed, and types of endoscope, needle, and anesthetic. There have been a number of consecutive series reported, and more recently attempts at randomized controlled trials, and these areas will be discussed. While reviewing the voluminous data, one must keep in mind the sentiment expressed by Raskin in a recent editorial in *Gastrointestinal Endoscopy*— "Endoscopic Sclerotherapy is Becoming Increasingly Popular. Are we not again running into the time-honoured tradition of relying on data from uncontrolled studies or comparing uncontrolled studies to each other?"[1]

2.1. History

In 1936 Crafoord and Frenckner[2] performed repeated endoscopic intravariceal injections of quinine–uretan on alternate days for a month, starting from the top of the esophagus and ending at the gastroesophageal junction. The subsequent report that the patient had been free of bleeding for 3 years evidently became lost in the otolaryngologic literature. Subsequent series reported by Moersch in 1941 and 1947,[3,4] Patterson and

Rouse in 1947,[5] and Macbeth in 1955[6] were all guardedly enthusiastic, but did not stimulate wide acceptance, presumably because of the enthusiasm for total shunt procedures at that time. In 1973 Johnston and Rodgers[7] reported an impressive series of 117 patients whose acute hemorrhage had been controlled in 93% by the use of injection sclerotherapy through a rigid esophagoscope. They reported a hospital admission mortality of 18%, and because of a high rebleeding rate (the typical repeated injections now performed were not used), Johnston gradually became more enthusiastic about circular stapling of the lower esophagus as an emergent and definitive method of stopping and controlling hemorrhage. Raschke and Paquet[8] were the most accomplished sclerotherapists in Europe, and they reported similar success rates in 640 patients. In addition to early control, they had impressive long-term survival using a different technique of injection.

Since these reports, endoscopic injection sclerotherapy has been carried out widely, often in an uncontrolled fashion. However, in the last 5 years, there have been significant attempts at randomized trials to widen our understanding of the procedure and its effects. These seven trials will be detailed in the section on long-term results.

2.2. Rationale and Pathological Changes

The venous supply of the lower esophagus offers an ideal communication between the subdiaphragmatic portal system and the supradiaphragmatic azygous–caval system. The lower esophagus appears to have extramural, intramural subepithelial, and intramural submucosal plexuses.[9] The latter in portal hypertension becomes grossly distended and can produce varices in some situations from the gastroesophageal junction virtually to the cricopharyngeus. However, most patients present with either varices or at least bleeding from varices relatively close to the gastroesophageal junction. Theoretically, if only those submucosal varicosities threatening the patient's life could be eradicated, the other veins might continue to offer enough portal decompression that recurrent submucosal varices would not form. In addition, it is presumed that the effect of sclerosis of these esophageal veins does not depress total hepatic blood flow as do shunt procedures, so that the feared sequelae of portasystemic encephalopathy will be minimized.

Sclerosing solutions are inflammatory, vasoconstrictive, and induce tissue necrosis and subsequent thrombosis after only 1 sec of contact.[10,11] Evans et al.[12] have shown, in a human postmortem study of patients having undergone sclerotherapy, that thrombosis and tissue necrosis were present within 1 day of sclerotherapy, followed by ulceration after 1 week and fibrosis at a month. These changes are seen after *intra*variceal injection. Depending on the concentration and volume of sclerosant injection, significant ulceration, perforation, and mediastinitis can occur, in addition to the intended effects of thrombosis of the vessel.

Wodak[13] proposed an entirely different method of controlling and preventing bleeding: esophageal wall sclerosis or *Osophaguswandsklerosierung*. He used multiple *para*variceal injections of dilute sclerosant in a helical fashion so as to achieve a fibrous column around the varices rather than early thrombosis and ulceration. This method has been more recently popularized by Paquet.[8,14]

In an interesting postsclerotherapy study of esophageal function in patients, Reilly *et al.*[15] demonstrated that although there was no effect on lower esophageal sphincter pressure, gastroesophageal reflux was even more prevalent after treatment than before. It occurred in 60% of postsclerotherapy patients, and striking disturbances were seen in esophageal motility. Similar changes were demonstrated by Sauerbruch and co-workers.[16]

2.3. Sclerosants Used

The substances used for endoscopic injection sclerotherapy have been previously employed for sclerosis of hemorrhoids and peripheral varicose veins.[17] Polidocanol (Aethoxysclerol) is the agent used by Paquet for his paravariceal injections.[14] For the intravariceal injections, ethanolamine oleate is the substance most frequently used in England and is also available in Canada. Various studies testing different concentrations of ethanol, sodium tetradecyl sulphate (thrombovar in Canada), and sodium morrhuate have been reported. Jensen[17] has found that a solution of TES (1% tetradecyl, 33% ethanol, and saline) proves to be efficacious (70% success) with a relatively low incidence of esophageal damage (10% ulcers).

The fatty-acid-base sclerosants (morrhuate and ethanolamine) seem to cause more postoperative symptoms such as chest pain and fever, in comparison with the aqueous agents ethanol and tetradecyl. Blenkinsopp[18] tested the rate of sclerosis of rat veins, comparing 5% ethanolamine to tetradecyl, and found that the latter led to a higher thrombosis rate. In turn, tetradecyl was more efficacious than morrhuate in Reiner's study.[19]

At present the choice of sclerosant seems to depend on availability and preference based on personal communications. The use of morrhuate, however, according to Gibbert *et al.*,[20] appears to be followed by more complications than use of other solutions.

2.4. Method

The methods of sclerotherapy, in addition to the intra- and paravariceal options, are varied. Rigid endoscopy was initially used, generally by surgeons, and is still favored by some groups especially in the emergent situation when the endoscope is actually used to effect tamponade. A 50-cm, rigid Negus esophagoscope has been modified with a slot at the distal end so that after injection with a rigid needle, the varix can be tamponaded by simple rotation of the scope at which time an additional varix can prolapse into the slot.[21] Additional advantages, according to Terblanche et al.,[22,23] are the proximal light source, which does not become obscured in the emergent situation when active bleeding is encountered, and the long, wide-bore sucker, which is clearly more efficient than the suction channel of flexible fiberoptic scopes. A modified Macbeth or a modified Roberts needle is used.[24] Clear disadvantages of the rigid Negus scope are the requirement of general anesthesia and the fact that substantially more expertise is required in comparison with flexible scopes. Initially Terblanche injects 6–8 ml of ethanolamine oleate. He believes that sodium tetradecyl is too dangerous when it extravasates.[24] Subsequent injections complete the sclerosis just proximal to the gastroesophageal junction, but other endoscopists continue repeated injections of lesser amounts of sclerosants more proximally. Reinsertion of the Sengstaken–Blakemore tube, which is removed just prior to the procedure, is not recommended.

Fiberoptic endoscopy and sclerosis, using a variety of flexible needles, has the advantage that it can be performed under local anesthesia with less expertise than is needed for rigid endoscopy.[25] Although a windowed sheath has been designed to be used especially in the emergent situation so that varices can be compressed after injection,[25] the practical use of it is somewhat cumbersome. Many have used fiberendoscopy after the initial hemorrhage has been stopped at least temporarily with a combination of intravenous Pitressin and balloon tamponade. In almost all cases, the bleeding stops long enough for the veins to be injected without the use of any rigid or flexible instrument for compression. Other ingenious methods to tamponade variceal inflow from the portal system have been described, varying from specially designed balloon catheters[26] to modified rubber condoms.[27]

If the intravariceal method is used, multiple 2-ml injections will be made at various levels in the esophagus, using from 15 to 30 ml total as injections progress proximally. Using the paravariceal technique, Paquet and Oberhammer[14] inject strictly paravariceally and subepithelially; 0.5–1.4 ml of Polidocanol is injected (in Paquet's case through a rigid esophagoscope and also a rigid 60-cm fiberscope) to raise a pale weal at the point of injection. This is repeated 30–50 times in the distal esophagus, producing a helical arrangement of weals as the esophagoscope is withdrawn. Paquet[28] believes that the ruptured varix is mechanically occluded by the massive edema from the confluent weals. The terminal column of esophageal fibrosis is achieved by a total of 80–160 injections during two to four sessions over 5–8 days. Paquet also avoids the use of balloon tamponade after sclerotherapy. If the hemorrhage is quite active, 2–10 paravariceal injections to the left and right of the bleeding point are used.

The frequency of injections is controversial. It seems that large veins require more injections, and they tend to bleed[29] and to rebleed[30] more often. The rebleeding rates, and in fact the mortality rates, are highest at the beginning of treatment,[30] and therefore, most physicians have gravitated toward the plan of early frequent therapy followed by reendoscopy and resclerosis until the varices are obliterated. In general, advocates of the intravariceal method perform two to three scleroses in the first admission within approximately 2 weeks, with follow-up injections every 7–14 days until obliteration, and then at 6-month intervals afterward.

A recent randomized trial of different treatment schedules carried out by the King's College group suggested that weekly injections, leading to obliteration at approximately 10 weeks, provided a better overall result than 3-week injections.[31] Patients in the weekly treated group returned earlier to normal activity and work even though the frequency of rebleeding and the number of courses of injection required for obliteration were not different. Mucosal ulceration was, in fact, observed more frequently in the weekly treated group. At present, the King's College group recommends a maximum of three courses at weekly intervals followed by a period of 3 weeks of observation before reassessing the need for further injection.

To date there have been no large studies comparing intravariceal to paravariceal regimens, but a study of 20 patients by Rose, Crane, and Smith[30] suggested that intravenous sclerosant was significantly more effective in producing thrombosis. However, as the paravariceal method is extremely painstaking, the actual method of paravariceal injection may have been different from that of Paquet.

2.5. Complications

When a group of patients is generally extremely ill with acute gastrointestinal bleeding and underlying severe liver disease, coagulotherapy, and other organ system failure, it is important to separate the complications of a specific procedure from the complications and mortality

of the overall disease process. The morbidity and mortality of a first variceal hemorrhage is high, no matter what treatment is given. Death
directly related to variceal sclerotherapy probably occurs in 1–2%, but the
admission mortality for bleeding esophageal varices when sclerotherapy
is used is 15–25%.[7,14,22] Complication rates have varied tremendously,
with Johnston and Rodgers[7] reporting a complication rate of 0.9%, and
Terblanche et al. 49%.[22] All are agreed, however, on the most common
problems seen—fever, tachycardia and chest pain,[22,32,33] pleural effusion,[26]
and ulceration and sloughing of the esophageal mucosa sometimes leading to minor recurrent bleeds.[22,34,35] Esophageal perforation,[22] mediastinitis, empyema, and even bronchoesophageal fistula have been reported,
but are fortunately infrequent. As stated, the natural history of esophageal
ulceration is that of fibrosis, and esophageal stricture may be a resultant
late complication. However, this is usually easily treated by dilation.

In the paravariceal group, Paquet[28] reported a 11.5% complication
rate over half of which were esophageal ulcerations, with 1.5% of patients
developing mediastinitis and 2% developing esophageal stenosis.

2.6. Efficacy of Sclerotherapy: Rebleeding and Long-Term Survival

Especially in earlier nonrandomized series,[7,14] attention focused on
the incidence of control of active variceal hemorrhage and the incidence
of rebleeding during the treatment schedule, whether that schedule
involved observation or frequent reinjection. There seems no doubt that
early control of active bleeding, although difficult, is achieved in approximately 90% with aggressive use of injection sclerotherapy, whether the
paravariceal or intravariceal method is used. However, one is tempted to
think that relatively few of the so-called "emergent" injections are
actually carried out with varices actively bleeding. In fact, the vast majority, probably 80–90% of patients with bleeding esophageal varices, have
either stopped at the initial endoscopy (the group that Terblanche[24] feels
should be classified as patients with a more favorable outcome) or can be
controlled at least temporarily with a combination of intravenous Pitressin and balloon tamponade therapy.[24,36]

No matter what treatment regimen is used, which scope, which sclerosing solution, whether the para- or intravariceal method, patients with
varices who have been treated with injection sclerotherapy do rebleed.
However, the bleeding is often less massive and life-threatening in comparison with the first hemorrhage.[24] Rebleeding, therefore, may not be as
important a variable to follow in these patients as ultimate quantity and
quality of survival itself.

To date, there have been seven prospective randomized trials,[37-47] most of which have been reported in the last 3 years. To quote Conn, a "maximal methodologic diversity" has been demonstrated.[48] All seven have a mean follow-up of approximately 7–25 months, so that definitive conclusions are somewhat difficult to draw. In general, the incidence of rebleeding has been frequently decreased as compared to the control group (Table 1). However, the use of "medical" treatment as the control group, consisting of early management with supportive measures such as Pitressin, balloon tamponade, blood transfusion, and simple follow-up, may be somewhat inappropriate today, with more conventional medical and surgical options available. Perhaps the best known trial was reported by Clark et al.[37] and later McDougall et al.,[38] who studied 107 patients randomized between repeated sclerotherapy and medical treatment, with a mean follow-up of approximately 24 months. Rebleeding was decreased from 75% to 43% in the test group, and survival was increased from 58% to 75% over the 2-year test period. Terblanche's trial, in fact, showed a decrease in rebleeding from 73% to 43% in the sclerotherapy group, but ultimately led to no increased survival.[40] His conclusion may have been complicated, however, by the fact that his control group of patients actually received sclerotherapy as initial treatment before being randomized. Yassin and Sherif[46] randomized 108 patients between sclerotherapy and conventional treatment at their center which included medical and

Table 1. Randomized Controlled Trials of Sclerotherapy (Scl)

Author	Year	No. pt.	Control group	Follow-up (mo)	Percent rebleeding		Percent survival	
					Scl	Control	Scl	Control
Clark et al.[37]	1980	64	Medical	12	33	68	65	46
MacDougall et al.[38]	1982	107	Medical	24	43	75	75	58
Terblanche et al.[40]	1982	75	Scl and medical	25	43	73	35	35
Larson and Chapman[44]	1982	33	Medical	6	0.16/pt mo	0.49[a]	85	70
Korula et al.[47]	1983	120	Medical	14	0.29/pt mo	1.1	NS	
Paquet[42]	1982	65	Medical	24	6	66	94	58
Barsoum et al.[43]	1982	100	Tamponade	30	26	58	74	58
Cello et al.[45]	1982	12	Transection	7	33	0	33	0
Yassin and Sherif[46]	1983	108	Medical ± OR	17	13	29	91	78

[a] Data expressed in number of bleeding episodes per patient per month.

surgical options. Although the follow-up was short, the rebleeding rate was decreased in the sclerosis group with a suggestion of improved survival. However, results from this study can probably not be extrapolated to the North American experience because of the preponderance of patients with nonalcoholic liver disease. Barsoum's trial[43] randomized 100 patients to either sclerotherapy or balloon tamponade groups and showed a significant reduction in rebleeding rates, but no difference in survival statistics. The same caution concerning nonalcoholic liver disease could be exercised with this series of patients. Cello et al.[45] reported a smaller series of sclerotherapy versus transection and compared these results to a historical shunt series, but the results were somewhat difficult to interpret as none of the transection patients survived. Another series published in abstract form by Korula et al.[47] with a medical control group and a follow-up of approximately 1 year again showed a decreased incidence of rebleeding but no significant difference in survival.

Paquet[42] studied the use of *prophylactic* sclerotherapy in patients with varices that have not bled. Interestingly, this group of 65 patients had a significantly decreased rate of bleeding and a survival of 94% over the 2-year follow-up period. This has been the only study looking at treatment in the prophylactic setting, a group of patients that was abandoned long ago as far as shunting procedures are concerned.

There seems no doubt that sclerotherapy, performed in an early and then repeated fashion, leads to decreased episodes of rebleeding as compared to control therapy (frequently nontherapy). However, there remains real doubt as to whether overall survival is improved when compared to reasonable control groups. Results of on-going studies using conventional surgical management of bleeding varices as the control group will be awaited with interest (L. Rikkers, personal communication).

2.7. Cost/Benefit Ratio

The foregoing review has been an attempt to outline the benefits of sclerotherapy and the cost to the patient as far as complication and rebleeding are concerned. At present, the implications of any treatment as far as cost to the medical care delivery system are becoming increasingly more important. Chung and Lewis,[49] in a retrospective analysis, attempted to evaluate the costs of initial hospitalization, readmission, and total treatment of four different groups (portasystemic shunt, medical therapy, ligation therapy, and endoscopic injection sclerotherapy). Although their review was retrospective and the groups of patients uncontrolled (in fact, the endoscopic sclerotherapy patients were the sickest of the four groups), the findings are worthy of discussion. The total cost of medical treatment per 2-year survivor was approximately $12,300 for the endoscopic injection sclerotherapy group, $23,400 for the medically treated group, $44,200 for the portasystemic shunting group, and $52,700 for the ligation group. The survival at 2 years for these uncontrolled groups was, in fact, 67%, 46%, 33%, and 43%, respectively. Readmission rate was lowest in the endoscopic sclerotherapy group in Lewis et al.'s review.[26] Another review, by O'Donnell et al.,[50] also showed that nonsurgical treatment was less expensive.

2.8. Summary of Endoscopic Sclerotherapy

Endoscopic sclerotherapy may be one of the most exciting rebirths seen in recent medical history. If it does prove, in fact, to be the most effective treatment for the most numbers of patients with bleeding varices, it will certainly be welcomed by gastroenterologists, who can learn the method quickly and easily, by surgeons, who may not have to carry out long, arduous shunting procedures in the middle of the night, and by administrators, who are becoming increasingly concerned with skyrocketing medical costs, especially for patients who are notorious for long, expensive admissions. However, because of the unbridled enthusiasm for this procedure, there is a danger that patients will be treated in a haphazard manner using a large number of methods, so that relatively small numbers will be available for study in randomized controlled trials. Every doctor who treats bleeding esophageal varices seems to have a bias toward his or her particular pet procedure; in the case of endoscopic injection sclerotherapy, it is not hard to develop a bias for a procedure that seems relatively simple, safe, efficacious, and cheap. However, more prospective studies examining the various conflicting results to date will be necessary to eventually decide selection of patients best suited for sclerotherapy and the best overall method.

3. ENDOSCOPIC SPHINCTEROTOMY

A natural extension of visualization of the biliary and pancreatic ducts by endoscopic retrograde cholangiopancreatography was surgical intervention into those ducts, i.e., sphincterotomy. Developed in Japan[51] and Germany,[52] the procedure has been learned throughout the world, and it is estimated that by the end of its first decade, sphincterotomy will have been carried out 20,000 times worldwide.[53] Over that period, the indications for sphincterotomy have widened considerably, variations devised, and contraindications defined.

Endoscopic sphincterotomy has proven most useful in the nonoperative treatment of choledocholithiasis in the elective situation. However, its scope has not been extended to include choledocholithiasis in various clinical situations, biliary strictures, acute gallstone pancreatitis, chronic pancreatitis, and palliative treatment for ampullary carcinoma. Each of these indications will be described separately.

3.1. Method

Endoscopic sphincterotomy is carried out either on an inpatient or on an outpatient who is prepared for endoscopic retrograde cholangiopancreatography (ERCP), and who will be admitted for observation after an endoscopic sphincterotomy if necessary. A diagnostic ERCP is carried out in the standard fashion under Valium sedation and local anesthetic spray. Usually, some form of duodenal relaxant such as Buscopan or glucagon is used as well. The procedure is performed in an endoscopy/radiology suite where high-quality radiographs can be obtained quickly. A wide variety of side-viewing duodenoscopes manufactured by the Olympus, ACMI, and Fuginon Companies have all been used successfully. After a diagnosis (e.g., choledocholithiasis) requiring endoscopic sphincterotomy is radiologically confirmed, a papillotome is placed into the common bile duct. The most commonly used papillotome is one that on tension produces a bowstring effect such as the Erlangen or Seuberth instruments.[54] An alternative cutting instrument, which produces a "caterpillar" effect on pressure, was designed by Sohma and Kawai and is especially useful in cannulation of the ampulla when approached from below in a patient with a previous Billroth II gastrectomy.

Once the papillotome is confirmed to be in the common bile duct either by its positon on the fluoroscopy screen or by a confirmatory injection of Hypaque dye, the sphincterotomy can begin. Approximately 25% of the bowstring wire outside the cannula should be seen outside the papilla, and the cannulated papillotome should be angled at 11–12 o'clock as seen on the medial wall of the duodenum by the endoscopist. The choice of cutting, coagulation, or blended current is up to the endoscopist, but it seems that a pure cutting current is probably most dangerous as far as bleeding is concerned because of the very fast division of tissues failing to coagulate small arteries. On the other hand, simple coagulation for a long period of time may well create more edema and ultimate risk of pancreatic duct obstruction and pancreatitis. It seems that a blended current is consequently safest. An incision of approximately 15–20 mm is made into the common duct,[53] at which time a rush of bile is usually seen, unless the duct is decompressed from above with a T tube or transhepatic tube. A small amount of bleeding is common, but this stops quickly. Various modifications of the procedure may begin at this time and will be discussed under the different indications for sphincterotomy.

Postoperative treatment consists of keeping the patient NPO for a few hours or overnight and beginning on fluids the following day. Most patients with an uncomplicated sphincterotomy can return home within 24 hr of the procedure.

Most treatment failures of sphincterotomies are caused by the presence of a duodenal diverticulum, especially one that actually contains the papilla in its apex or one that is situated immediately adjacent to the papilla. The Billroth II gastrectomy can present significant obstacles for the endoscopist, but employing forward-viewing instruments, these are not insurmountable.[55]

In patients with extremely tight papillae, which do not allow the papillotome (which is considerably more bulky than the regular ERCP cannula) to pass into the common bile duct, a "precut" is sometimes performed.[54,56] However, most endoscopists use this maneuver with great care, as burning not directed precisely into the bile duct may be putting the pancreas at much greater risk. It is generally thought that this should be reserved for patients in whom the alternative, a laparotomy, is unacceptably dangerous. Another alternative to the very tight papilla is transhepatic introduction by the radiologist of a guide wire and balloon to dilate the papilla at the lower end of the common duct so that the endoscopist can properly place the papillotome.

3.2. Indications

3.2.1. Choledocholithiasis

Choledocholithiasis is the most common indication for endoscopic sphincterotomy. If the presence of choledocholithiasis is confirmed on ERCP, an endoscopic sphincterotomy is carried out as described earlier. Many endoscopists treat all patients with antibiotics when common duct stones are confirmed, but other, such as Safrany and Cotton[57] and Zimmon et al.,[58] treat selectively with antibiotics, such as patients who have had previous cholangitis or are undergoing sphincterotomy with their gallbladders still in place. The sphincterotomy is performed, and bile is taken for culture and sensitivity, so that septic complications, if they occur, can be specifically treated. Stones can either be left to pass spontaneously or be extracted from the duct by means of balloon catheters, or Dormia baskets. Stones less than 1 cm usually pass spontaneously, sometimes producing a sharp, transient pain in the right upper quadrant.[54]

However, if the patient has had recent cholangitis, or particularly if it is difficult for the patient to return for a follow-up endoscopy because of geographical problems, the stones should be immediately removed from the duct by whatever technique is favored by the endoscopist. The balloon catheters are, in fact, expensive and break easily, but they are most efficacious for multiple small stones floating in the duct.[57] Basketing is more effective for larger stones, but can be quite frustrating and time consuming.

Large stones and multiple small stones present the greatest problems for the endoscopist. Since the conventional endoscopic Dormia basket can exert pressure of only 0.1 Kp/mm^2, it is usually not possible to crush common bile duct stones, even ones of the typical mushy primary variety.[53] In fact, attempts to do this may trap the basket in the common bile duct and lead to surgical removal of the stone and its accompanying basket. Demling's[53] group has devised a mechanical lithotripter which exerts 17 times the above pressure via the "capturing arms" and effectively crushes the stone into pieces small enough to pass through the sphincterotomy. If this type of lithotripter is not available for use endoscopically, the radiologist can pass shorter, stouter instruments through the liver via percutaneous transhepatic cholangiography to crush the larger stones after endoscopic sphincterotomy has been performed.[54] Other means of stone crushing are the use of ultrasonic drills[59] and electrohydrolysis.[60]

An alternative method for the difficult case of larger or multiple stones is nasobiliary drainage.[61-63] This theoretically has the advantage of decompressing the common duct, monitoring the passage of stones with repeated cholangiography without the need for ERCP, and may also be used for instillation of dissolving substances such as monooctonoin.[64-67] There is no question that results have been encouraging with monooctonoin in dissolving common duct stones, but with prolonged instrumentation and delay of adequate clearance of the duct, it must be recognized that the patient is at risk for development of potentially severe cholangitis.[54]

The success rate of sphincterotomy in choledocholithiasis is approximately 95%, and the rate for clearance of the duct without any further surgery approximates 90% in most series.

3.2.2. Choledocholithiasis—Special Cases

3.2.2a. Gallbladder in Situ. Increasing experience especially in the European literature has been reported with endoscopic sphincterotomy for choledocholithiasis and cholelithiasis with the gallbladder still *in situ.*[68-72] This was originally advocated for patients who were elderly and otherwise at high risk for surgery. The controversy concerning the need for operation once the jaundice and/or cholangitis has cleared is still not settled. There is a growing body of evidence, however, suggesting that a relatively small number of patients may require cholecystectomy for acute cholecystitis if endoscopic sphincterotomy has resulted in total clearance of the common duct. In a large follow-up of 260 patients (mean age 76) for 1–6 years after endoscopic spincterotomy, only 10% of patients required cholecystectomy for biliary symptoms.[57] Enthusiasm for this approach has increased, and in 1981, 40% of Safrany's endoscopic sphincterotomies were carried out for choledocholithiasis with gallbladders *in situ*.[57] Riemann *et al.*[70] state that as a result, the rate of elective cholecystectomy at his institution has clearly diminished without any increase of emergency cholecystectomy occurring. Almost all patients treated are older, and it may be dangerous to suggest that the same approach be adopted for young and fit patients. At the moment, most in the younger age group are encouraged to undergo cholecystectomy, as the long-term results of endoscopic sphincterotomy may not be known for some years.

3.2.2b. Choledocholithiasis with Recent Cholecystectomy, T Tube in Place. The conventional treatment for this problem is relatively easily soluble by a radiologist or a clinician experienced in manipulation of baskets through the T-tube tract, as described by Burhenne,[73] or variations of this technique, such as introduction of a choledochoscope percutaneously through the T-tube tract. However, if this method fails because of a small, undilatable tract, a too tortuous or too straight tract, or simple failure of the radiologist to retrieve a floating or impacted stone, endoscopic sphincterotomy may be carried out. With increasing numbers of patients being sent to referral centers from long distances, it may also be impractical for a patient to wait the 4–6 weeks necessary for the T-tube tract to mature. After the endoscopic sphincterotomy, if stones cannot be removed from below, the radiologist can often be of help by pushing the stones through the sphincterotomized lower end.[54]

The use of the Nd:YAG laser introduced through choledochoscopy to break up large stones has been described,[74] and its application in the endoscopic setting after sphincterotomy may prove useful.

3.2.2c. Choledocholithiasis—Impacted Stones. Impacted stones can usually be dislodged by the endoscopist and retrieved after sphincterotomy. However, endoscopic choledochoduodenostomy or "fistulotomy" above an obstructed papilla has been described to handle instances in which the endoscopist is not able to perform the sphincterotomy through the papilla.[53,75]

3.2.2d. *Acute Gallstone Pancreatitis*. There is renewed surgical interest in the early aggressive treatment of gallstone pancreatitis with reported rapid improvement in both the patient and his pancreas after clearance of common duct stones.[76] It seems reasonable to extrapolate this finding to the endoscopic field, and correspondingly, a number of series have been reported in which emergent endoscopic sphincterotomy has been carried out for acute gallstone pancreatitis. Roesch and Demling,[78] Safrany *et al.*,[78,79] and Van der Spuy[80] all reported rapid resolution of the clinical problem with complication rates that were no higher than after the less emergent types of endoscopic sphincterotomy.

Although the number of patients with acute gallstone pancreatitis that does not settle down quickly must be small, this approach may be a significant advance for a selected group.

3.2.3. Biliary Strictures

Endoscopic dilatation of biliary strictures with or without sphincterotomy has been described.[63] Strictures at previous choledochoduodenostomy sites may be dilated endoscopically with a Grundzig balloon, but these techniques can be expected to give only temporary relief. The addition of endoprostheses, to be described in Section 3.2.6, may be appropriate in selected cases with very high benign strictures or malignant strictures inappropriate for surgery.

3.2.4. Chronic Pancreatitis

The experience using endoscopic sphincterotomy for patients with chronic pancreatitis is limited to anecdotal reports. Wurbs[81] reported use of an endoscopic sphincterotomy into Wirsung's duct to free an impacted biliary stone, and Cremer *et al.*[82] described improvement in a patient with pancreatic insufficiency in whom they had performed endoscopic sphincterotomy and removal of a pancreatic concretion. The application of the procedure for this particular indication, however, must be viewed with caution.

3.2.5. Ampullary Carcinoma

Ampullary carcinoma remains a potentially curable disease, but in the elderly or infirm, the operation required for removal may be too formidable. It is wise to remember, however, that more reports of local excision of ampullary tumors are now becoming available.[83] If the patient is a candidate for palliative therapy, however, either endoscopic sphincterotomy and/or the insertion of stents across the periampullary tumor may be appropriate.[84,85]

3.2.6. Drains, Stents, and Daughter Scopes

As discussed previously, nasobiliary drains introduced through the endoscope are now used in certain cases after endoscopic sphincterotomy for monitoring and possible treatment of common duct stones. These can occasionally be used without endoscopic sphincterotomy, as long as the drain is left in place for decompression until stone dissolution takes place.

There is renewed enthusiasm for the concept of preoperative biliary decompression.[86–90] More recent literature suggests that the operative mortality rate is, in fact, decreased in patients who have had effective decompression and normalization of liver tests. Indwelling stents placed endoscopically may also be indicated for more long-term relief of obstruction from a tumor or a bile duct stricture in patients inappropriate for laparotomy.

Technique of Insertion of Stents or "Conduit." A modified Seldinger technique is used[63,91] in which a guide wire is passed through an ERCP cannula into the entrahepatic ducts, whereupon the cannula is removed. At that point either a drain or a stent can be placed. If a drain is chosen, a 300-cm pigtail drain with multiple side holes is threaded over the guide wire and the wire is then removed. The endoscope is removed while the drain is advanced into the duodenum and then transposed to a nasal position at the proximal end.

If a stent is used, usually a double pigtail stent is placed over the guide wire and pushed into position over the guide wire by a biliary catheter or ERCP cannula. This stent likewise has multiple side holes. The ideal use for the stents is in periampullary tumors, but they have been used for temporary decompression of common bile duct stones when the latter have been too large to remove. The major problem with stents and drains, however, is that they do plug frequently in the sizes that are presently used. Larger sizes are being developed.

The concept of fine fiberoptic endoscopes being introduced through the biopsy channel of a "mother" scope is not new. The theoretical advantages of endoscoping the bile and pancreatic ducts after endoscopic sphincterotomy have thus far not been borne out in practice.

3.2.7. Papillary Stenosis

The diagnosis of papillary stenosis accounts for approximately 5% of endoscopic sphincterotomies carried out.[70] This remains an elusive disease, with even the most enthusiastic endoscopists hesitating to conclude that a sphincterotomy will cure the patient's clinical illness. A combination of abdominal pain, altered biochemical liver tests, and a papilla very resistant to cannulation presents a vague syndrome at best. Consequently, the previously high incidence of this indication for endoscopic sphincterotomy is now decreasing.

3.3. Complication Rates

The complication rates for endoscopic sphincterotomy vary between 7 and 10% with a mortality rate of 0.5–2%.[92–95] Complications consist of bleeding at the sphincterotomy site, cholangitis, retroperitoneal perforation, hyperamylasemia and pancreatitis, and trapped Dormia baskets requiring surgical exploration. The mortality and morbidity rates are undoubtedly inversely proportional to experience, as Safrany and Cotton reported only 17 deaths in their first 2000 cases and operative mortality of 0.85%.[57]

Although there has been controversy in the literature from aggressive surgeons who draw attention to the not insignificant mortality of endoscopic sphincterotomy, it seems that the mortality rate of common bile duct exploration for stones is higher.[96–99] When one considers that the proportion of elderly sick patients is probably higher in the endoscopic sphincterotomy group, there seems no doubt about the preferred treatment.

The long-term results of the endoscopic procedure will be awaited with interest. To this date, restenosis of an endoscopic sphincterotomy site is rare. Why this should be, when surgical spincterotomy in the past led to stenosis frequently, is unclear; however, it may be that the extensive coagulation in performing the sphincterotomy may actually produce a fused mucosa-to-mucosa apposition, which then heals in contrast to the previous surgical sphincterotomy. Because the long-term effects on repeated biliary contamination are not known, some endoscopists are hesitant to perform sphincterotomy on young patients with gallbladders *in situ,* who have a safe alternative of cholecystectomy and choledochotomy.[57,68–72] Seifert *et al.*[100] compiled collective statistics in Germany and found good long-term, symptomatic relief for patients who had had endoscopic sphincterotomy. The rate of recurrent stones was approximately 6%, which is more encouraging than Riemann's own long-term results reporting a 19% recurrence rate.[70]

Endoscopic sphincterotomy has been a major advance in the treatment of choledocholithiasis, and to a lesser extent other problems of the biliary tree. It can be performed safely with little cost, and both the early and long-term results are excellent. Morbidity and mortality are minimized with greater experience.

4. LASERS

The concept of light amplification by the stimulated emission of radiation (LASER) was first proposed by Einstein.[101] By the late 1960s, development of lasers had progressed far enough to be applied to the endoscopy field.[102-104] Numerous contributions in the medical field have been in ophthalmology, neurosurgery, urology, oral medicine, and general surgery. The number of uses within the latter field is growing, as the CO_2 laser in particular can be used virtually when a knife is used. Experience with liver resection, intestinal anastomoses, pelvic surgery, pancreatic resection, reduction mammoplasty, various procedures about the head and neck, and even vascular anastomoses is growing.

The principal contributions of the laser to endoscopic work are in photocoagulation of alimentary tract bleeding of both the upper and lower gastrointestinal (GI) tract and in the phototherapy of tumors.

4.1. Effect of Laser on Tissue

Light produced by any laser source is absorbed by tissue with the conversion of light energy to heat. Heating of the tissue occurs between 37°C and 60°C followed by denaturation of proteins and loss of cell membrane integrity above that temperature. At 100°C, cells explode as their water boils, and above that temperature vaporization and charring occur. Whether control of hemorrhage is caused by vessel shrinkage or perivascular edema is debatable. The difference between the three lasers available, CO_2, argon, and Nd:YAG, is the volume of tissue that can be heated before vaporization of superficial cells occurs. Generally, photocoagulation necrosis is similar to an electrical burn, and the various wave lengths available with different laser types determine their mode of action, i.e., cutting effect with the CO_2 laser or predictable thermal damage of a much lesser degree as is required in hemostasis of bleeding lesions with the argon and Nd:YAG lasers.

4.1.1. Argon Laser

The argon laser emits energy in the blue-green range of the visible spectrum and can be focused through a fine endoscopic quartz fiber with very little divergence. This laser is effective in producing hemostasis of bleeding gastric ulcers, but because its light is absorbed by red blood cells, active bleeding, which cannot be cleared at the time of therapy, is a major problem. This is solved by instillation of carbon dioxide gas to blow away the overlying blood, and consequently a mechanism for immediate removal of the gas to prevent overdistention must be used.

Power used is usually in the range of 5 W and is administered at full power after an initial low-power argon beam used to focus the energy on the bleeding site.

4.1.2. Neodymium–Yttrium Aluminum Garnet (Nd:YAG)

Depth of effect of this invisible laser is greater than that of the argon instrument. Potential effect on tissue is therefore greater and potential dangers correspondingly increased. Its energy is more widely scattered in tissue than the argon laser, so that in the presence of hemorrhage, the Nd:YAG laser is more effective. Usual power levels are between 60 and 90 W with short bursts of 0.3–0.7 sec for hemostasis without severe ulceration or perforation. For bleeding lesions in the upper GI tract, the Nd:YAG laser also has the advantage that the short bursts are not affected by motility of the stomach, whereas the 1- to 3-sec exposure required for the argon source application may be complicated by a moving target. Whereas the argon laser is aimed with a low-power output of its own source, the Nd:YAG laser has to be aimed with an additional visible spectrum laser. The invisibility of the Nd:YAG laser also may potentially lead to greater incidence of endoscopist eye injury, as the operator cannot detect the injury taking place.

Cost of lasers is a serious impediment to their universal use. At present, the cost for a Nd:YAG laser in North America is approximately $100,000, and in addition, the installation of a three-phase electrical supply, high-flow water-cooling system, importability, and high maintenance costs are all major disadvantages. Specialized two-channel endoscopes are most convenient, and the additional cost of $10,000–$15,000 if these are used must be considered.

4.2. Alimentary Tract Bleeding

There is no question that, properly used, the argon and Nd:YAG lasers are effective in stopping upper and lower GI bleeding. Their use in upper GI bleeding has been for a wide range of lesions including peptic ulcers, gastric erosions, tumors, and even bleeding esophageal varices.[105-108] The use through the colonoscope, however, has been limited to the phototherapy of minor bleeding or lesions whose bleeding has stopped, e.g., cecal angiodysplasia or arteriovenous malformations.[109,110]

It is generally recognized that the mortality rate of upper GI bleeding has not improved over the last 25–30 years.[111-113] Intuitively, this may seem surprising despite the enthusiasm for early endoscopy and consequently early diagnosis and selection of patients who are at high risk to rebleed. Rebleeding is the crucial factor as far as mortality is concerned.[114] When one considers uncontrolled series of laser photocoagulation of actively bleeding gastric and duodenal sources, one must consider that 80–90% of these lesions will stop bleeding spontaneously without any treatment. Frühmorgen et al.,[106] using the argon laser, reported a success rate of 95% in 100 patients. Brunetaud et al.[107] and Cotton's[108] group also reported, in consecutive series, cessation of bleeding in over 80% of cases using the argon instrument. Kiefhaber has been the main early proponent of the Nd:YAG laser for cessation of upper GI bleeding and reported success in 93% of 600 patients, 40% of whom had bleeding esophageal varices.[115,116] Perforations have occurred in approximately 1% of cases with the Nd:YAG laser and have not been reported with the argon method.

A number of prospective control trials have been conducted using either the argon or Nd:YAG lasers.[117-122] Ideally, one would like to have results of efficacy of stopping hemorrhage, incidence of rebleeding, and ultimate mortality rate. Few of these studies, however, have all of this information available. In addition, the test group, i.e., the group of patients admitted with endoscopically proven upper GI bleeding thought to be at high risk, varies from "active peptic ulcer bleeding" to "visible vessel" to "stigmata of recent hemorrhage." In general, as one can see from Table 2, the rebleeding rates of the nontreated groups are higher in most cases than those treated with laser phototherapy. However, the statistics of eventual mortality are not convincing, as most series did not show statistical improvement.

If significant differences are to be shown for the acute treatment of bleeding lesions, the appropriate high-risk group must be selected. At present, the most acceptable is the "SRH group" including visible vessel, red or blue spots, or recent clot in the base of an ulcer.[123-125] Despite the use of this group, which is presumably at greater risk for rebleeding, very large numbers of patients will be required to reach statistical significance. In addition, the actual methods of usage and expertise of therapy undoubtedly vary so that the results from one group may not be extrapolatable to others.

Table 2. Randomized Controlled Trials of Laser Coagulation of Upper Gastrointestinal Bleeding

Author	Year	No. pt.	Type	Group	Percent early control of bleeding		Percent rebleeding		Percent mortality	
					Laser	Control	Laser	Control	Laser	Control
Vallon et al.[117]	1981	136	Argon	SRH[a]	67	31	29	34	7	15
Swain et al.[118]	1981	52	Argon	Visible vessel	—	—	33	61	0	25
Swain[119]	1983	82	Argon	SRH	—	—	7	44	2	12
Ihre et al.[120]	1981	135	Nd:YAG	Active bleeding	93	74	27	19	14	10
Rutgeerts et al.[121]	1982	129	Nd:YAG	SRH	100	77	5	38	13	15
MacLeod et al.[122]	1982	12	Nd:YAG	Visible	100	0	17	—	17	33

[a]SRH, stigmata of recent hemorrhage.

4.3. Complications with Laser Photocoagulation of Bleeding Sites

The major complication, especially with the Nd:YAG laser, is gastric perforation.[126,127] In addition, the technique of coagulating around a visible vessel is well known in order to avoid actually "drilling" into the vessel and causing greater hemorrhage than one started with.[117,120] Delayed hemorrhage has also been reported.[128]

As stated, the invisibility of the Nd:YAG laser ray can lead to inadvertent endoscopist eye trauma.[129] The Nd:YAG laser scatters up to 40% more of the light energy in a backward direction toward the endoscopist's eye and, being in the invisible range, does not stimulate blinking.[119] One of the more significant complications of laser usage, it must be remembered, is the financial burden inflicted on the institution that buys and maintains it.

4.4. Tumor Phototherapy

The CO_2 laser remains popular as a cutting surgical instrument used by the surgeon, and the argon and the Nd:YAG lasers can be used through the endoscope for surgery on gastrointestinal and other tumors.[130] The endoscopic lasers are also capable of heating larger volumes of tissue. At the moment, experience with endoscopic phototherapy of tumors is limited to palliative "recanalization" and, in a few instances, curative procedures in patients unsuitable for surgery.

Broncial neoplasms have been recanalized successfully with good palliative results.[131] In the GI tract, the laser beam is fired at nodules of tumor protruding into the lumen where it is narrowest with care being taken to avoid firing perpendicular to the esophageal or gastric wall.[130] Multiple treatments are needed, and in Swain et al.'s[132] series of six patients, good palliation and survival of 5–16 weeks were achieved. The other alternative to such treatment, i.e., a Celestin or Mousseau–Barbin tube, has not been compared to the laser option.

In addition to the debulking of esophageal or gastric tumors, the argon and Nd:YAG laser have been used with colonic polyposis[133,134] and early gastric cancer in patients at high risk for major surgery.[135]

Most of the tumor therapy has been external; i.e., the laser beam is fired at a distance of 5–15 mm from the target. A larger quantity of energy can be introduced into the tumor if the laser tip is actually inserted into the tissue. This is termed interstitial therapy. Use of lasers in this way is in the experimental stage.[130]

Selective destruction of malignant tumors can be enhanced by the use of a hematoporphyrin derivative (HpD) for which neoplastic and traumatized tissues have a great affinity. The laser light from whatever source activates the HpD in the tissue, converting triplet 02 to excited singlet 02, which is cytotoxic to the cell membrane, specifically those cells containing the greatest concentration of HpD. Animal studies[136,137] have confirmed that this theoretical selective photosensitization can in fact be demonstrated. Series in humans[138,139] have suggested encouraging results in the field of breast surgery, malignant melanomas, and brain surgery, but have been limited to bronchial carcinomas[140,141] in the endoscopic field. However, one series reported problems with massive delayed hemorrhage after treatment.[141]

The use of endoscopic laser therapy of tumors continues to find its place in relatively few centers.

5. CONCLUSION

Interventional endoscopy is a rapidly expanding field. Technological progress combined with endoscopists' inventiveness and daring have created better instruments with increasing applications in the clinical setting. The judicious use of these aggressive maneuvers should lead to more efficient care of the patient with little morbidity and mortality as compared to the surgical alternatives.

REFERENCES

1. Raskin JB: Emergency endoscopic sclerotherapy for variceal hemorrhage: Is it superior to balloon tamponade? *Gastrointestinal Endoscopy* 1984;29(1):60 (editorial).
2. Crafoord C, Frenckner P: New surgical treatment of varicose veins of the esophagus. *Acta Otolaryngol* 1939;27:422–429.
3. Moersch HJ: Further studies on the treatment of esophageal varices by injection of a sclerosing solution. *Ann Otol Rhinol Laryngol* 1941;50:1233–1244.
4. Moersch HJ: Treatment of esophageal varices by injection of a sclerosing solution. *JAMA* 1947;135:754–757.
5. Patterson CO, Rouse MO: The sclerosing therapy of esophageal varices. *Gastroenterology* 1947;9:391–395.
6. Macbeth R: Treatment of esophageal varices in portal hypertension by means of sclerosing injections. *Br Med J* 1955;2:877–880.
7. Johnston GW, Rodgers HW: A review of 15 years' experience in the use of sclerotherapy in the control of acute hemorrhage for esophageal varices. *Br J Surg* 1973;60:797–800.
8. Raschke E, Paquet KJ: Management of hemorrhage from esophageal varices using esophagoscopic sclerosing method. *Ann Surg* 1973;177:99–102.
9. Stelzner S, Lierse W: Der angiomuskulare Verschlub der speiserohre. *Langenbecks Arch Klin Chir* 1981;321:35–64.

10. Dietrich HP, Sinapius D: Experimentelle Endothelschadigung durch Variezenvero-dungsmittel. *Arzneim Forsch* 1968;18:116–120.

11. Blenkinsopp WK: Effect of injected sclerosant (tetradecyl sulphate of sodium) on rat veins. *Angiologica* 1968;5:386–396.

12. Evans DMD, Jones DB, Cleary DK, Smith PM: Oesophageal varices treated by scle-rotherapy: a histopathological study. *Gut* 1982;23:615–620.

13. Wodak E: Osophagusvarizen—Blutung bei portaler Hypertension; ihre Therapie und Prophylaxe. *Wien med Wochenschr* 1960;110:581–583.

14. Paquet KJ, Oberhammer E: Sclerotherapy of bleeding esophageal varices by means of endoscopy. *Endoscopy* 1978;10:7–12.

15. Reilly JJ, Schade RR, Van Thiel DS: Esophageal function after injection sclerotherapy: Pathogenesis of esophageal stricture. *Am J Surg* 1984;147:85–88.

16. Sauerbruch T, Wirsching R, Leisner B, Weinzierl M, Pfahler M, Paumgartner G: Esophageal function after sclerotherapy of bleeding varices. *Scand J Gastroenterol* 1982;17:745–751.

17. Jensen DM: Sclerosants for injection sclerosis of esophageal varices. *Gastrointest Endosc* 1983;29:315–317.

18. Blenkinsopp WK: Comparison of tetradecyl sulfate of sodium with other sclerosants in rats. *Br J Exp Pathol* 1968;59:197–201.

19. Reiner L: The activity of anionic surface active compounds in producing vascular obliteration. *Proc Soc Exp Biol Med* 1946;62:49–54.

20. Gibbert V, Feinstat T, Burns M, Trudeau WA: Comparison of the sclerosing agents sodium tetradecyl sulfate and sodium morrhuate in endoscopic injection sclerosis of esophageal varices (abstract). *Gastrointest Endosc* 1982;28:147.

21. Bailey ME, Dawson JL: Modified oesophagoscope for injection oesophageal varices. *Br Med J* 1975;2:540–541.

22. Terblanche J, Northover JMA, Bornman P, et al: A prospective evaluation of injection sclerotherapy in the treatment of acute bleeding from esophageal varices. *Surgery* 1979;85:239–245.

23. Terblanche J: Treatment of oesophageal varices (editorial). *J R Soc Med* 1979;72:163–166.

24. Terblanche J: Treatment of esophageal varices by injection sclerotherapy. *Surg Annu* 1981;257–291.

25. Williams KGD, Dawson JL: Fibreoptic injection of oesophageal varices. *Br Med J* 1979;2:766–767.

26. Lewis J, Chung RS, Allison J: Sclerotherapy of oesophageal varices. *Arch Surg* 1980;225:476–480.

27. Brooks WS: Adapting flexible endoscopes for sclerosis of oesophageal varices. *Lancet* 1980;1:266 (Letter to the editor).

28. Paquet KJ: Endoscopic paravariceal injection sclerotherapy of the esophagus—Indi-cations, technique and complications: Results of a period of 14 years. *Gastrointest Endosc* 1983;29:310–315.

29. Lebrec D, De Fleury P, Rueff B, Bahum H, Benhamou JP: Portal hypertension, size of esophageal varices and risk of gastrointestinal bleeding in alcoholic cirrhosis. *Gas-troenterology* 1980;79:1139–1144.

30. Rose JDR, Crane MD, Smith PM: Factors affecting successful endoscopic sclerother-apy for esophageal varices. *Gut* 1983;24:946–949.

31. Westaby D, Melia WM, MacDougall BRD, Hegarty, Williams R: Injection sclerother-apy for esophageal varices: A prospective randomized trial of different treatment schedules. *Gut* 1984;25:129–132.

32. Barsoum MS, Morro Ha-W, Bolous FL, Ramzy AF, Rizk-Allah MA, Mahmood FI: The complications of injection sclerotherapy of bleeding oesophageal varices. *Br J Surg* 1982;69:79–81.
33. Sivak MV, Stout DJ, Skipper G: Endoscopic injection sclerosis (EIS) of esophageal varices. *Gastrointest Endosc* 1981;27:52–57.
34. Palani CK, Abuabara S, Kraft AR, Jonasson O: Endoscopic sclerotherapy in acute variceal hemorrhage. *Am J Surg* 1981;141:164–168.
35. Ayers SJ, Goff JS, Warren GH, Schaffer JW: Esophageal ulceration and bleeding after flexible fiberoptic esophageal vein sclerosis. *Gastroenterology* 1982;83:131–136.
36. Terblanche J, Yakoob HI, Bornman PC, et al: Acute bleeding varices: A five year prospective evaluation of tamponade and sclerotherapy. *Ann Surg* 1981;194:521–529.
37. Clark AE, Westaby D, Silk DBA, et al: Prospective controlled trial of injection sclerotherapy in patients with cirrhosis and recent variceal hemorrhage *Lancet* 1980;2:552–554.
38. MacDougall BRD, Westaby D, Theadossi A: Increased long term survival in variceal hemorrhage using injection sclerotherapy. *Lancet* 1982;1:124–127.
39. Terblanche J, Northover JMA, Borman P, et al: A prospective controlled trial of sclerotherapy in the long-term management of patients after esophageal variceal bleeding. *Surg Gynecol Obstet* 1979;148:323–333.
40. Terblanche J, Bornman PC, Kahn D, et al: Failure of repeated injection sclerotherapy to improve long-term survival after esophageal variceal bleeding. A five year prospective controlled clinical trial. *Lancet* 1983;2:1328–1331.
41. Terblanche J, Jonker MAT, Bornman PC, et al: A 5-year prospective randomized controlled clinical trial of sclerotherapy after oesophageal variceal bleeding. *S AFr J Surg* 1982;20:176–177.
42. Paquet KJ: Prophylactic endoscopic sclerosing treatment of the esophageal wall in varices—A prospective controlled randomized trial. *Endoscopy* 1982;14:4–5.
43. Barsoum MS, Bolous FI, El-Rooby AA, Rizk-Allah MA, Ibrahim AS: Sclerotherapy in the management of bleeding oesophageal varices. *Br J Surg* 1982;69:76–78.
44. Larson AW, Chapman DJ: Acute esophageal variceal sclerotherapy. Results of a prospective controlled trial. *Clin Res* 1982;30:36A (abstract).
45. Cello JP, Crass R, Trunkey DP: Endoscopic sclerotherapy versus esophageal transection of Child's class C patients with variceal hemorrhage. Comparison with results of portacaval shunt. *Surgery* 1982;91:333–338.
46. Yassin YM, Sherif SM: Randomized controlled trial of injection sclerotherapy for bleeding oesophageal varices—An interim report. *Br J Surg* 1983;70:20–22.
47. Korula J, Yamada S, Balart LA, et al: A prospective randomized controlled trial of chronic esophageal variceal sclerotherapy. *Hepatology* 1983;3:825 (abstract).
48. Conn HO: Endoscopic sclerotherapy. An analysis of variants. *Hepatology* 1983;3:769–771.
49. Chung R, Lewis JW: Cost of treatment of bleeding esophageal varices. *Arch Surg* 1983;118:482–485.
50. O'Donnell TF, Gembarowicz RM, Callow AD, Parker SG, Kelly JJ, Deterling RA: The economic impact of acute variceal bleeding: Cost-effectiveness implications for medical and surgical therapy. *Surgery* 1980;88:693–701.
51. Kawai K, Akasaka Y, Murakimi K, Tada M, Kohli Y, Nakajima M: Endoscopic sphincterotomy of the ampulla of Vater. *Gastrointest Endosc* 1974;20:148–151.
52. Classen M, Demling L: Endoskopishe sphinkterotomie der papilla vateri und steinextrakzien aus dim ductus choledochus. *Deutsche Med Wochenscr* 1974;99:496–497.
53. Demling L: Papillotomy—Indications and technique. *Endoscopy* 1983;15:162–164.

54. Taylor BR, Ho CS: Nonsurgical treatment of common bile duct stones. *Can J Surg* 1984;27:28–32.
55. Safrany L, Neuhaus B, Portocarrero G, Krause S: Endoscopic sphincterotomy in patients with Billroth II gastrectomy. *Endoscopy* 1980;12:16–22.
56. Passi RB, Raval B: Endoscopic papillotomy. *Surgery* 1982;92:581–588.
57. Safrany L, Cotton PB: Endoscopic management of choledocholithiasis. *Surg Clin North Am* 1982;62:825–836.
58. Zimmon DS, Falkenstein DB, Kessler RE: Management of biliary calculi by retrograde endoscopic instrumentation (lithocenosis). *Gastrointest Endosc* 1976;23:82–86.
59. Davies H, Bean WIJ, Barnes FS: Breaking up residual gallstones with an ultrasonic drill. *Lancet* 1977;2:278–279.
60. Koch H, Rosch W, Walz V: Endoscopic lithotripsy in the common bile duct. *Gastrointest Endosc* 1980;26:16–18.
61. Nagai N, Toli F, Oi I: Continuous endoscopic pancreatocholedochal catheterization. *Gastroinest Endosc* 1976;23(2):78–81.
62. Cotton PB, Burney PGJ, Mason RR: Transnasal bile duct catheterization after endoscopic sphincterotomy. *Gut* 1979;20:285–287.
63. Zimmon DS, Clemett AR: Endoscopic stents and drains in the management of pancreatic and bile duct obstruction. *Surg Clin North Am.* 1982;62:837–844.
64. Thistle JL, Carlson GL, Jofmann AF, et al: Monooctanoin, a dissolution agent for retained cholesterol bile duct stones: Physical properties and clinical application. *Gastroenterology* 1980;78:1016–1022.
65. Sharp KW, Gadacz TR: Selection of patients for dissolution of retained common duct stones with monooctanoin. *Ann Surg* 1982;196:137–139.
66. Cotton PB, Vallon AG, Mason RR: Intra-ductal infusion of monooctanoin for duct stones. *Lancet* 1981;1:436–437.
67. Jarratt LN, Balfour TW, Bell GD, Knapp DR, Rose DH: Intraductal infusion of monooctanoin. *Lancet* 1981;1:68–70.
68. Cremer M, Toussaint J, Dunham H, Jeanmart J: Endoscopic sphincterotomy with gallbladder in situ. *Gastrointest Endosc* 1981;27:141 (abstract).
69. Cotton PB, Vallon AG: Doudenoscopic sphincterotomy for removal of bile duct stones in patients with gallbladders. *Surgery* 1982;91:628–630.
70. Riemann JD, Lux G, Foresten P, Altendorf A: Long-term results after endoscopic papillotomy. *Endoscopy* 1983;15:165–168.
71. Geenen JE, Bennes JA, Sulvis SE: Resume of a seminar on endoscopic retrograde sphincterotomy (ERS). *Gastrointest Endosc* 1982;27:31–38.
72. Neoptolemos JP, Carr-Locke DL, Fraser I, Fossand DP: The management of common bile duct calculi by endoscopic sphincterotomy in patients with gallbladders in situ. *Br J Surg* 1984;71:69–71.
73. Burhenne JH: Nonoperative retained biliary tract stone extraction. A new roentgenologic technique. *Am J Roentgenol Radium Ther Nucl Med* 1973;117:388–398.
74. Orii K, Nakahara A, Takese Y, Ozaki A, Sakita T, Iwasaki Y: Choledocholithotomy by YAG laser with a cholecochopterscope: Case reports of two patients. *Surgery* 1981;90:120–122.
75. Osacs M: Endoscopic choledocho-duodenostomy for common bile duct obstructions. *Lancet* 1979;1:1059–1060.
76. Acosta JM, Rossi R, Galli OMR, Pellegrini CA, Skinner DB: Early surgery for acute gallstone pancreatitis: Evaluation of a systemic approach. *Surgery* 1978;83:367–370.
77. Roesch W, Demling L: Endoscopic management of pancreatitis. *Surg Clin North Am* 1982;62:845–852.

78. Safrany L, Cotton PB: A preliminary report: Urgent duodenoscopic sphincterotomy for acute gallstone-related pancreatitis. *Surgery* 1981;89:424–428.
79. Safrany L, Neuhaus B, Krause S, Portocarrero G, Schott B: Endoskopische papillotomie bei akuter, biliar bedingter pankreatitis. *Dtsch Med Wschr* 1980;105:115–119.
80. Van der Spuy S: Endoscopic sphincterotomy in the management of gallstone pancreatitis. *Endoscopy* 1981;13:25–26.
81. Wurbs D: Gallensteinextraktion aus dem Pankerasgang, in Henning H: *Fortschritte der gastroenterologischen endoskopie*. Baden-Baden, Witzstrock, 1979.
82. Cremer M, de Toeuf J, Hermanus A: Eiste-il des indications de la sphinterotomie dans les pancreatites chronoilues primitives? III. International Symposium of Digestive Endoscopy, Brussels, 1977.
83. Jones BA, Langer B, Taylor B, Girotti M: Periampullary tumors—which ones should be resected? *Am J Surg* 1985;149:46–52.
84. Laurence BH, Cotton PB: Decompression of malignant biliary obstruction by duodenoscopic intubation of bile duct. *Br Med J* 1980;280:522–523.
85. Classen M, Osseberg FW, Wurbs D, Dammerman R, Hagenmüller F: Pancreatitis— An indication for endoscopic papillotomy? *Endoscopy* 1978;10:223 (abstract).
86. Nakayama T, Ikeda A, Okuda K: Percutaneous transhepatic drainage of the biliary tract: technique and results in 104 cases. *Gastroenterology* 1978;74:554–559.
87. Zimmon DS, Clemett AR: Visualization of the bile ducts, in Popper H, Schaffner F (eds): *Progress in Liver Disease*, Vol. VI. New York, Grune & Stratton, 1979.
88. Denning DS, Ellison EC, Carey LC: Preoperative percutaneous transhepatic biliary decompression lowers operative morbidity in patients with obstructuve jaundice. *Am J Surg* 1981;141:61–65.
89. Hatfield ARW, Murrary RS: Pre-operative biliary drainage in patients with obstructive jaundice. A comparison of the percutaneous transhepatic and endoscopic transpapillary routes. *S Afr Med J* 1981;60:737–742.
90. Koyama K, Takagi Y, Ito K, Sato T: Experimental and clinical studies on the effect of biliary drainage in obstructive jaundice. *Am J Surg* 1981;142:293–299.
91. Kozarek RA: Endoscopically placed pancreatico biliary conduits: Diagnostic and therapeutic uses. *J Clin Gastroenterol* 1982;4:497–501.
92. Allen B, Sharpiro H, Way L: Management of recurrent and residual common duct stones. *Am J Surg* 1981;142:41–47.
93. Mee AS, Vallon AG, Croker JR, Cotton PB: Non-operative removal of bile duct stones by duodenoscopic sphincterotomy in the elderly. *Br Med J* 1981;283:521–523.
94. Reiter J, Bayer H, Mennicken C, Manegold B: Results of endoscopic papillotomy: A collective experience from nine endoscopic centers in West Germany. *World J Surg* 1978;2:505–511.
95. Safrany L: Duodenoscopic sphincterotomy and gallstone removal. *Gastroenterology* 1977;72:338–343.
96. Blumgart LH, Wood CB: Endoscopic treatment of biliary-tract disease. *Lancet* 1978;2:1249 (letter to editor).
97. Cotton PB: Endoscopic treatment of biliary-tract disease. *Lancet* 1979; 1:150 (letter to editor).
98. Glenn F, McSherry CK: Calculous biliary tract disease. *Curr Probl Surg* 1975;June, 1–38.
99. Kune CA: *Current Practice of Biliary Surgery*. Boston, Little Brown, 1972.
100. Seifert EK, Gail K, Weismuller J: Langzeitresultate nach endoskopischeer sphinkterotomie. *Dtsch Med Wschr* 1982;107:610–614.
101. Einstein A: *Zur Quantum Theorie der Strahlung*, 1917.

102. Maiman TH: Stimulated optical radiation in ruby. *Nature* 1960;187:493–494.
103. Lahida EF, Gordon FI, Miller RC: Continuous duty argon ion lasers. *IEEE J Quant Electron* 1965;1:273–279.
104. Gensic JE, Marcos HM, van Uitert LG: Laser oscillations in Nd-doped Yttrium aluminium, Yttrium gallium and Gadolinium garnet. *Appl Physics Lett* 1964;4:182–184.
105. Frühmorgen P, Bodem F, Reidenbach HD, Kaduk B, Demling L: Endoscopic laser photocoagulation of bleeding gastrointestinal lesions with report of the first therapeutic application in man. *Gastrointest Endosc* 1976;23:73–75.
106. Frühmorgen P, Bodem F, Reidenbach HR, Kaduk B, Demling L: Endoscopic photocoagulation by laser irradiation in the gastrointestinal tract of man. *Acta Heptaogastroenterol (Stuttg)* 1978;25:1–5.
107. Brunetaud JM, Enger A, Flamert JB, Berjot M, Moschette Y: Utilisation d'un laser a argon conise en endoscopie digestive: photocoagulation des lesions hemorragiques. *Rev Physique Appl* 1979;14:385–390.
108. Laurence BH, Cotton PB, Vallon AG, et al: Endoscopic laser photocoagulation for bleeding peptic ulcers. *Lancet* 1980;1:124–125.
109. Waitman AM, Grant DZ, Chateau F: Argon laser photocoagulation treatment of patients with acute and chronic bleeding secondary to telangiectasia. *Gastrointest Endosc* 1982;28:153 (abstract).
110. Jensen D, Machicado G, Tapia J, Beilin D: Endoscopic treatment of hemangiomata with argon laser in patients with gastrointestinal bleeding. *Scand J Gastroenterol* 1982; 17(suppl 78):182 (abstract).
111. Schiller KFR, Truelove SC, Williams GD: Haematemesis and melaena with special reference to factors influencing the outcome. *Br Med J* 1970;2:7–14.
112. Peterson WL, Barnett CC, Smith HJ, Allen MH, Corbett DB: Routine early endoscopy in upper gastrointestinal tract bleeding: A randomized controlled trial. *N Engl J Med* 1981;304:925–929.
113. Conn HO: To scope or not to scope? *N Engl J Med* 1981;304:967–969.
114. Avery-Jones F: Hematemesis and melena with special reference to causation and to the factors influencing the mortality from bleeding peptic ulcers. *Gastroenterology* 1956;30:166–190.
115. Kiefhaber P, Nath G, Moritz K: Endoscopic control of massive gastrointestinal hemorrhage by irradiation with a high power Nd YAG laser. *Prog Surg* 1977;15:140–155.
116. Kiefhaber P, Moritz K, Schildberg FW, Feifel G, Herfarth C: Endoscopic Neodymium YAG laser irradiation for control of bleeding acute and chronic ulcers. *Langenbecks Arch Chir* 1978;347:567–571.
117. Vallon AG, Cotton PB, Laurence BH, Armengol Miro JR, Salord Oses JC: Randomized trial of endoscopic argon laser photocoagulation in bleeding peptic ulcers. *Gut* 1981;22:228–233.
118. Swain CP, Brown SG, Storey DW, Northfield TC, Kirkham JS, Salmon PR: Controlled trial of argon laser photocoagulation in bleeding peptic ulcers. *Lancet* 1981;2:1313–1316.
119. Swain CP: Laser photocoagulation in alimentary bleeding. *World J Surg* 1983;7:710–718.
120. Ihre T, Johansson C, Seligson U, Törngren S: Endoscopic YAG laser treatment in massive upper gastrointestinal bleeding. Report of a controlled randomized study. *Scand J Gastroenterol* 1981;16:633–640.
121. Rutgeerts P, vanTrappen G, Broeckhaert L, et al: Controlled trial of YAG laser treatment of upper digestive hemorrhage. *Gastroenterology* 1982;83:410–416.

122. MacLeod IA, Mills PR, MacKenzie JF, Russell RI, Carter DC: A prospective controlled trial of Neodymium YAG laser photocoagulation for major acute upper gastrointestinal hemorrhage. *Scand J Gastroenterol* 1982;17(suppl 78):237 (abstract).

123. Griffiths WJ, Neumann DA, Welsh JD: The visible vessel as an indicator of uncontrolled or recurrent gastrointestinal hemorrhage. *N Engl J Med* 1979;300:1411–1413.

124. Foster DN, Miloszewski KJA, Losowsky MS: Stigmata of recent hemorrhage in diagnosis and prognosis of upper gastrointestinal bleeding. *Br Med J* 1978;1:1173–1177.

125. Storey DW, Bown SG, Swain CP, Salmon PR, Kirkham JS, Northfield TC: Endoscopic prediction of recurrent bleeding in peptic ulcers. *N Engl J Med* 1981;305:915–916.

126. Mallow A, Chabot L: *Laser Safety Handbook.* New York, Van Nostrand Reinhold Company, 1978.

127. Laser Institute of America: Laser Safety Guide, 5th ed. Toledo, OH, Laser Institute of America, 1982 (abstract).

128. Johnston JH: Complications following endoscopic laser therapy. *Gastrointest Endosc* 1982;28:135 (abstract).

129. Becker CD: An accident victim's view. *Laser Focus* 1977;13(6):6.

130. Bown SG: Phototherapy of tumours. *World J Surg* 1983;7:700–709.

131. Toty L, Personne C, Colchen A, Vourc'h G: Brochoscopic management of tracheal lesions using the Nd YAG laser. *Thorax* 1981;36:175–178.

132. Swain CP, Bown SG, Edwards DAW, Kirkham JS, Salmon PR, Clark CG: Laser reconalization of obstructing for gut cancer. *Br J Surg* 1984;71:112–115.

133. Dixon JA, Burt RW, Rotemy RH, McClosky DW: Endoscopic argon laser photocoagulation of small sessile colonic polyps. *Gastrointest Endosc* 1982;28:162–165.

134. Spinelli P, Pizzetti P, Mirabile V, et al: Nd YAG laser treatment of the rectal remnant after colectomy for familia polyposis. *Laser Tokyo* 1981;Section 23, 49–50.

135. Kasugai T, Sugira H, Ito Y, Kano T, Matsuura A, Hiroaka Y: Endoscopic laser treatment for mucosal tumours of the gastrointestinal tract. *Scand J Gastroenterol* 1982;17(suppl 78):192 (abstract).

136. Gregorie HB Jr, Edgar OH, Ward HL, et al: Hematoporphyrin derivative fluorescence in malignant neoplasms. *Ann Surg* 1968;167:820–828.

137. Berenbaum MC, Bonnett R, Scourides PA: *In vivo* activity of components of haematoporphyrin derivative. *Br J Cancer* 1982;45:571–581.

138. Forbes IJ, Cowled PA, Leong AsY, et al: Phototherapy of human tumors using hematoporphyrin derivative. *Med J Aust* 1980;2:489–493.

139. *Proceedings of the Workshop on Porphyrin Sensitization, September 1981, Washington, DC.* New York, Plenum Press, 1983.

140. Cortese DA, Kinsey JH: Endoscopic management of lung cancer with hematoporphyrin derivative phototherapy. *Mayo Clin Proc* 1982;57:543–547.

141. Hayata Y, Kato H, Konaka C, Ono J, Takizawa N: Hematoporphyrin derivative and laser photoradiation in the treatment of lung cancer. *Chest* 1982;81:269–277.

6

Diarrhea and Malabsorption Syndromes

Grant Gall

1. INTRODUCTION

Chronic diarrhea is a common problem in both children and adults.[1] Diarrhea is defined as the excess loss of water and electrolytes in the feces, leading to the increased frequency, fluidity, and volume of bowel movements. This discussion will focus on the mechanism of diarrhea and the clinical and laboratory approach to the diagnosis. Although the discussion will be primarily aimed at the problem in the pediatric age group, the overall approach is relevant to the adult patient. A complete discussion of all the causes of chronic diarrhea in children and adults is not feasible here, but Table 1 lists the extensive differential diagnoses for chronic diarrhea and malabsorption in infancy and childhood. Many of these conditions are rare. In many children and adults with chronic diarrhea, despite extensive investigation, no specific entity can be identified.

2. NORMAL PHYSIOLOGY

Before the abnormal is discussed, one needs some understanding of the normal pattern for the intestinal handling of water and electrolytes. The gut handles an enormous volume of fluid.[2] In the normal child about 5 liters of fluid enters the upper small intestine each day. Of this volume

Grant Gall ● Department of Medicine, University of Calgary, Calgary, Alberta, Canada T2N 1N4.

Table 1. Causes of Chronic Diarrhea and Malabsorption in Children

1. Watery diarrhea
   Osmotic
     Disaccharidase deficiency
       Lactase
       Sucrase–isomaltase
     Glucose–galactose malabsorption
     Excessive intake, e.g., sorbitol
   Abnormal water and electrolyte
     transport
   Infective
     Viral
     Enterotoxigenic bacteria
     Giardia lamblia
   Allergic gastroenteropathy
     Cow's milk protein
     Soy protein
   Short gut
     Congenital
     Postsurgical
   Bacterial overgrowth
     Motility disorder
     Anatomical obstruction
   Laxative abuse
   Immune deficiency disorders
   Congenital chloride-losing
   diarrhea
   Acrodermatitis enteropathica
         Functioning tumors
       Pancreatic islet cell tumors
       Neural crest tumors
       Medullary carcinoma of thyroid
   Bile salt malabsorption
   Endocrine disease
     Adrenal insufficiency
     Diabetes mellitus

2. Steatorrhea
   Pancreatic insufficiency
     Cystic fibrosis
     Shwachman's syndrome
     Malnutrition

2. Steatorrhea (*continued*)
   Pancreatic insufficiency (*continued*)
     Chronic pancreatitis
     Lipase, colipase deficiency
   Inadequate bile salt concentration
     Biliary atresia
     Cirrhosis
     Cholestatic syndromes
       Acquired
       Familial
     Bacterial overgrowth syndromes
     Disease or resection of ileum
   Inadequate absorptive area
     Celiac disease
     Short gut syndrome
     Cow's milk protein and soy protein
       intolerance
     Whipple's disease
     Immune deficiency disorders
   Intracellular defect
     Abetalipoproteinemia
   Impaired lymphatic drainage
     Lymphoma
     Intestinal lymphangiectasia
     Constructive pericarditis

3. Bloody Diarrhea
   Infection
     Campylobacter
     Shigella
     Salmonella
     Yersinia
     Invasive *Escherichia coli*
     Cytomegalovirus colitis
   Chronic inflammatory bowel disease
   Pseudomembranous colitis
   Milk protein intolerance (infants)
   Necrotizing enterocolitis
   Amebiasis
   Hirschsprung's enterocolitis
   Diarrhea associated with anal lesions

only about 1–2 liters is derived from oral intake. The remainder is from the endogenous secretions of saliva, gastric juices, bile, pancreatic juice, and small intestinal secretions. To this volume must be added variable quantities of fat, carbohydrate, and protein derived from the diet and protein from digestive secretions and sloughed intestinal cells. The majority of the total volume is absorbed in the small intestine; only about 500–1000 ml passes the ileocecal valve. Stool volumes range from 75 to 200 g, of which 65–80% is water. Thus, the reabsorption of this luminal fluid is exceedingly efficient, but even small increases in stool volume may cause the patient to complain of diarrhea.

Fluid entering the jejunum is essentially isotonic despite the wide variation in osmolality of ingested food. Meals are modified to some extent by hypotonic saliva and isotonic gastric secretions, but regardless of intragastric osmolality, meals leaving the duodenum are rendered isotonic. This is accomplished by varying the rate of gastric emptying and by altering the movement of water and electrolytes into or out of the lumen of the intestine. The epithelia of the gastrointestinal tract vary considerably in their ionic permeability. Those that are leaky, for example, the small intestine, have a very high passive permeability to small ions and water, low electrical transepithelial potential difference, and are capable of absorbing large volumes of salt and water as isotonic fluid. Epithelia that are moderately leaky, for example, colonic epithelia, are capable of generating differences in ionic composition and osmolality but have a more limited capacity for salt and water absorption. Thus, large volumes of essentially isotonic fluid are absorbed in the small intestine, whereas the colon has a large reserve capacity and also the ability to concentrate the remaining intestinal output.

Transcellular absorption of sodium chloride by the intestine appears to be accomplished by three cellular processes: electrogenic active sodium absorption that is accompanied by passive diffusion of chloride; sodium absorption coupled with the absorption of organic solutes such as glucose, amino acids, and bile salts; and finally, neutral sodium chloride absorption. Adequate digestion and absorption of dietary constituents are also essential for normal intestinal function. Readers are referred to recent reviews of the enzymatic and physiochemical events required for absorption of fat, carbohydrate, protein, and other nutrients.[3-5]

3. MECHANISMS OF DIARRHEA

Three major defects may contribute to the production of diarrhea: (1) osmotic retardation of water absorption, (2) abnormal water and electrolyte transport, and (3) disordered transit. In the majority of clinical conditions that lead to chronic diarrhea, more than one mechanism is involved.

3.1. Osmotic Retardation

The presence of unabsorbed dietary components in the bowel constitutes an abnormal osmotic load which leads to retardation of water absorption. This can result from dietary overloading (e.g., sorbitol- or fructose-induced diarrhea) or from malabsorption of ingested nutrients, usually carbohydrates. Malabsorbed carbohydrates undergo fermentation by colonic bacteria to organic acids. This further increases the osmotic load, and some of these organic acids may also stimulate the colon to secrete fluid. The flux of water into the bowel exceeds absorptive capacity, and watery diarrhea results. In osmotic diarrhea, the stools are low in sodium concentration, and stool osmolality exceeds that predicted from two times the sum of the sodium and potassium concentrations. This "osmotic gap" reflects the load of unabsorbed solute causing the diarrhea.

3.2. Abnormal Water and Electrolyte Transport

Derangement of water and electrolyte transport can be induced by direct mucosal injury or can be secondary to the effect of intraluminal or circulating factors. The response of the patient depends on the region and extent of the intestine involved. Since about 90% of fluid and electrolyte absorption is normally completed by the small intestine, relatively minor abnormalities here may cause diarrhea.

Intraluminal agents that impair water and electrolyte absorption and induce secretion include bacterial enterotoxins (cholera and enterotoxigenic *Escherichia coli*), humoral agents, deconjugated bile salts, and hydroxylated fatty acids. Bacterial deconjugation of bile acids occurs in bacterial overgrowth of the small bowel and when malabsorbed bile salts are acted upon by colonic bacteria. Hydroxy fatty acids are produced from the actions of colonic microflora on unabsorbed dietary fat. Deconjugated bile acids and hydroxy fatty acids are potent secretagogues. Functioning tumors such as carcinoids, pancreatic islet cell tumors, neural crest tumors, and medullary carcinoma of the thyroid secrete humoral agents that stimulate water and electrolyte secretion. With this type of diarrhea the sum of the electrolyte concentrations in the stool equals the osmolality of the stool.

3.3. Disorders of Transit

An adequate length of small bowel is necessary for the normal digestion and absorption of food. Congenital or acquired short gut may result in inadequate mucosal exposure of intraluminal contents and diminished absorption of nutrients. An intact ileocecal valve is important in controlling intestinal transit and preventing bacterial contamination of the distal small bowel.

Disorders of motility may result in chronic diarrhea and malabsorption. Normal motility is important to maintain the normal bacterial flora of the small intestine. Hypomotility allows bacterial overgrowth of the small intestine with resultant absorptive defects. Hypomotility is seen in intestinal pseudoobstruction, partial anatomical obstruction, Hirschsprung's disease, scleroderma, and diabetes. Hypermotility can be seen in intestinal infection, laxative abuse, thyrotoxicosis, and with certain functioning endocrine tumors.

4. DIFFERENTIAL DIAGNOSIS

The spectrum of disease causing chronic diarrhea and malabsorption ranges from benign problems to life-threatening illness and includes a long list of possible disorders. One way to classify and thereby narrow down the differential diagnosis is by considering the characteristics of the stool: Are the stools fatty or watery, and if watery do they contain blood?

4.1. Watery Diarrhea

Watery diarrhea usually indicates small bowel disease.

4.1.1. Carbohydrate Malabsorption

In children chronic watery diarrhea is frequently related to carbohydrate malabsorption from secondary disaccharidase deficiency. This injury is most commonly caused by viral enteritis, but other examples include giardiasis, celiac disease, milk or soy protein intolerance, short gut syndrome, and bacterial overgrowth syndrome. In addition, young infants on occasion will develop secondary monosaccharide intolerance after a severe or repeated bouts of viral enteritis.

Primary lactase deficiency is not uncommon in non-Caucasians and may manifest in later childhood or adulthood as chronic watery diarrhea. Other inherited disorders of carbohydrate absorption are rare. Sucrase-isomaltase deficiency presents in infancy after the introduction of sucrose-containing foods. Glucose–galactose malabsorption is a life-threatening disease presenting in the neonatal period. In younger patients with sugar malabsorption, the ingestion of the offending sugar leads to explosive watery diarrhea.

4.1.2. Abnormal Water and Electrolyte Transport

Secretory diarrhea is likely in patients with continuing watery diarrhea despite complete bowel rest. The diarrhea is related to decreased absorption, active secretion, or a combination of both. Numerous toxic, humoral, chemical, and mucosal factors have been implicated in secretory diarrheas. Bacterial enterotoxins are a common cause (e.g., *E. coli* enterotoxin in traveler's diarrhea), but the disease is usually acute and self-limited. In patients with severe diarrhea that persists and in whom stool osmolality is explained by the electrolyte concentrations, consider laxative abuse[6] or hormone-producing disorders.

4.2. Steatorrhea

Fat malabsorption results from inadequate pancreatic lipase or colipase, insufficient intraluminal bile salt concentration, insufficient absorptive surface, cellular defects, or obstructed lymphatic drainage.

4.2.1. Pancreatic Insufficiency

Cystic fibrosis is the most common cause of pancreatic insufficiency in childhood in developed countries. Many of these patients now survive to adulthood and require care by internists. Cystic fibrosis is the most frequent lethal gene in Caucasians. Inheritance is autosomal recessive. Most patients present in the first year of life with pulmonary disease, chronic diarrhea, and failure to thrive. However, patients with milder disease may present at a later age, even occasionally as adults. The disease affects many systems. The major clinical manifestations are related to dysfunction of the respiratory and gastrointestinal tracts. Nearly all aspects of the gastrointestinal system are involved including pancreas, liver, biliary tract, and both small and large intestine.[7,8]

Although pancreatic disease is a major manifestation, not all patients have pancreatic insufficiency. Approximately 10% of patients with cystic fibrosis retain sufficient pancreatic function for normal absorption. The latter patients with nearly normal pancreatic function are at risk for recurrent episodes of pancreatitis. Progressive destruction of pancreatic tissue in patients with cystic fibrosis can involve islets of Langerhans and can lead to abnormalities of carbohydrate metabolism. About 40% of patients have abnormal glucose tolerance tests, but diabetes occurs in only 1%. Intestinal complications of cystic fibrosis include meconium ileus, rectal prolapse, meconium ileus equivalent, and intussusception. Meconium ileus equivalent refers to the clinical problem of abdominal pain and intestinal obstruction occurring after the neonatal period. In patients with cystic fibrosis who are more than 12 years of age, the frequency of meconium ileus equivalent is estimated to be about 25%. The etiology of this condition appears to be related to impaction of food residues in the terminal ileum and right colon.

Pathological liver changes are also frequent in patients with cystic fibrosis. The highest incidence of clinical symptoms referrable to liver disease is seen in the adolescent and older age group. As more individuals with cystic fibrosis are surviving to adulthood, we can expect to see increased numbers of these patients presenting complications related to liver dysfunction. The initial lesion of focal biliary cirrhosis is common and can be seen early in life. In some patients, this lesion progresses to multilobular biliary cirrhosis. One of the features of liver disease in cystic fibrosis is the lack of early signs and symptoms. The first indication of severe liver disease is often a massive bleed from esophageal varices or the finding of splenomegaly secondary to portal hypertension. Biliary tract disease is also common in the older patient with cystic fibrosis. Cholesterol gallstones are common, variably estimated to occur in 4–10% of patients. Roy and co-workers[8] have demonstrated that bile from cystic fibrosis patients is lithogenic, presumably owing to fecal bile salt loss and liver dysfunction.

Other causes of pancreatic insufficiency include Shwachman's syndrome and chronic pancreatitis. Pancreatic exocrine insufficiency in Shwachman's syndrome is associated with bone marrow hypoplasia, short stature, and, less commonly, metaphyseal dysostosis.

4.2.2. Celiac Disease (Gluten Enteropathy)

Celiac disease usually presents in the first 2 years of life after introduction of cereals into the diet, but these patients can present at any age. Irritability, diarrhea, and failure to thrive are common symptoms. Abdominal distention, wasting, and growth failure are usually evident on examination. In general, if a child with chronic diarrhea is thriving, celiac disease is an unlikely diagnosis.

4.2.3. Other Conditions

Short gut syndrome, whether congenital or acquired, causes steatorrhea because of inadequate surface area for absorption. Steatorrhea, from inadequate intraluminal levels of conjugated bile salts, can result from bacterial contamination of the small bowel, disease of the terminal ileum, and severe liver disease. Rare mucosal defects producing steatorrhea include abetalipoproteinemia and intestinal lymphangiectasia.

4.3. Bloody Diarrhea

Bloody diarrhea usually indicates colonic disease. In infective colitis and chronic idiopathic inflammatory bowel disease, involving the colon, pus cells are readily apparent on microscopy of the stool. Diarrhea associated with anal lesions may on occasion mimic bloody diarrhea.

4.3.1. Infective

Intestinal infections are usually associated with acute diarrhea, but occasionally infections by *Campylobacter, Salmonella,* and *Yersinia* and infestation by *Giardia lamblia* can lead to chronic symptoms. *Yersinia enterocolitica* and *Campylobacter jejuni* require special techniques for their identification.

Amebic dysentery should be considered in any patient who has traveled to the southern United States or to the tropics or who has been in contact with individuals who have recently returned from the tropics. Pseudomembranous colitis and *Clostridium difficile* infection should be considered in patients who develop profuse diarrhea following antibiotic therapy. In the majority of cases, proctosigmoidoscopic examination reveals colonic musosa covered with adherent yellowish–white plaques or membranes. The diagnosis is confirmed by isolation of *C. difficile* from the stool and identification of the specific toxin.

4.3.2. Chronic Inflammatory Bowel Disease

Idiopathic ulcerative colitis and Crohn's disease occur in children as well as adults. In ulcerative colitis, severe bloody diarrhea, abdominal discomfort, urgency to stool, and tenesmus are the usual presenting symptoms. Frequent passage of small stools is the hallmark of rectal inflammation. Patients with Crohn's disease may have a similar presentation, but more commonly complaints of abdominal pain, anorexia, and systemic manifestations, including malnutrition, growth failure, and delayed puberty, dominate the clinical picture. Chronic inflammatory bowel disease should be suspected in patients with chronic symptoms with negative stool cultures.

4.3.3. Protein Intolerance

Chronic diarrhea can be a manifestation of cow and soy protein intolerance. In the very young infant, protein intolerance often presents as colitis. The presence of blood and eosinophils in the diarrheal stool suggests the diagnosis. The improvement of symptoms following withdrawal of the offending protein and exacerbation with rechallenge is diagnostic.

5. APPROACH TO THE DIAGNOSIS

The challenge to the physician is to separate the patient in whom chronic diarrhea is a manifestation of underlying intestinal disease from the well individual who has chronic loose stools. The diagnosis can be established in the majority of patients with a thorough clinical assessment and stool examination.

5.1. Clinical Assessment

The initial assessment will reveal whether the patient is ill. If so, immediate attention and investigation may be warranted. If not, a "wait and see" approach may be far more rewarding than an immediate and costly investigation.

Assessment of appetite, well-being, and, in the child, growth is important. Patients with pancreatic insufficiency may have voracious appetites. The converse is usually true of patients with celiac disease, who often display anorexia and irritability. If the patient is not thriving, a thorough dietary history should be taken. Patients with chronic diarrhea often have frequent manipulations of their diet with accompanying severe caloric restriction in an attempt by frustrated parents, patients, and physicians to control stool output. Such manipulations are usually without success. A chronological record of dietary milestones may suggest a diagnosis: Celiac disease frequently presents within 3–6 months of the introduction of cereals.

The consistency, frequency, and type of stool may indicate the presence of underlying disease and may localize pathology to a specific part of the intestinal tract. The presence of blood and mucus usually indicates a colonic problem: Steatorrhea and water diarrhea suggest a problem in the small intestine.

Assessment of general health is important as many gastrointestinal disorders display extraintestinal manifestations. Frequent sinopulmonary infections suggest cystic fibrosis, disorders of immune deficiency, or neutropenia (Shwachman's syndrome). Fever, anemia, arthritis, and skin rashes occur in chronic inflammatory bowel disease and bacterial enteritis. Delay in pubertal development can occur with many chronic diseases but should alert one to the possibility of Crohn's disease.

The physical examination includes assessment of growth percentiles in children, nutritional status, and pubertal development. Plotting of height, weight, and head cricumference is mandatory for the assessment of any child with chronic diarrhea. A patient who is growing normally is unlikely to be suffering from significant gastrointestinal disease. The plotting of longitudinal percentiles can give important information about timing and severity of disease and may even suggest a diagnosis. Other indicators of malabsorption and abnormal nutritional status include loss of subcutaneous fat and muscle bulk, peripheral edema (hypoproteinemia), and bruising (vitamin K deficiency). Recurrent aphthous ulcers are seen frequently with chronic intestinal disease such as Crohn's disease. Finger clubbing suggests chronic disease and is frequently seen in cystic fibrosis, celiac disease, and Crohn's disease. On rectal examination one must specifically look for evidence of perianal disease, fissures, and fecal impaction. This procedure also affords an opportunity to assess the severity of the diarrhea and to inspect and examine a stool specimen.

5.2. Stool Examination

The importance of stool examination is frequently overlooked, but it should be considered a routine part of the examination in a patient with chronic diarrhea. The presence of numerous red and white cells on microscopy is seen in chronic infections and chronic inflammatory bowel disease but rarely in diarrhea originating in the small bowel. Cysts or trophozoites of *G. lamblia* on occasion may be found, but diagnosis, at best, can be made in only 50% of cases by stool examination. Undigested fat is seen as globules of neutral fat that stain orange with oil red 0 or sudan red. Outside the newborn period the presence of neutral fat is always abnormal and indicates pancreatic insufficiency. In a child this suggests the diagnosis of cystic fibrosis or, less likely, Shwachman's syndrome. Care must be taken since lubricants and ointments are indistinguishable from fat on microscopy. The presence of meat fibers also indicates pancreatic insufficiency. Excess fatty acids, which are apparent at high power as refractile crystals, suggest a mucosal problem such as celiac disease.

The presence of sugar in the stool can be detected by the use of Clinitest tablets. A small amount of liquid stool is diluted with twice the volume of water, and 15 drops of this solution together with the Clinitest tablet are placed in a separate tube. The resultant color change is compared with the chart provided. The test needs to be performed immediately upon obtaining the stool sample in order to prevent further fermentation of sugars by colonic bacteria. Sucrose is not a reducing substance; if its presence is suspected, it may be necessary to first hydrolyze the sugar with acid before testing. Greater than 250 mg/dl of reducing substances indicates carbohydrate malabsorption. The exception is the breast-fed infant whose stools frequently contain excess lactose in the absence of underlying disease.

5.3. Laboratory Investigations[9]

Clinical assessment and stool examination will, in the majority of patients, indicate whether the person is ill and, if so, will often point to a likely diagnosis. Initial assessment may lead to routine blood tests for anemia and inflammation, stool cultures, examination of stools for parasites, and measurement of sweat electrolytes if cystic fibrosis is a possibility. Serum electrolytes and urea, though frequently performed, are rarely of diagnostic help. Total serum protein and albumin levels provide a rough index of nutritional status and intestinal protein loss. At this point, enough information is usually available to the physician to justify a wait-and-see approach or, if the presence of underlying disease is suspected, to guide the subsequent line of investigation.

5.3.1. Assessment of Watery Diarrhea

The first step in the assessment of water diarrhea is repeated testing of the stool for reducing substances by Clinitest tablets, as previously described. In patients with persisting watery stools, which do not appear to contain excess carbohydrate and are culture negative, the estimation of daily stool output and fecal electrolyte content and osmolality is indicated. In patients with secretory diarrhea, normal stool electrolyte concentrations are altered, with a marked increase in the sodium and potassium content. The stool osmolality can be accounted for by the ionic constituents; twice the sum of the stool concentrations of sodium and potassium will approximate the stool osmolality. This is distinct from an osmotic diarrhea. In an osmotic diarrhea, the ionic constituents do not account for the stool osmolality; instead an osmotic gap is apparent, reflecting the load of unabsorbed solute causing the diarrhea. If the patient does have an osmotic diarrhea, breath hydrogen analysis following oral challenge with the suspected sugar such as lactose or sucrose may be a useful test despite the absence of obvious carbohydrate malabsorption.[10] Breath hydrogen testing is also useful in patients with suspected bacterial overgrowth syndrome or abnormality of intestinal transit. The breath hydrogen analysis is based on the principle that one of the end products of colonic fermentation of malabsorbed carbohydrate is hydrogen. Hydrogen gas is normally present in very low concentrations in expired alveolar air. The hydrogen produced by fermentation of carbohydrate in the colon is absorbed into the blood stream and eliminated through the lungs. In about 2% of otherwise normal individuals, hydrogen-producing colonic bacteria are absent, and this test may give a false negative result. This is especially true of newborn infants and in children for a variable period of time following a bout of acute gastroenteritis.

In the breath hydrogen test, the patient is given the substrate (lactose, sucrose, starch, or lactulose) at a dose of 2 g/kg, to a maximum of 50 g orally after at least an 8-hr fast. Expired tidal air is collected before and then at 30-min intervals through a nasal prong attached to a syringe. Samples are usually collected for 3–4 hr, but if starch absorption is being assessed, samples need to be collected for a longer period, up to 8 hr. The ability of the patient to ferment malabsorbed carbohydrate can be confirmed by repeating the test, if necessary, with lactulose, a nonabsorbable carbohydrate. Lactulose is also used when one suspects bacterial overgrowth or when assessing small intestinal transit time. The CO_2 content of the sample is also determined to ensure that the collected sample accurately reflects end-expired tidal air. The CO_2 and hydrogen concentration are determined by gas liquid chromatography. This technical requirement limits the general application of this useful test.

In patients with unexplained osmotic or secretory diarrhea, one must always consider the possibility of laxative abuse. Four general categories of laxatives are recognized: indigestible fiber, lubricants, osmotic agents, and stimulants. The stimulant laxatives have most commonly been recognized as agents of abuse, although osmotic agents such as magnesium salts have occasionally been incriminated. The stimulant group includes naturally occurring substances, castor oil, senna, and cascara, as well as synthetic agents, such as phenolphthalein, bisacodyl, danthron, and dioctyl sodium succinate. These compounds stimulate cyclic AMP-mediated secretion or inhibit absorption. The diarrhea produced by stimulant laxatives is characteristic of a secretory diarrhea: The stools are voluminous, watery, and free of blood, pus, or abnormal amounts of fat. The diarrhea continues despite the cessation of oral intake, and stool electrolyte concentrations are increased and account for the stool osmolality. Once laxative abuse is suspected, it is relatively easy to establish a diagnosis. Alkalinization of stool or urine containing phenolphthalein or aloe produces a color change to red, pink, or mauve. This is demonstrated by a slow addition of 0.1 N sodium hydroxide to stool or urine. Senna can be detected by the addition of sulfuric acid and carbon tetrachloride to urine. Chromatographic methods can detect phenolic and anthraquinone laxatives in urine up to 32 hr after their ingestion. Magnesium can be measured in stool water.

Consider humoral factors in patients with severe diarrhea that persists despite restricting oral intake, and in which stool osmolality is explained by the electrolyte content. Studies are aimed at identifying the specific hormonal agent, such as vasoactive intestinal peptide and gastrin in serum and catecholemines in serum and urine.

Specific investigations can be diagnostic in patients with clinical features suggestive of an unusual disorder. For example, low serum zinc points to a diagnosis of acrodermatitis enteropathica in a patient presenting with failure to thrive, mucocutaneous lesions, and alopecia. Acanthocytic red cells, low serum cholesterol, and abnormal lipoprotein electrophoresis confirm a diagnosis of abetalipoproteinemia. Differential white-cell count and immunoglobulin estimation may lead to a diagnosis of immunodeficiency disease or intestinal lymphangiectasia.

5.3.2. Assessment of Steatorrhea

As indicated in Section 5.2, simple light microscopy can be very helpful as a semiquantitative assessment of fat malabsorption. Additional investigation is, however, required to confirm the presence of fat malabsorption. The distaste of handling and examining stool specimens has led to the development of numerous screening tests for malabsorption. Indirect tests to document malabsorption such as fasting serum carotene levels, vitamin A tolerance tests, and D-xylose tolerance tests have proven to be unreliable. Breath tests utilizing radiolabeled triglycerides and measurement of the label in expired air have been successfully employed for the assessment of fat absorption. In many of these breath tests, ^{14}C-labeled products have been used as substrates. Although the radioactivity is low, the long biological half-life of ^{14}C makes these tests inappropriate for use in children. The recent availability of stable isotopes such as ^{13}C avoids the need for radioactive labels, but the need for the sophisticated methodology of mass spectrometry limits their use.

The most practical and accurate method for quantitative assessment of absorptive function and confirmation of steatorrhea is measurement of fecal fat excretion. The stool collection should last at least 3 days while the patient consumes an adequate amount of fat before and during the collection. In an infant the fat intake should be 20–30 g/day, in an older child 50 g or more, and in an adult 100 g of fat should be taken each day.

Results are best expressed as a percentage excretion of fat intake. Normal values vary considerably with age. Prematures normally excrete 20–30% of their fat intake, full-term newborns 10–20%, children 1–3 years less than 10%, and older children and adults less than 5%.

In patients with steatorrhea and suspected pancreatic insufficiency, exocrine pancreatic function is best evaluated by measurement of pancreatic enzymes and electrolytes in duodenal juice following stimulation with cholecystokinin and secretin using a quantitative marker perfusion technique. Fecal chymotrypsin determination, which provides a semi-quantitative assessment of pancreatic function, can be helpful in assessing infants with steatorrhea but has proven to be unreliable in older children and adults. In general, however, in the pediatric patient the problem is approached more directly by measuring chloride, sodium, or both in sweat, since cystic fibrosis is the major cause of pancreatic insufficiency in childhood. Elevated sweat electrolytes are a constant feature of cystic fibrosis, and their measurement is the procedure of choice for diagnosis. The test, although not difficult to perform, can be associated with numerous errors in the hands of the inexperienced. In pediatric centers where the test is being performed regularly, false positives or false negatives are rare. This, unfortunately, is not the case at centers where the test is done infrequently. The reliability of the test depends on obtaining adequate amounts of sweat, at least 100 mg, which is best accomplished by stimulation of local sweating with pilocarpine or urecholine prior to collection. Indirect methods such as chloride electrodes and measurement of sweat osmolality have proven to be temperamental and frequently unreliable.

In normal children sweat sodium and chloride levels are less than 60 meq/liter and usually are less than 40 meq/liter. In patients with cystic fibrosis levels are greater than 60 meq/liter and frequently are as high as 90 meq/liter or more. In infants and young children levels between 50 and 60 meq/liter should be carefully reexamined. After puberty sweat electrolyte concentrations may exceed levels of 60 meq/liter in normal individuals, and the test is no longer as discriminating in the diagnosis of cystic fibrosis.

In patients with fat malabsorption and a suspected mucosal defect, peroral biopsy of the small intestine remains the most reliable and efficient means for assessment. Histological definition of mucosal injury is a must for the diagnosis of celiac disease. Histological features will aid in the diagnosis of many other conditions, for example, Whipple disease, abetalipoproteinemia, and intestinal lymphangiectasia. The diagnostic value of a small intestinal biopsy is not limited to histological assessment.

Additional information can be obtained from enzymatic, metabolic, immunological, and microbiological studies of the biopsy material.

5.3.3. Assessment of Bloody Diarrhea

In the patient with bloody diarrhea the approach is aimed at excluding infective agents by culture and direct microscopy of stool, and in demonstrating anatomical lesions suggestive of an underlying disorder, such as chronic ulcerative colitis or Crohn's disease, by direct visualization (proctosigmoidoscopy, colonoscopy), biopsy, and radiological investigations.

6. SUMMARY

In the majority of patients, severe disease can be excluded or a diagnosis established with thorough clinical assessment, stool examination, simple tests performed in the office, and, when necessary, more detailed investigations as indicated. However, many patients with chronic diarrhea have no identifiable disease and are grouped into diagnostic conglomerates such as chronic nonspecific diarrhea and spastic bowel syndrome. In children the onset of chronic nonspecific diarrhea may follow an episode of acute enteritis and is usually a problem in those younger than 3 years of age. Stools are loose but not watery and may occur 4–10 times per day. Despite the frequency of stools, most patients are robust and thriving. The problem is benign and self-limited and is usually of greater concern to the parent than the child. There is no specific therapy. The course, however, may be complicated by multiple inappropriate dietary manipulations and caloric restriction. In patients who are failing to thrive, caloric restrictions should be corrected before intensive investigation, unless clinical assessment strongly suggests underlying disease.

REFERENCES

1. Anderson CM: Malabsorption in children. *Clin Gastroenterol* 1977;6:355–376.
2. Phillips SF: Diarrhea: A current view of the pathophysiology. *Gastroenterology* 1972;63:495–518.
3. Freeman HJ, Kim YS: Digestion and absorption of protein. *Annu Rev Med* 1978;29:99–116.
4. Friedman HI, Nylund B: Intestinal fat digestion, absorption and transport. *Am J Clin Nutr* 1980;33:1108–1139.

5. Silk DBA, Dawson AM: Intestinal absorption of carbohydrate and protein in man, in Crane RK (ed): *International Review of Physiology. Gastrointestinal Physiology III,* Vol. 19. Baltimore: University Park Press, 1979, pp. 151–204.

6. Morris AI, Turnberg LA: Surreptitious laxative abuse. *Gastroenterology* 1979;77:780–786.

7. Gaskin KJ, Durie PR, Lee L, Hill R, Forstner GG: Colipase and lipase secretion in childhood-onset pancreatic insufficiency. *Gastroenterology* 1984;86:1–7.

8. Roy CC: Gastrointestinal and hepatobiliary complications: changing patterns with age, in Sturgess JM (ed): *Perspectives in Cystic Fibrosis.* Mississavga, Ontario: Imperial Press, 1980, p. 190.

9. Russell RI, Lee FD: Tests of small intestinal function: Digestion, absorption, secretion. *Clin Gastroenterol* 1978;7:277–316.

10. Barr RG, Perman JA, Schoeller DAS, Watkins JB: Breath tests in pediatric gastrointestinal disorders: New diagnostic possibilities. *Pediatrics* 1978;62:393–401.

7

Inflammatory Bowel Disease
The Distinction between Crohn's Disease and Ulcerative Colitis

Hugh James Freeman

1. INTRODUCTION

Ulcerative colitis, since its original description in 1865 in the Union Army,[1] has emerged as a heterogeneous collection of inflammatory bowel disorders recognized and separated from the parent group by the identification of a variety of clinicopathological features and most important by the exclusion of specific infectious agents. Today, ulcerative colitis remains an idiopathic entity requiring for diagnosis the exclusion of specific etiological agents and the evaluation of a combination of clinical, radiographic, endoscopic, and histological features.[2]

In 1960, this diagnostic problem was especially accentuated by the recognition of Crohn's disease of the colon as a clinical entity.[3-5] Given that two different patterns of idiopathic inflammatory disease may be recognized, is there a need to make this distinction?

2. DIAGNOSIS OF ULCERATIVE COLITIS AND CROHN'S DISEASE

Ulcerative colitis is characterized clinically by rectal bleeding, diarrhea, abdominal pain, fever, and weight loss and pathologically by diffuse

Hugh James Freeman • The University of British Columbia, Health Sciences Centre Hospital, Vancouver, British Columbia, Canada V6T 1W5.

mucosal inflammatory change. The rectum is invariably involved with proximal extension for variable distances. Rectal biopsy mirrors these endoscopic findings with diffuse changes extending across the mucosa, i.e., transmucosal disease. Crypt abscesses are frequently present as markers of inflammation. However, crypt abscesses are certainly not pathognomonic of ulcerative colitis: other entities, especially infectious causes of colitis, may produce similar changes, particularly during the initial or acute presentation. Thus, diagnosis of ulcerative colitis or Crohn's disease depends on exclusion of other causes of colitis producing indistinguishable clinical and pathological features.

Crohn's disease is characterized clinically by fever, abdominal pain, diarrhea, weight loss, as well as slowing of growth in children.[6] Bleeding occurs in up to two-thirds of patients. Although bleeding is less frequent than in ulcerative colitis, this symptom is of no differential value. Pathologically, changes are more often focal or segmental. Radiologically, maximal involvement is most often localized to the distal ileum and proximal colon. For example, in the National Cooperative Crohn's Disease Study, 46% of patients had documented ileocolonic involvement.[6] A focal aphthoid ulcer may be visualized, and the mucosa between ulcers or between involved bowel segments may appear normal. This appearance may be paralleled by a histological pattern of inflammation characterized by patchy or focal inflammatory change. Crypt abscesses may also be seen in Crohn's disease. Occasionally, microgranulomata containing epithelioid or giant cells are seen. These are usually observed in the mucosa rather than in the submucosa because of the limited depth of endoscopic biopsy specimens. Many investigators believe granulomata are characteristic, if not diagnostic, for Crohn's disease. However, detection of microscopic granulomata depends, to some degree, on the care and interest of individuals obtaining, processing, and interpreting the biopsies. With a single-step section of a rectal biopsy, 7% of patients with Crohn's disease had granulomas.[7] With careful study of serial sections from two biopsies, however, the yield of granuloma may be up to 28%. Interestingly, these granulomas may be seen as frequently in grossly normal as in grossly abnormal mucosa.[8] Although less frequent, similar observations may be made in upper endoscopic gastric and duodenal biopsies. Even granulomatous oral lesions (or cheilitis) have been described, sometimes antedating by several years the appearance of bowel disease.[9] These findings, particularly from "radiographically negative" sites, provide strong evidence that Crohn's disease is a far more extensive process than was formerly appreciated.[10]

In recent years, a broadening spectrum of disorders has emerged, many with similar patterns of inflammatory change.[2] In part, increased awareness has resulted from developments in endoscopy and biopsy methodology,[11] as well as improved microbiological methods for defining the presence of specific infectious agents. These entitites deserve special emphasis because in previous years, there may have been a lack of recognition and emphasis of their importance.

3. TWO PATHOGENS OF PARTICULAR INTEREST

Two groups of pathogens of particular interest include *Yersinia* and *Campylobacter*. *Yersinia enterocolitica* is a gram-negative rod that has become better recognized with increasing frequency worldwide as a human pathogen. In children, *Yersinia* infections usually cause acute enteritis with fever and diarrhea. In adolescents and adults, acute terminal ileitis and mesenteric adenitis seem to occur more frequently with *Yersinia* infections. Other features of the disease include erythema nodosum, polyarthritis, septicemia, and metastatic abscesses. Recent studies using endoscopy and radiography document a high frequency of colonic as well as small bowel disease. Although treatment is usually effective, a significant percentage of patients may have persistent ileitis.[12]

In 1980, based on different biochemical features,[13] this agent was reclassified to include *Y. enterocolitica sensu stricto* and a variety of "new," formerly labeled atypical *Yersinia* specimens. Detection of *Yersinia* has also been substantially improved recently with the development of highly selected *Yersinia* growth media that yield "red-target" colonies, and with the use of cold incubation enrichment methods.

One of these biochemically atypical species, *Yersinia frederiksenii*, differs in its ability to ferment rhamnose. Recent studies[14,15] indicate that this agent may be associated with a syndrome of diarrhea, frequently bloody, abdominal pain, and joint symptoms, including mono- and polyarthritis. The disease appears to be self-limited, but inflammatory changes may be observed in mucosal biopsies, and some patients have giant cell granulomata detected in serially sectioned mucosal biopsies.

Another particularly interesting infection is that caused by the "newly recognized" *Campylobacter jejuni*.[16] In less than a decade, this organism has emerged from obscurity as a veterinary pathogen to a leading recognized cause of enteritis in humans. It is a curved or spiral, motile, gram-negative rod with very fastidious growth characteristics (42°C, 5–10% oxygen, and 3–10% carbon dioxide). In many patients, clinical features are similar to those of ulcerative colitis[17] or Crohn's disease.[18] Patients with *C. jejuni* infection present with an acute illness with fever, abdominal pain, diarrhea, and sometimes rectal bleeding. Symptomatic relapses may occur,[19] and toxic megacolon,[20] as well as massive hemorrhage,[21] has been recorded. The diagnosis may be made by direct stool examination using dark-field or phase-contrast microscopy and may be confirmed by positive stool cultures.[22] The vast majority of patients improve without therapy. When symptoms are severe or prolonged, erythromycin is recommended. Thus, patients with unrecognized *Campylobacter* infections may show a dramatic "response" to treatment (including steroids) and may have been provided with an incorrect diagnosis and an uncertain prognosis.

4. NATURAL HISTORY AND MORTALITY

Direct comparisons between ulcerative colitis and Crohn's disease are difficult because of the variable definitions and methods of expressing clinical data, as well as the changing therapeutic modalities. In Canada, the onset of clinical disease defined in a survey of members of the Canadian Foundation for Ileitis and Colitis was apparently represented by a single peak in young adults for both diseases, with a slight predominance of females, especially in the province of Quebec.[23] Similar observations were made in the National Cooperative Crohn's Disease Study, i.e., age of onset showing a single peak between the second and fourth decades with approximately equivalent sex distribution.[6]

The course and prognosis of both diseases is highly variable.[24-30] Significant differences occur, especially in clinical severity, even among individuals with apparently similar extent of disease, or from year to year even for a given patient. Some generalizations, however, can be made. Most often, a relapsing and remitting course is observed, although some patients may remain continuously symptomatic. Both Crohn's disease and ulcerative colitis are typically chronic disorders, although acute, even fulminating courses are occasionally observed. In patients with acute fulminating disease, exclusion of specific infectious agents is especially important.

The severity of clinical symptoms and signs and, to a lesser degree, the extent of disease generally define the therapy in ulcerative colitis. The majority of patients have mild or moderately severe disease and respond to medical therapy (i.e., steroids and/or salazopyrin) in 80–90% of cases. About 10–15% of all patients will require surgery over a 10-year period. In about half of patients with idiopathic inflammatory bowel disease, the surgery will be required within the first year after diagnosis.[30] Patients with left-sided disease have an approximately 20% probability of developing more extensive disease or pancolitis.[27] In children or elderly patients, the clinical course tends to be more severe.

The assessment of the clinical symptoms in patients with Crohn's disease due to disease activity per se may be made more difficult because of the tendency toward bowel obstruction and septic complications. Furthermore, Crohn's disease is more frequently complicated by anal and perianal disease, fistulae, and abscesses. These may be unsuspected,[31] especially if colonic and/or rectal disease is present, and may require specific treatment, including surgery. Catheter drainage for abscesses may be considered, especially with ultrasound or other imaging guidance.[32,33] The absence of perianal disease was considered an important predictive factor for favorable outcome in the National Cooperative Crohn's Disease Study.[6] Another important feature of Crohn's disease is the frequency of operative procedures. The need for operation appears greater for patients with ileocolonic disease compared to those with disease localized only in the small or large bowel.[29,34]

Survival with inflammatory bowel disease appears to be approaching survival of the general population.[30] Recent data from Birmingham in 513 patients with Crohn's disease[35] and 676 patients with ulcerative colitis[36] demonstrates an approximately twofold increased mortality risk for these diseases. For both diseases, excess mortality was attributed to digestive diseases. There was an excess mortality in young patients soon after the initial diagnosis as well as from digestive tract cancer. No sexual differences were apparent in the mortality rate, and excess mortality from other diseases was not observed. Interestingly, males with ulcerative colitis, especially with disease onset before age 40 and treated with proctocolectomy, had a reduced incidence of deaths from circulatory system diseases and lung cancer.[36]

5. COMPLICATING FACTORS

Whereas anal and perianal disease[37] as well as fistulae and abscesses occur more commonly in Crohn's disease than in ulcerative colitis, some hepatobiliary tract complications, particularly primary sclerosing cholangitis, more frequently accompany ulcerative colitis.[38] Although the diagnosis of these associated conditions may lead to the exclusion of underlying and even occult inflammatory bowel disease, no specific intestinal or extraintestinal complication will clearly discriminate between ulcerative colitis and Crohn's disease. The incidence of clinically observed extraintestinal complications in 700 patients with Crohn's disease and ulcerative colitis has been extensively enumerated.[39] The frequencies of joint, skin, and ocular manifestations were similar. Interestingly, a significantly increased frequency of pyoderma gangrenosum and erythema nodosum was observed in ulcerative colitis and Crohn's colitis, respectively.[39]

A variety of pathophysiological complications occur in Crohn's disease owing to small bowel disease or resection. Malabsorption of vitamin B_{12} and fat is common, and the malabsorption of bile acids is associated with a high incidence of gallstone formation. Hyperoxaluria and oxalate stones result from increased absorption of luminal oxalates. Although urinary tract stones may result in hydronephrosis, especially on the right side, most often this complication is due to extension of the inflammatory process from the ileum and right colon in Crohn's disease. Sometimes periureteral inflammation is clinically silent and may involve both ureters.

6. PREGNANCY AND FERTILITY

Neither ulcerative colitis nor Crohn's disease has an adverse effect on the outcome of pregnancy. Usually a normal full-term infant is delivered,[40] although the birth weight of the child may be lower.[41] No effects on the incidence of stillbirths, prematurity, spontaneous abortion, or congenital defects have been definitely documented. Logically, inactive disease is considered more optimal than active disease.[42] Conversely, pregnancy has no significant adverse effect on the course of either ulcerative colitis or Crohn's disease.[43] Relapse may occur during pregnancy, more often during the first trimester or during the postpartum period, but the relapse is usually mild. Pregnancy following ileostomy for inflammatory bowel disease has as good a prognosis as pregnancy in inflammatory bowel disease without an ileostomy.[40]

Fertility in the female is generally regarded as normal in ulcerative colitis. Infertility in females has been reported in patients with Crohn's disease, but this appears to be temporary, frequently resolving after surgery, nutritional repletion, or vitamin B_{12} therapy. In some patients, bilateral fallopian tube obstruction has been recorded, possibly due to the direct extension of the intestinal inflammatory process.[44]

Recently, salazopyrin has been reported to cause reversible male infertility, but the mechanism requires elucidation.[45,46] Importantly, it is worth noting that there are no reported studies on the effect of ulcerative colitis or Crohn's disease per se on male fertility. Proctocolectomy still poses a potential risk for impaired sexual function in the male; no studies are available for females.

7. FAMILIAL AND GENETIC ASPECTS

Earlier studies recorded the familial occurrence of inflammatory bowel disease.[47,48] Recently, positive family histories were obtained in approximately one-third of 838 patients with either Crohn's disease or ulcerative colitis. For both disorders, parents, siblings, relatives, and grandparents were similarly affected, and up to 10% of multiple members in a single family may be affected. Disease was seen especially in pairs of different siblings rather than in pairs of parents and siblings. Such information must be viewed with caution because of the limitations of recall data and the dependence on accurate diagnoses, sometimes in distant or deceased relatives.[49] Identical twins with inflammatory bowel disease are rare but occur.[50] Inflammatory bowel disease may rarely develop in cohabiting spouses.[51].

Several studies have examined the frequency of various markers, such as histocompatibility (HLA) antigens. Most earlier studies did not define increased antigen frequency in ulcerative colitis or Crohn's disease,[52–54] although sharing of HLA identical haplotypes was recorded in affected pairs of siblings.[55] Recently, HLA-A, B, C, and DR antigens were examined in 27 Viennese patients with Crohn's disease and in 30 patients with ulcerative colitis.[56] A significant increase in HLA-B12 was observed in Crohn's disease but was also observed in controls and ulcerative colitis. Interestingly, in HLA-B12-positive patients with Crohn's disease, there was a concomitant occurrence of HLA-CW5, and HLA-DR2 antigen frequency was reported in 70% of Japanese patients with ulcerative colitis.[57] No comparison has been reported of HLA haplotypes in family members with and without inflammatory bowel disease. Taken together, these studies suggest that genes coding for HLA antigens or possibly other marker proteins[58] may play a role in the pathogenesis of these disorders.

8. MALIGNANCY

Prior studies have firmly established that the incidence and cumulative risk of colorectal cancer is increased in hospitalized patients with ulcerative colitis.[59,60] Although this risk seems to be greatest for individuals with pancolitis, especially with disease onset in childhood,[59] it is now becoming better appreciated that there is a substantial risk of cancer even in patients with only left-sided colitis.[60] Indeed, the incidence of cancer in left-sided colitis virtually parallels that observed in universal disease, with the frequency curve shifted about 10 years to the right.[60] Interestingly, a recent report from a private-practice setting suggests that the magnitude of cancer risk may have been overemphasized in previous reports from referral centers.[61]

Besides the increased risk of colorectal cancer in patients with ulcerative colitis, a smaller but definite risk for intestinal cancer also occurs in patients with Crohn's disease.[62] At present, the magnitude of this risk is unknown. In a recent survey of 126 members of the Scientific Advisory Committee of the National Foundation for Ileitis and Colitis,[63] the most commonly reported site was colorectum (54%), followed by ileum (23%). Multiple tumors were reported in 35% of colons with carcinoma. A predilection for bypassed intestine was observed, similar to earlier reports.[64,65] Recent animal studies using a chemically induced intestinal cancer model have also demonstrated an increased incidence of colorectal cancer after intestinal bypass,[66] although this may reflect, in part, the presence of suture materials.[67]

In recent years, interest has especially focused on the detection of atypical histological mucosal changes (i.e., dysplasia) in ulcerative colitis as a possible marker of precancerous epithelium.[68,69] Similar changes have also been reported in Crohn's disease.[70,71] Early detection of these changes might enable colectomy to be initiated before the development of cancer.

9. RECURRENCE AND REOPERATION

Perhaps the most important and controversial issue related to differentiating between these two disorders is the anticipated prognosis after initial resective surgery. By definition, ulcerative colitis is limited to the large bowel. Thus, it follows that if the large bowel is removed, surgery is curative. However, in Crohn's disease clinically recognizable ileitis after proctocolectomy may be a major problem. Because Crohn's disease is defined as a disease of the entire gastrointestinal tract, it is not surprising that "recurrence" after proctocolectomy can occur in this disease. It can be argued that disease was present and simply not recognized prior to surgery, since pathological studies have amply documented evidence of focal microscopic disease in grossly normal intestine. It is the definition, however, that is so crucial. If inflammation "recurs" in a patient initially thought to have ulcerative colitis, then the diagnosis will probably be altered to Crohn's disease. Using this approach, no patient with ulcerative colitis can possibly have "recurrent" ileal disease.

The postoperative course of patients with ulcerative colitis and Crohn's disease has been compared in many studies. Glotzer et al.[72] reported that the number of ileostomy revisions done for obstructive symptoms in Crohn's colitis (33%) was not significantly different from ulcerative colitis (18%). In contrast, Korelitz et al.[73] recorded a higher recurrence rate. However, Nugent et al.[74] reported that following protocolectomy in Crohn's colitis, only 3% of patients developed evidence of ileal granulomata, deep fissures, or transmural inflammation and fibrosis. A further 7 of 44 patients with Crohn's colitis had 14 ileostomy revisions (similar to the frequency in their ulcerative colitis group, 9 of 53 patients with 17 revisions) for nongranulomatous ileal stomatitis.

In a subsequent report from Birmingham,[75] the sequelae of colectomy and ileostomy were compared in Crohn's colitis and in ulcerative colitis. The immediate and late mortality, as well as the septic complications, were similar in both ulcerative colitis and Crohn's disease. However, the need for reoperation was greater in Crohn's colitis for both ileostomy reconstruction and recurrent disease. In this study, recurrence was defined histologically, but granulomata were not considered to be a necessary histological criterion to diagnose recurrent Crohn's disease. This was different from Nugent's study. In the National Cooperative Crohn's Disease Study, the type of initial surgery also appeared to be an important determinant of the need for later surgery[76]; more surgery was required if the initial procedure was a bypass rather than a resection.

In addition, the site of involvement was important in defining the time when initial surgery was required; the time from onset of symptoms to surgery was shortest in ileocolitis, longer for disease only in the small bowel, and longest for those with colon-only disease. Similarly, Vender et al.[77] reported that site of Crohn disease involvement was important; the incidence of ileostomy revision or recurrent gastrointestinal symptoms such as diarrhea, pain, and bleeding after colectomy for Crohn's colitis was higher in those patients with ileal disease compared to those with no ileal disease. "Recurrent" disease, defined histologically, was observed in 18% of Crohn's colitis patients after colectomy, with a mean follow-up of 7.6 years. Interestingly, this occurred most often in those with transmural (50%) rather than superficial mucosal disease (10%). Lock et al.[78] recorded similar results but noted a linearly increasing requirement for reoperation with increasing time after the initial surgery. In addition, surgery was performed more frequently if the small bowel was involved. More recently, using clinical criteria for the diagnosis of Crohn's disease, Wolfson et al.[79] claimed that recurrence was not influenced by the presence or absence of granulomata.

The risk following colectomy in Crohn's colitis may have been overemphasized in the past, largely because of variable criteria used to define Crohn's disease per se and "recurrence." The desire to make this distinction has been even further emphasized in recent years because of increasing numbers of patients seeking ileostomy alternatives. In these patients, "recurrent disease" may necessarily lead to further resection and loss of significant lengths of small bowel used to create the pouch. For this reason, most regard Crohn's disease as a contraindication to this procedure. At present, data do suggest an increased risk for clinically significant and histologically confirmed Crohn's disease of the ileum after colectomy. However, more studies using uniformly defined criteria are required.

REFERENCES

1. Fein HD: The history of Crohn's disease, in Korelitz BI (ed): *Inflammatory Bowel Diseases. Experience and Controversy.* Littleton, MA, John Wright-PSG, 1982, pp. 1–3.
2. Freeman HJ: Crohn's disease. Emerging pathologic and bacterial spectrum. *Can J Surg* 1984;27:431–433.
3. Brooke BN: Granulomatous disease of intestine. *Lancet* 1959;1:745–749.
4. Lockart-Mummery HE, Morson BC: Crohn's disease (regional enteritis) of the large intestine and its distinction from ulcerative colitis. *Gut* 1960;1:87–105.
5. Lockart-Mummery HE, Morson BC: Crohn's disease of the large intestine. *Gut* 1964;5:483–509.
6. Mekhjian HS, Switz DM, Melnyk CS, Rankin GB, Brooks RK: Clinical features and natural history of Crohn's disease. *Gastroenterology* 1979;77:898–906.
7. Hill RB, Kent TH, Hansen RN: Clinical usefulness of rectal biopsy in Crohn's disease. *Gastroenterology* 1979;77:938–944.
8. Surawicz CM, Meisel JL, Ylvisaker T, Saunders DR, Rubin CE: Rectal biopsy in diagnosis of Crohn's disease: Value of multiple biopsies and serial sectioning. *Gastroenterology* 1981;80:66–71.
9. Talbot T, Jewel L, Schloss E, Yakimets W, Thomson ABR: Cheilitis antedating Crohn's disease: Case report and literature uptake of oral lesions. *J Clin Gastroenterol* 1984;6:349–354.
10. Korelitz BI. Evidence for Crohn's disease as an extensive process, in Korelitz BI (ed): *Inflammatory Bowel Disease. Experience and Controversy.* Littleton, MA, John Wright-PSG, 1982, pp. 9–14.
11. Freeman HJ, Shnitka TK, Piercey JR, Weinstein WM: Cytomegalovirus infection of the gastrointestinal tract in a patient with late onset immunodeficiency syndrome. *Gastroenterology* 1977;73:1397–1403.
12. VanTrappen G, Penette E, Geboes K, Bertrand P: Yersinia enteritis and enterocolitis: Gastroenterological aspects. *Gastroenterology* 1977;72:220–227.
13. Ursing J, Brenner DJ, Bercovier H, et al: *Yersinia frederiksenii:* A new series of Enterobacteriaceae composed of rhamnose-positive strains. *Curr Microbiol* 1980;4:213–217.
14. Scholey J, Freeman H: *Yersinia frederiksenii:* a newly recognized agent in an inflammatory bowel disease syndrome (abstr). *Clin Invest Med* 1983;6:51.
15. Scholey J, Freeman H: Diarrhea and *Yersinia frederiksenii:* demonstration of heat-stable enterotoxin activity in a human-derived strain (abstr). *Clin Invest Med* 1983;6:51.
16. Blaser MN, Reller LB: *Campylobacter* enteritis. *N Engl J Med* 1981;305:1444–1452.
17. Blaser MJ, Parsons RB, Wang WL: Acute colitis caused by *Campylobacter fetus* ss *jejuni. Gastroenterology* 1980;78:448–453.
18. Loss RW Jr, Mangla JC, Pereira M: *Campylobacter* colitis presenting as inflammatory bowel disease with segmental colonic ulcerations. *Gastroenterology* 1980;79:138–140.

19. Lambert ME, Scholfield PF, Ironside AG, Mandal BK: *Campylobacter* colitis. *Br Med J* 1979;1:857–859.

20. McKinley MJ, Taylor M, Sangree MH: Toxic megacolon with campylobacter colitis. *Conn Med* 1980;44:496–497.

21. Michalak DM, Perrault J, Gilchrist MJ, Dozois RR, Carney JA, Sheedy PF II: *Campylobacter fetus* ss *jejuni:* A cause of massive lower gastrointestinal hemorrhage. *Gastroenterology* 1980;79:742–745.

22. Butzler JP, Skirrow MB: *Campylobacter* enteritis. *Clin Gastroenterol* 1979;8:737–765.

23. Grace M, Priest G: The epidemiology of inflammatory bowel disease, in Thomson ABR (ed): *Idiopathic Inflammatory Bowel Disease, Crohn's Disease and Chronic Ulcerative Colitis.* Ottawa, Ontario, Canadian Public Health Association, 1982, pp. 52–65.

24. Edwards FC, Truelove SC: The course and prognosis of ulcerative colitis. *Gut* 1963;4:299–315.

25. Edwards FC, Truelove SC: The course and prognosis of ulcerative colitis. *Gut* 1964;5:1–22.

26. Bonnevie O, Bindor V, Anthonisen P, Riis P: Prognosis of ulcerative colitis. *Scand J Gastroenterol* 1974;9:81–92.

27. Ritchie JK, Powell-Tuck J, Lennard-Jones JE: Clinical outcome of the first ten years of ulcerative colitis and proctitis. *Lancet* 1978;1:1140–1143.

28. Truelove SC, Pena AS: Course and prognosis of Crohn's disease. *Gut* 1976;17:192–201.

29. Farmer RG, Hawk WA, Turnbull RB: Clinical patterns in Crohn's disease: a statistical study of 615 cases. *Gastroenterology* 1975;68:627–635.

30. Prokipchuk EJ. Course and prognosis, in Thomson ABR (ed): *Idiopathic Inflammatory Bowel Disease, Crohn's Disease and Chronic Ulcerative Colitis.* Ottawa, Ontario, Canadian Public Health Association, 1982, pp. 180–192.

31. Keighley MRB, Eastwood D, Ambrose NS, Allan RN, Burdon DW: Incidence and microbiology of abdominal and pelvic diseases in Crohn's disease. *Gastroenterology* 1982;83:1271–1275.

32. Gerzof SG, Robbins AH, Johnson WC, Birkett D, Nabseth DC: Percutaneous catheter drainage of abdominal abscesses. *N Engl J Med* 1981; 305:653–657.

33. Sonnenberg A, Erckenbrecht J, Peter P, Niderau C: Detection of Crohn's disease by ultrasound. *Gastroenterology* 1982;83:430–434.

34. Farmer RG, Hawk WA, Turnbull RB: Indications for surgery in Crohn's disease. Analysis of 500 cases. *Gastroenterology* 1976;71:245–250.

35. Prior P, Gyde S, Cooke WT, Waterhouse JAH, Allan RN: Mortality in Crohn's disease. *Gastroenterology* 1981;80:307–312.

36. Gyde S, Prior P, Dew MJ, Saunders V, Waterhouse JAH, Allan RN: Mortality in ulcerative colitis. *Gastroenterology* 1982;83:36–43.

37. Lockhart-Mummery HE: Anal lesions in Crohn's disease. *Clin Gastroenterol* 1972;1:377–382.

38. Wiesner RH, Larusso NF: Clinicopathologic features of the syndrome of primary sclerosing cholangitis. *Gastroenterology* 1980;79:200–206.

39. Greenstein AJ, Janowitz HD, Sachar DB: The extra-intestinal complications of Crohn's disease and ulcerative colitis: A study of 700 patients. *Medicine* 1976;55:401–412.

40. Fielding JF: Pregnancy and inflammatory bowel disease. *Irish J Med Sci* 1982;151:194–202.

41. Schade RR, Van Thiel DH, Gavaler JS: Chronic idiopathic ulcerative colitis. Pregnancy and fetal outcome. *Dig Dis Sci* 1984;29:614–619.

42. Willoughby CP, Truelove SC: Ulcerative colitis and pregnancy. *Gut* 1980;21:469–474.

43. Vender RJ, Spiro HM: Inflammatory bowel disease and pregnancy. *J Clin Gastroenterol* 1982;4:231–249.
44. Fielding JF, Cooke WT: Pregnancy and Crohn's disease. *Br Med J* 1970;2:76–77.
45. Toovey S, Hudson E, Hendry WF, Levi A: Sulphasalazine and male infertility: Reversibility and possible mechanism. *Gut* 1981;22:445–451.
46. Birnie GG, McLeod TIF, Watkinson G: Incidence of sulphasalazine-induced male infertility. *Gut* 1981;22:452–455.
47. Kirsner JB, Spencer JA: Family occurrences of ulcerative colitis, regional enteritis and ileocolitis. *Ann Intern Med* 1963;59:133–144.
48. Almy TP, Sherlock P: Genetic aspects of ulcerative colitis and regional enteritis. *Gastroenterology* 1966;51:757–763.
49. Farmer RG, Michener WM, Mortimer EA: Studies of family history among patients with inflammatory bowel disease. *Clin Gastroenterol* 1980;9:271–278.
50. Klein GL, Ament ME, Sparkes RS: Monozygotic twins with Crohn's disease: A case report. *Gastroenterology* 1980;79:931–933.
51. Murray CJW, Thomson ABR: Marital idiopathic inflammatory bowel disease: Crohn's disease in a husband and wife. *J Clin Gastroenterol* 1986 (in press).
52. Gleeson MH, Walker JS, Wentzel JA, Chapman JA, Harris R: Human leukocyte antigens in Crohn's disease and ulcerative colitis. *Gut* 1972;13:438–440.
53. Leukonia RM, Woodrow JC, McConnell RB, Evans DAP: HL-A antigens in inflammatory bowel disease. *Lancet* 1974;1:574–575.
54. Bergman L, Lindblom JB, Safwenberg J, Krause U: HL-A frequencies in Crohn's disease and ulcerative colitis. *Tissue Antigens* 1976;7:145–150.
55. Schwartz SE, Siegelbaum SP, Faziotl, Hubbell C, Henry JB: Regional enteritis: evidence for genetic transmission by HLA typing. *Ann Intern Med* 1980;93:424–427.
56. Smolen JS, Gangl A, Polterauer P, Menzel EJ, Mayr WR: HLA antigens in inflammatory bowel disease. *Gastroenterology* 1982;82:34–38.
57. Asakura H, Tsuchiya M, Aiso S, et al: Association of the human lymphocyte-DR2 antigen with Japanese ulcerative colitis. *Gastroenterology* 1982;82:34–38.
58. Kagnoff MF, Brown RJ, Schanfield MS: Association between Crohn's disease and immunoglobulin heavy chain (GM) allotypes. *Gastroenterology* 1983;85:1044–1047.
59. Devroede GJ, Taylor WF, Sauer WG, Jackman RJ, Stickler GB: Cancer risk and life expectancy of children with ulcerative colitis. *N Engl J Med* 1971;285:17–21.
60. Greenstein AJ, Sachar DB, Smith H, et al: Cancer in universal and left-sided ulcerative colitis: Factors determining risk. *Gastroenterology* 1979;77:290–294.
61. Katzka I, Brody RS, Morris E, Katz S: Assessment of colorectal cancer risk in patients with ulcerative colitis: Experience from a private practice. *Gastroenterology* 1983;85:22–29.
62. Weedon DD, Shorter RG, Ilstrup DM, Huizenga KA, Taylor WF: Crohn's disease and cancer. *N Engl J Med* 1973;289:1099–1102.
63. Korelitz BI: Carcinoma of the intestinal tract in Crohn's disease: Results of a survey conducted by the National Foundation for Ileitis and Colitis. Am J Gastroenterol 1983;78:44–46.
64. Lightdale CJ, Sternberg SS, Posner G, Sherlock P: Carcinoma complicating Crohn's disease. *Am J Med* 1984;59:262–268.
65. Greenstein AJ, Sachar D, Pucillo A, et al: Cancer in Crohn's disease after diversionary surgery. *Am J Surg* 1983;84:725–731.
66. Scudamore CH, Freeman HJ: Effects of small bowel transection, resection, or bypass in 1,2-dimethylhydrazine-induced rat intestinal neoplasia. *Gastroenterology* 1983;84:725–731.

67. Calderisi RN, Freeman HJ: Differential effects of surgical suture materials in 1,2-dimethylhydrazine-induced rat intestinal neoplasia. *Cancer Res* 1984;44:2827–2830.

68. Morson BC, Pang LSC: Rectal biopsy as an aid to cancer control in ulcerative colitis. *Gut* 1967;8:423–434.

69. Riddell RH, Goldman H, Ransohoff DF, et al: Dysplasia in inflammatory bowel disease. Standardized classification with provisional clinical applications. *Human Pathol* 1983;14:931–968.

70. Craft CF, Mendelsohn G, Cooper HS, Yardley HS: Colonic "precancer" in Crohn's disease. *Gastroenterology* 1981;80:578–584.

71. Simpson S, Traube J, Riddell RH: This histologic appearance of dysplasis (precarcinomatous change) in Crohn's disease of the small and large intestine. *Gastroenterology* 1981;81:492–501.

72. Glotzer DH, Gardner RC, Goldman H, Hinrichs HR, Rosen H, Zetzel L: Comparative features and course of ulcerative and granulomatous colitis. *N Engl J Med* 1970;282:582–587.

73. Korelitz BI, Present DH, Alpert LI: Recurrent ileitis after ileostomy and colectomy for granulomatous colitis. *N Engl J Med* 1972;287:110–115.

74. Nugent FW, Viedenheimer MC, Meissner WA, Haggitt RC: Prognosis after colonic resection for Crohn's disease of the colon. *Gastroenterology* 1983;65:398–402.

75. Steinberg DM, Allan RN, Boroke BN, Cooke WT, Alexander-Williams J: Sequelae of colectomy and ileostomy: comparison between Crohn's colitis and ulcerative colitis. *Gastroenterology* 1975;68:33–39.

76. Mekhjian HS, Switz DM, Watts D, Deren JJ, Katon RM, Beman FM: National Cooperative Crohn's Disease Study: Factors determining recurrence of Crohn's disease after surgery. *Gastroenterology* 1979;77:907–913.

77. Vender RJ, Richert RR, Spiro HM: The outlook after total colectomy in patients with Crohn's colitis and ulcerative colitis. *J Clin Gastroenterol* 1979;1:209–217.

78. Lock MR, Farmer RG, Fazio VW, Jagelman DG, Lavery IC, Weakley FL: Recurrence and reoperation for Crohn's disease. The role of disease location in prognosis. *N Engl J Med* 1981;304:1586–1588.

79. Wolfson DM, Sachar DB, Cohen A, et al: Granulomas do not affect postoperative recurrence rates in Crohn's disease. *Gastroenterology* 1982;83:405–409.

8

Nutritional Support for the Gastroenterology Patient
Total Parenteral Nutrition, Enteral Feeding, or "Home Cooking"?

Josef E. Fischer

1. INTRODUCTION

The evolution of nutritional support and the enthusiasm that originally greeted total parenteral nutrition (TPN) has by now given way to a more balanced view of what nutritional support entails and its indications, risks, and benefits as well as its efficacy. Included in the rethinking of this important therapeutic modality is the concept now commonly accepted that nutritional support given by gut is probably more appropriate than nutritional support given by vein. There are at least eight different areas in which advantages for enteral nutritional support are apparent, although many of them are still conjectural:

   1. Absorption is more normal when foodstuffs are given through the gastrointestinal tract. Some of the processes of absorption are poorly understood, and there may be other purposes served by these and other functions of the gut.

Josef E. Fischer ● Department of Surgery, University of Cincinnati Medical Center, Cincinnati, Ohio 45267.

2. We know that certain metabolic functions, such as transamination of amino acids, take place in the wall of the gut. When nutrients are given by vein instead of by the more normal enteral route, transamination still takes place in the wall of the gut. To a certain extent, this may be responsible for the increase in energy expenditure and gastrointestinal blood flow that follow the administration of certain amino acids by vein.

3. Under normal circumstances all blood from the gut passes through the liver, and hepatocytes sitting astride the portal vein have as one of their primary functions the absorption, assimilation, metabolism, and storage of various nutrients. It has been estimated that between 75 and 100% of some of the more critical nutrients, such as certain amino acids or carbohydrate, is cleared by the liver in one pass. The liver also stores for future release, in response to hormonal or neurogenic signals, various nutrients for distribution to the periphery in an orderly fashion. Obviously, if the primary path of nutrients is via the periphery, the liver is deprived of its fair share of the nutrients which it generally receives through the gut. Whether or not this is deleterious is not clear, but certainly normal physiological function is bypassed. It is also not clear whether the other implication of this phenomenon, that the liver *requires* this huge normal flow of nutritional substances to maintain its integrity, is true. What should follow as a corollary of this assumption, if it were true, is that there is less hepatic derangement following enteral nutrition than parenteral nutrition. Although an attractive hypothesis, current evidence does not support this concept.

4. It is clear that food passing through the gut provides trophic effects on the gastrointestinal mucosa and the gastrointestinal tract under the influence of certain hormones.

5. The gut produces large amounts of various globulins. Several authorities have ascribed some immunological function to the gut, and some experimental as well as clinical evidence suggests that there may be some immunological functions which are lost when the gut is bypassed in favor of intravenous nutrition.

6. We certainly do not understand the myriad of hormonal signals generated when food passes through the gut or their importance in the overall economy. However, almost certainly this aspect of hormonal control, whatever the effects, is bypassed by the intravenous route.

7. Enteral nutrition is clearly cheaper.

8. Not all of the functions of the gut are understood. Our understanding of many of them, such as immunological functions, is yet in its infancy. Presumably, there are other functions which the gut normally performs which we have not yet fathomed.

Despite all its advantages, the adage that enteral nutrition is safer than parenteral nutrition is simply not true. A single episode of fatality from aspiration of tube feeding is greater than the mortality of a well-run parenteral nutrition program for 2 or 3 years. Many of the patients receiving enteral nutrition have altered states of consciousness and an ineffective gag reflex. Under these circumstances, aspiration remains a distinct possibility. Moreover, sudden changes in gastric and enteral motility with the sudden onset of sepsis will result in aspiration, especially with a tube through the gastric cardia rendering it incompetent.

Most authorities in the nutritional field agree that the patient with gastrointestinal disease is far better off being nourished by the enteral route as compared to the parenteral route. However, in many situations this proves impractical. Patients with a variety of gastrointestinal diseases simply cannot take sufficient enteral nutrition to keep themselves alive. Under these circumstances, total parenteral nutrition is essential.

2. COMPARISON OF ENTERAL AND PARENTERAL NUTRITION

Various investigators have examined the efficacy of enteral and parenteral nutrition in both experimental animals and in patients. It should be pointed out, however, that in comparison to the sophistication of the functions that may differentiate between the efficacy of enteral and parenteral nutrition, the functions that have been examined by various authors are relatively crude and are limited to, for example, nitrogen balance and amino acid profile, rather than such sophisticated functions such as immunological function. As I will point out, a few papers have examined these functions, but the results are clouded.

2.1. Results in Experimental Animals

Beginning in the mid 1970s, investigators began comparing the efficacy of enteral and parenteral nutrition. Lickely and her collaborators suggested that enteral nutrition seemed to give marginally better nitrogen balance as compared with parenteral nutrition in rats.[1] More recently, Maiz and his collaborators suggested that enteral nutrition was associated with better hepatic protein synthesis,[2] a finding widely anticipated but remarkably difficult to establish. Kudsk, in several papers, suggested that enteral nutrition is more protective against immunological disturbances (in this case the challenge of hemoglobin adjuvant peritonitis) than is parenteral nutrition.[3,4] In experiments using protein-depleted rats, Kudsk *et al.* demonstrated that nutritional repletion using TPN did not protect as well against hemoglobin adjuvant peritonitis as did enteral nutrition.[3,4]

Alexander (personal communication, 1984) has pointed out that there appears to be a nonspecific immunological response to abdominal operative procedures, such as gastrostomy used for feeding, which will cloud these results, although he and his co-workers have been able to demonstrate similar findings in guinea pigs.[5] However, in a study in burned children it did appear as though those children who received a higher dose of protein, and received it enterally instead of parenterally, appeared to fare better from the standpoint of infection, with increased survival.[6] These data are open to a variety of interpretations, one of which is that patients receiving enteral nutrition have better immunological function than those who do not.

A number of discrepancies, however, have arisen in these studies. Our own laboratory has been unable to repeat these studies, but the discrepancies can be explained if animals with catheter sepsis are eliminated. Catheter sepsis in rats, particularly, is very difficult to detect. In our own studies we have only been able to detect animal catheter sepsis using serial mediastinal histological sections and mediastinal smears and cultures. When animals were considered as a group and animals with catheter sepsis were not eliminated, enteral nutrition was clearly superior to parenteral nutrition.[7] However, when experimental animals with catheter sepsis were eliminated, enteral and parenteral nutrition were equivalent. In most of the other studies in which parenteral nutrition was not equivalent to enteral nutrition, catheter sepsis was not looked for nor were those animals eliminated.

2.2. Results of Studies in Patients

There are not a great many studies that properly compare enteral and parenteral nutrition. A number of studies compare gastrostomy feeding and parenteral nutrition in the preparation of patients for operation. Lim et al. for example, found that a gastrostomy was superior to parenteral nutrition, but the patients in that study were neither isocaloric nor isonitrogenous.[8] On the other hand, Rowlands et al., using an isocaloric and isonitrogenous regimen, gave different levels of calories and nitrogen to patients undergoing abdominal surgery and found that although none of the regimens brought patients into nitrogen equilibrium, patients with gastrostomy feedings showed generally superior results.[9] Burt et al., utilizing patients with neoplastic disease, found that parenteral feedings were slighly superior with respect to nitrogen retention as compared with enteral feedings, but the differences were slight.[10]

Our own studies (recently published) were carried out in matched pairs of patients following upper abdominal surgery in which either needle catheter jejunostomy or standard parenteral nutrition was utilized, and isocaloric and isonitrogenous feedings were carried out in matched fasion over 7–10 days.[11] Both groups maintained initial body weights and achieved positive nitrogen balance by day 5, and there were no differences in urinary 3-methylhistidine excretion, which rose after surgery and declined as time progressed without complications. Surprisingly, there were no differences in plasma levels of albumin, transferrin, or thyroxine-binding prealbumin, whereas retinol-binding protein rose slightly in the TPN group by day 6. Insulin increased similarly in both groups, and pancreatic glucagon and total glucagon were unchanged. The most surprising difference between the groups, which otherwise were indistinguishable, was the rise in alkaline phosphatase in the group receiving enteral nutrition while falling in the group receiving TPN. Thus, a series of carefully studied parameters in matched patients failed to reveal any advantages to patients receiving enteral nutrition.

I have previously alluded to a study carried out at the University of Cincinnati and Shriner's Burn Institute by Alexander, myself, and our colleagues, in which burned children were randomized for either a high-protein diet (25% calories as protein) or a standard diet containing 15% of calories as protein, intended to analyze the role of protein in various immunological responses.[6] The high-protein group showed a statistically significant improvement in survival. It should be pointed out that review of the data retrospectively showed that a higher percentage of patients in the high-protein group received more of their calories enterally than parenterally. Some have interpreted these data as showing that enteral nutrition supports immunological functions, such as neutrophil bactericidal index and opsonic index, better than parenteral nutrition. This is by no means clear, as it is possible that the patients receiving a standard protein diet were sicker and therefore would not eat and had to receive their nutrition by the parenteral route. This intriguing possibility remains to be investigated.

3. NUTRITION IN INFLAMMATORY BOWEL DISEASE

3.1. Crohn's Disease

Crohn, Ginzburg, and Oppenheimer are generally credited with the first description of what has come to be known as Crohn's disease or granulomatous inflammatory bowel disease (GIBD).[12] We now know it to be a disease that can occur anywhere from the mouth to the anus, and although regional enteritis remains a synonym because of the affectation of the ileum, primarily by early disease, it may present anywhere. Clinical manifestations, pathology, and diagnosis are beyond the scope of this chapter, and the present discussion will be limited principally to the controversial role of nutritional support, mainly parenteral nutrition, in the management of this disease.

It has been estimated that the majority (up to 75%) of patients with inflammatory bowel disease who are considered for surgery may be suffering from some degree of malnutrition, variously defined. Causation includes catabolism secondary to ongoing active or chronic inflammatory processes, the use of steroids as a treatment, and protein loss secondary to ulceration or inflammation of the involved bowel. Malabsorption secondary to diarrhea with rapid transit time results in massive losses of nutrients,. which is further augmented by repeated resections resulting in the short bowel syndrome. Since these patients feel ill, almost all of them are anorectic, resulting in inadequate dietary intake.

Nutritional support has become important for both the medical and surgical management of GIBD, and many authorities in the field advocate the use of elemental diets for patients with this disease. Although I have seen an occasional patient who has responded to elemental diets, a bland, soft, low-roughage diet is generally better tolerated, is certainly more palatable, and is much more likely to have the patient continue on it than on enteral nutrition using either a modular or synthetic amino acid mixture or hydrolystate. Although enteral nutrition, using a defined formula diet, may be useful either for supplementation or for long-term outpatient therapy, my experience with these patients suggests that it is a rare patient who will stay on such defined formula diets for any period of time. Others have advocated repeated use of elemental diets for limited periods of time for controlling flareups and have reported success, although published reports are few. Success probably varies directly with the enthusiasm of the observer. Under such circumstances, especially when patients are within the hospital, parenteral nutrition has been utilized.

Parenteral nutrition may be utilized in one of three ways:

1. To replete nutritional deficits as a part of ongoing medical therapy.
2. To allow complete bowel rest for healing or repair of the diseased bowel in an attempt to place patients into remission.
3. If surgery is required, at least theoretically to provide for perioperative nutritional support in an attempt to minimize complications, morbidity, and mortality.

The rationale for bowel rest using parenteral nutrition is to decrease the mechanical, hormonal, and chemical stimuli to small bowel while providing adequate nutrition to allow healing and regeneration. Studies in animals are supportive of this concept, demonstrating fewer intestinal myoelectric potential, decreased gastric, intestinal, and pancreatic fluid and enzyme secretion, as well as mucosal atrophy presumably brought about by lack of stimulation and bypass of the gut using TPN.[13] It should be emphasized here that complete bowel rest on 5% dextrose and water is not likely to result in bowel healing if such starvation goes on for any period of time. The development of the associated protein/calorie malnutrition not only inhibits healing of diseased bowel wounds and fistulae, but may contribute to deranged immunological competence as well.

Since an early published report by Fischer *et al.* in 1973 indicating that hospital remissions could be expected in up to two-thirds of patients with both colonic and small bowel GIBD,[14] a numer of other studies have been published[15-30] (Table 1). In general, the results are consistent, and favorable rates of response, especially in patients with largely small bowel disease, may be expected. Although a few of the studies, such as those of Mullen *et al.*,[23] Dean *et al.*,[21] and Bos and Westerman,[28] have remission rates in the range of 40%, these may represent unfavorable hospitalized

Table 1. Results of TPN and Bowel Rest in Patients with GIBD

Study	No. patients	Duration of TPN (days)	Nutritional response (%)	Hospital remission (%)	Late remission (%)
Fischer *et al.* (1973)[14]				67	
Vogel *et al.* (1974)[15]	14	9–50	78	100	50
Eisenberg *et al.* (1974)[16]	46	5–46			
Reilly *et al.* (1976)[17]	23	29–36	74	61	
Fazio *et al.* (1976)[18]	67	20		77	
Greenberg *et al.* (1976)[19]	43	25		77	67
Dudrick *et al.* (1976)[20]	52			54	
Dean *et al.* (1976)[21]	16			43	
Harford and Fazio (1978)[22]					21
Mullen *et al.* (1978)[23]	50	26–37		38	
Driscoll and Rosenberg (1978)[24]	16		100	75	50
Holm *et al.* (1981)[25]	6	60–98		86	86
Elson *et al.* (1980)[26]	20	36	100	65	25
Dickinson *et al.* (1980)[27]	9	18–24		66	16
Bos and Weterman (1980)[28]	115	41		41	
Shiloni and Freund (1983)[29]	19	21–150	100	56	37.5
Muller *et al.* (1983)[30]	30	84		83	43

patients at one end of the spectrum, and most investigators report remission rates between 60 and 80%, presumably allowing discharge from the hospital. It is clear from all studies, as was noted by Reilly et al. in 1976,[17] that remission rates were likely to be higher in patients with disease confined to small bowel. It is also true that while steroids could be decreased, the ability to induce remission using TPN in such patients and completely discontinuing steroids was probably not wise, and that one would be better served by maintaining steroids at a low level of 5–10 mg/24 hr.[17]

The problem encountered with GIBD and parenteral nutrition has remained the same for the past decade, and that is the duration of remission and the degree of recurrence. Here again, Table 1 shows that there is a remarkable variability in the late remission rates, ranging from approximately 15–20% to 85%. It is likely that the mean remission rate in such patients remains about 30–40% after 1 year. It is also probably true that the duration of remission has a mean of approximately 11 months and that, although recurrences have been seen by myself as quickly as 24 hr following cessation of hyperalimentation, remission rates generally average 1 year, which, incidentally, is approximately the same mean duration of remission as following surgery.

Thus, in a patient with Crohn's disease in whom one has nothing left to offer but surgery, viewed from the perspective of a clinical surgeon with an active practice with patients with Crohn's disease, TPN is an appropriate way to avoid surgery, provided complications such as obstruction, bleeding, abscess, or gastrointestinal cutaneous fistula are not present. The remission rate will decrease over the first year, but some patients will remain in remission for prolonged periods of time. In addition, it is possible that smaller amounts of small bowel will need to be resected after activity is decreased with the use of parenteral nutrition in patients with granulomatous disease.

3.2. Ulcerative Colitis

Our initial results in treatment of patients with ulcerative colitis with TPN were rather poor. Only one patient of an initial dozen treated went into remission, this being a patient who had become extremely malnourished before discovery of the ulcerative colitis, and I believe that his response was to steroids, although TPN restored his nutritional state. Almost all of the other patients came to colectomy, except one patient who refused colectomy and died. Other authors have reported some long-term remissions, but overall, long-term remission in patients with ulcerative colitis is not impressive and probably less than 20% if all series are collated (Table 1). However, despite the lack of long-term remission in ulcerative colitis, I as well as others have found TPN to be useful in pre-

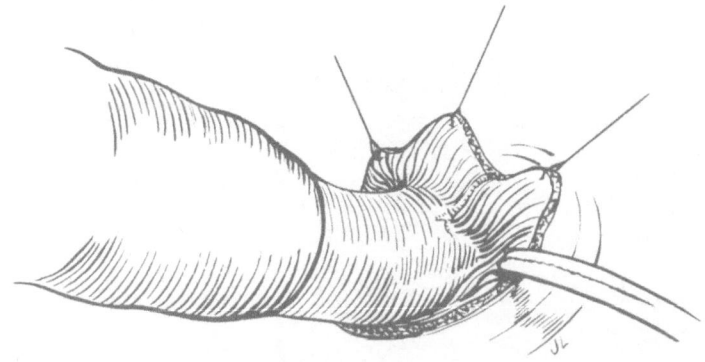

Figure 1. Rectal mucosal stripping for either ulcerative colitis or, in some cases, familial polyposis. With experience one can develop a plane between the mucosa and the muscularis, leaving the muscularis intact and stripping out the submucosa. Since the disease is confined to the mucosa in both ulcerative colitis and familial polyposis, this enables one to completely resect the disease while leaving the muscular plane to protect the anastomosis.

paring patients for pull-through operation.[31-33] Since ulcerative colitis is a disease limited to the mucosa, theoretically the mucosa can be stripped out surgically; a muscular sleeve remains (Fig. 1) through which the ileum can be anastomosed to a small remaining bit of rectal transitional epithelium (Fig. 2). A major problem with this operation is preparation of the rectal segment for stripping. Deep mucosal ulceration prevents adequate stripping because of inflammation, adherence, vascularity, and mechanical difficulty, increasing the possibility of leaving islands of rectal mucosa behind and exterior to the ileum, which will probably result in late failure of the operation. Thus, at the University of Cincinnati we have emphasized in-hospital TPN combined with nil p.o., antibiotics, bowel rest, systemic steroids as well as local steroids, and Azulfidine in an attempt to quiet the rectal mucosa to the point where it is feasible to strip the rectum. In our experience, this takes from 10 days to 6 weeks, although most patients require approximately 3 weeks for operation.

Using this careful approach, the results in our approximately 100 patients have been, even to ourselves, truly impressive.[33] Almost total continence has been the result. An occasional patient has a stricture requiring dilation under anesthesia. Few cases of pouchitis have been encountered, largely associated with pouch stasis. Although this approach requires a large investment of in-hospital preparation as well as a second operation to close an ileostomy (which we use to protect the numerous suture lines within the pelvis), the results have been truly gratifying.

Finally, the Soave operation (or Martin operation, as it should be called) for ulcerative colitis, as it does not require a permanent ileostomy,

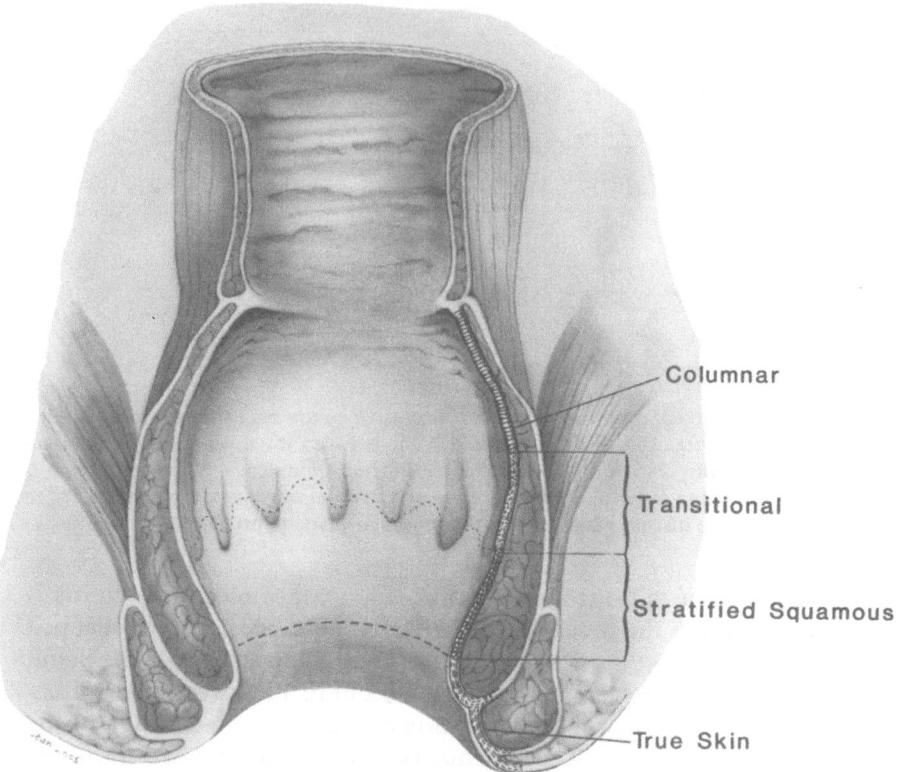

Figure 2. Transitional epithelium. It is important not to leave columnar epithelium because this will allow opportunities for recurrence. Transitional epithelium, however, is usually not involved in the disease and yet must be retained, in our opinion, to provide for rectal continence.

has changed the entire nature of surgery for this complication. Most patients, after they have had the ileostomy closed, state that they would not have persisted with their troublesome colitis had they known that the results of the operation would be this good, but would have had the operation much sooner. These operations are still being modified, but our longest-term patients are now approaching 10 years, and we believe that the operation is a good one.

3.3. Other Diseases of the Colon

Not all diseases of the colon are either granulomatous colitis or ulcerative colitis. We have seen a number of patients with bizarre diseases unresponsive to other forms of therapy other than TPN. When a disease is not clearly identified or, perhaps, a vasculitis or ischemic colitis is suspected, the use of TPN is probably beneficial and may enable patients to survive without operation, and the colon usually recovers.

Other uses of TPN in inflammatory bowel disease include the occasional patient in whom manifestation of inflammatory bowel disease is primarily that of a rectal fistula, but whose disease is otherwise mild. In these patients, placement of the patient on bowel rest, use of nonabsorbable antibiotics, and local excision and closure of the fistula, provided the patient is on 100% bowel rest, may result in an excellent functional result and the lack of necessity for a colectomy, for example, in granulomatous colitis.

4. PERIOPERATIVE PARENTERAL NUTRITION OR PREOPERATIVE NUTRITIONAL PREPARATION

The area of perioperative parenteral nutrition, particularly as it applies to patients with gastrointestinal disease, is controversial and one in which all of the data have not yet been collected. As one who has practiced parenteral nutrition for over 15 years, I have an intrinsic belief that patients who are parenterally nourished perioperatively tend to do better, look better, physiologically recover more quickly from operation (although their stay in the hospital may be slightly longer), and in general are well served by perioperative parenteral nutrition. Yet, I am the first to admit, and have argued for some time, that the evidence simply does not exist indicating that perioperative nutrition is a useful adjunct and worth the expense.[34]

4.1. The Concept of Risk

A number of investigators have attempted to establish whether patients who are severely malnourished are at increased risk for operation. The results have been quite mixed. As early as the 1930s it was pointed out that patients who underwent gastrectomy with a low serum albumin, presumably because of malnutrition, had a higher incidence of complications and a higher mortality than those who were well nourished.[35] A variety of studies have been done, many of them retrospective. At the University of Pennsylvania, Mullen and his co-workers studied a large series of patients at the Veterans Administration Hospital and at the University of Pennsylvania in retrospective fashion.[36,37] They initially attempted to define whether there were certain parameters which could be measured in preoperative patients and which would define a normal and abnormal patient population. Their initial attempt at the Veterans Administration Hospital revealed that only 3% of the population was normal with regard to all parameters and 35% of the population was abnormal with respect to three or more of the parameters studied.[36] Thus, this could not be accepted as a definition of malnutrition, since in the common surgical experience, even at the Veterans Administration Hospital, risk was not that high in this group of patients. They finally arrived at a formulation which they entitled "prognostic nutritional index" (PNI) and which, largely from retrospective studies, was given as follows[37]:

$$PNI (\%) = 158 - 16.6 (ALB) - 0.78 (TSF) - 0.20 (TFN) - 5.8 (DH)$$

where PNI is the risk (percent) of a complication occurring in an individual patient; ALB is the serum albumin level (grams per deciliter); TSF is the triceps skinfold (millimeters); TFN is the serum transferrin level (milligrams per deciliter); and DH is the cutaneous delayed hypersensitivity.

As can be seen from this equation, the weight of the formulation is in terms of the serum albumin, and our own statistical manipulations of this formula suggest that almost the same benefit is derived from the formulation if only serum albumin is considered.

The prognostic nutrition index and the studies from the University of Pennsylvania suggesting that patients do better when they are prepared preoperatively must be identified as being retrospective,[38] that is, that the groups are not strictly comparable. Almost anyone can walk through a given hospital and pick out patients who are at high risk, for example, those in the intensive-care unit as opposed to those having hernia repairs. The only properly done randomized, prospective trial is that in which patients are consecutive and submitted to randomization, with some hyperalimented and some not.

There are two other studies in which no parenteral nutrition was used. In a study of consecutive patients in the Mason Clinic, Ryan and Taft reported in the largest number of patients collected that there was no difference in such indicators as mortality rate and complication rate in a group of patients undergoing major surgical procedures. In this study they did not remove those patients who were severely at risk, that is, those individuals who lost more than 20% of their body weight.[39] Similarly, Higgens et al., in a recent study confined to patients with inflammatory bowel disease, also failed to reveal any evidence of increased mortality or morbidity in patients who lost more than 20% of their body weight.[40]

The obverse, that of preparing patients for operation with TPN in a randomized, prospective fashion, has been carried out by a number of institutions. Unfortunately, most of these studies involve patients with neoplastic disease. It is clear from Table 2 that in almost all studies in which TPN is used as adjunctive therapy in patients with neoplastic disease, there is no advantage to the patient and there may be some detriment to patients treated with radiation and chemotherapy, presumably due to the stimulatory effect on the growth of the tumor, which has been demonstrated recently by Popp and his co-workers in experimental animals.[41] The one exception to these lack of positive results has been where patients have been prepared for surgery with parenteral nutrition in neoplastic disease.

Lee showed a marginal improvement in outcome in patients prepared for gastrectomy with TPN as opposed to those who were not. The incidence of wound infections that could be attributed to malnutrition was decreased.[42] Holter and Fischer carried out a randomized, prospective trial comparing three groups of patients, one of which had been hyperalimented for 3 days preoperatively and postoperatively until 1500 calories were taken by mouth. There was a trend toward a decrease in major complications in patients given TPN who had lost weight as opposed to those who had lost weight and had not been given parenteral nutrition. Both groups fared worse than those patients who had not lost weight.[43] The results were not statistically significant, and it was estimated that an additional 200 patients would have had to enter the trial if such statistical significance was to be achieved. Muller and his co-workers treated patients with esophageal carcinoma preoperatively for 10 days with parenteral nutrition as compared to tube feedings and found a statistically significant improvement in patients treated with TPN, with deaths and infections decreased.[44] Yamamoto and his colleagues also reported improvement in outcome with patients treated with parenteral nutrition, even in patients with known disseminated disease treated with chemotherapy.[45]

These results suggest that although in neoplastic disease and surgery some case can be made for improvement in outcome in patients treated with TPN, in patients without neoplastic disease in two large consecutive series, including one with inflammatory bowel disease,[40] no difference in outcome has been reported between patients who have lost even large amounts of weight and those who have not lost weight.

5. HOME PARENTERAL NUTRITION

For patients with gastrointestinal disease who are unable to eat and cannot be controlled by any other means, home parenteral nutrition

Table 2. Studies of the Effects of Parenteral Nutrition (PN) on Patients with Cancer Undergoing Surgery, Radiation, or Chemotherapy

	No. pts.	Type of tumor	Type of therapy	Nutritional effects	Response to therapy (%)	Complications of therapy (%)		Survival (%)		Comments
						PN	Control	PN	Control	
Holter and Fischer (1977)[43]	56	GI cancer	Surgery	Decreased wt. loss and increased albumin level with PN	Same	13	19	93.4	92.4	Lower major complication rate with PN
Moghissi et al. (1977)[46]	15	Esophageal cancer	Surgery	Better N balance with PN	Same	0	20	NA	NA	Lower rate of wound infection
Issell et al. (1978)[47]	26	Squamous cell lung cancer	Chemotherapy	Improved wt. gain, arm circumference with PN	31 PN, 7 control	15	77	NA	NA	Less myelosuppression, less toxic effects of chemotherapy with PN
Heatley et al. (1979)[48]	74	Esophageal gastric cancer	Surgery	Same	Same	35	83	15	22	Significant reduction in postoperative wound infection
Sims et al. (1980)[49]	30	Esophageal gastric cancer	Surgery	Improved N balance and albumin level with PN	Same	NA	NA	10	10	
Lanzotti et al. (1980)[50]	56	Non-oat-cell lung	Chemotherapy	NA	10	23	NA	NA	Median 11 wk / 12 wk	
Sako et al. (1981)[51]	69	Head and neck cancer	Surgery	Wt. gain and better N balance with PN	Same	50	56	NA	NA	Significantly better long-term survival curve for PN
Valdivieso et al. (1981)[52]	49	Small cell bronchogenic cancer	Chemotherapy	Wt. gain with PN	85	59	NA	NA	Survival advantage for PN	PN did not ameliorate hematological, GI, or infection morbidity
Thompson et al. (1981)[53]	41	GI cancer	Surgery	Improved wt. gain with PN	Same	17	11	100	100	

Reference	No. of patients	Tumor	Therapy	Nutritional/metabolic effects	Outcome data	Comments
Popp et al. (1981)[54]	36	Diffuse lymphoma	Chemotherapy	Marked wt gain with PN; lean body mass anthropometry, albumin, transferrin, and total lymphocytes similar for both groups	11% subclavian vein thrombosis; 69; 66	No difference in drug tolerance or total drug dose between control and PN
Nixon et al. (1981)[55]	45	Metastatic colon cancer	Chemotherapy	Wt. gain with PN; no other differences	15; 12; 79 days	
Serrou et al. (1981)[56]	19	Anaplastic lung cancer	Chemotherapy	Same	83; 80; 84; 308 days	
Samuels et al. (1981)[57]	30	Metastatic testicular cancer	Chemotherapy	Less wt. loss with PN	Increased incidence of noncatheter infections with PN; 63; 79; 75; 79	
Lim et al. (1981)[8]	24	Esophageal cancer	Surgery	Better wt. gain and N balance with PN	6 Complications; 12; 90; 80	Preoperative TPN and gastrostomy feeding compared
Muller et al. (1982)[44]	125	GI cancer	Surgery	Improved wt. gain, visceral proteins, and immunological status with PN	17; 32; 96; 81	
Shamberger et al. (1983)[58]	27	Sarcomas	Chemotherapy		42; 33	Similar granulocyte and platelet recovery following chemotherapy-induced myelosuppression
Shamberger et al. (1984)[59]	32	Sarcomas	Chemotherapy	Improved N balance with PN, but similar visceral proteins	71; 86; Long-term survival	Shorter remissions for PN

remains an efficacious method of treating at least the results of such severe gastrointestinal disease as well as perhaps improving the disease itself. Home TPN is now approximately 12–13 years old and, although some authorities prefer a 24-hr method of treatment, at our nutritional support unit as well as in most others, the overnight mode is preferred. Although patients with massive enterectomy secondary to volvulus and mesenteric thrombosis make up the bulk of patients treated in most medical centers, regional enteritis represents a large group of patients who require home parenteral nutrition. In our own studies, this has included patients with massive, repeated small bowel resections due to regional enteritis (something we would almost never do in our own practice— these are patients who have been operated on elsewhere) and patients with fistulae that are resistant to therapy and closure. This group of patients is very highly motivated, and almost all of the patients that we treat with home parenteral nutrition are employed. In addition, such patients generally experience remission of the Crohn's disease from time to time, so that although most of them are dependent on TPN, some oral intake occurs which will help prevent fatty acid and trace metal deficiency (see Table 3).

The number of patients placed on home parenteral nutrition should be small in the adult group. In the pediatric age group, however, we consider stunting of growth a valid indication for TPN. A spurt of growth lasting 6 months generally follows hospitalization and TPN in a child. Consistent outpatient nutrition will enable normal growth and not doom such children, who often "outgrow" their disease, to a long-term social stigma of being a "runt." The effect on Crohn's disease in such patients is presumably salutory, but is secondary.

Table 3. Indications for Home Parenteral Nutrition

Short bowel syndrome
  Mesenteric vascular event
  Multiple or extensive bowel resections (malrotation and volvulus, internal hernia, Crohn's disease)
Gastrointestinal motor disturbances
  Chronic pseudoobstruction
  Scleroderma
Radiation enteritis
Crohn's disease
Mesenteric insufficiency
Recurrent multiple intraabdominal adhesions
Malignancy (rarely and must be concomitant with antineoplastic therapy)

6. SUMMARY

Enteral nutrition may be superior to parenteral nutrition with respect to convenience and cost, but proof of efficacy over TPN has not been forthcoming. On the other hand, patients who can experience amelioration of gastrointestinal disease with the use of chemically defined formulas should be so treated. The majority of patients, however, who are severely ill and require nutritional support will not tolerate such chemically defined formulas or any oral intake and will require TPN. The beneficial effects of TPN in Crohn's disease, albeit temporary, are useful. In severe cases in which patients cannot be supported by any other means, home parenteral nutrition should be considered. In ulcerative colitis, TPN should be used as an adjunct to preparing patients for sphincter-saving operation.

REFERENCES

1. Lickely HLA, Track NS, Vranic M, Bury KD: Metabolic responses to enteral and parenteral nutrition. *Am J Surg* 1978;135:172–176.
2. Maiz A, Sobrado J, Moldawer LL, Blackburn GL, Bistrian BR: Protein dynamics during refeeding of protein-depleted rats: Effects of increasing amino acid intake by TPN or enteral continuous feeding. *J Nutr* 1984;114:75–88.
3. Kudsk KA, Carpenter G, Petersen S, Sheldon GF: Effect of enteral and parenteral feeding in malnourished rats with *E. coli*–hemoglobulin adjuvant peritonitis. *J Surg Res* 1981;31:105–110.
4. Kudsk KA, Stone JM, Carpenter G, Sheldon GF: Enteral and parenteral feeding influences mortality after hemoglobin–*E. coli* peritonitis in normal rats. *J Trauma* 1983;23:605–609.
5. Saito H, Trocki O, Heyd T, Alexander JW: Effect of dietary unsaturated fatty acids and Indomethacin on metabolism and survival after burn. Proceedings American Burn Association 17th Annual Meeting, Orlando, FL, March 27–30, 1985;17:27.
6. Alexander JW, MacMillan BG, Stinnett JD, et al: Beneficial effects of aggressive protein feeding in severely burned children. *Ann Surg* 1980;192:505–517.
7. Gimmon Z, Nachbauer CA, Fischer JE: Comparative efficacy of parenteral vs enteral nutrition in the post-traumatic rat. *Gastroenterology* 1980;80:1156 (abstract).
8. Lim STK, Choa RC, Lam KH, Wong G, Ong GB: Total parenteral nutrition versus gastrostomy in the preoperative preparation of patients with carcinoma of the esophagus. *Br J Surg* 1981;68:69–72.
9. Rowlands BJ, Giddings AEB, Johnson AOB, Hindmarsh JT, Clark RG: Nitrogen-sparing effect of different feeding regimens in patients after operation. *Br J Anaesth* 1977;49:781–787.
10. Burt ME, Stein TP, Brennan MF: A controlled, randomized trial evaluating the effects of enteral and parenteral nutrition on protein metabolism in cancer-bearing man. *J Surg Res* 1983;34:303–314.

11. Muggia-Sullam M, Bower RH, Murphy RF, Joffe SN, et al: Postoperative enteral versus parenteral nutritional support in gastrointestinal surgery: a matched prospective study. *Am J Surg* 1985;149:106–112.
12. Crohn BB, Ginzburg L, Oppenheimer GD: Regional ileitis: a pathologic and clinical entity. *JAMA* 1932;99:1323–1329.
13. Copeland EM, Dudrick SJ: Intravenous hyperalimentation in inflammatory bowel disease, pancreatitis, and cancer. *Surg Annu* 1980;12:83–101.
14. Fischer JE, Foster GS, Abel RM, Abbott WM, Ryan JA: Hyperalimentation as primary therapy for inflammatory bowel disease. *Am J Surg* 1973;125:165–175.
15. Vogel CM, Corwin TR, Baue AE: Intravenous hyperalimentation in the treatment of inflammatory diseases of the bowel. *Arch Surg* 1974;108:460–467.
16. Eisenberg HW, Turnbull RB Jr, Weakley FL: Hyperalimentation as preparation for surgery in transmural colitis (Crohn's disease). *Dis Colon Rectum* 1974;17:469–475.
17. Reilly J, Ryan JA, Strole W, Fischer JE: Hyperalimentation in inflammatory bowel disease *Am J Surg* 1976;131:192–200.
18. Fazio VW, Kodner I, Jagelman DG, Turnbull RB Jr, Weakley FL: Inflammatory disease of the bowel: parenteral nutrition as primary or adjunctive treatment (symposium). *Dis Colon Rectum* 1976;19:574–578.
19. Greenberg GR, Haber GB, Jeejeebhoy KN: Total parenteral nutrition and bowel rest in the management of Crohn's disease. *Gut* 1976;17:828.
20. Dudrick SJ, MacFadyen BV, Daly JM: Management of inflammatory bowel disease with parenteral hyperalimentation, in Clearfield HR, Dinoso VP (eds): *Gastrointestinal Emergencies.* New York, Grune & Stratton, 1976, pp 193–199.
21. Dean RF, Campos MM, Barrett B: Hyperalimentation in the management of chronic inflammatory intestinal disease. *Dis Colon Rectum* 1976;19:601–604.
22. Harford FJ, Fazio VW: Total parenteral nutrition as primary therapy for inflammatory disease of the bowel. *Dis Colon Rectum* 1978;21:555–557.
23. Mullen JL, Hargrove WC, Dudrick SJ, Fitts WT, Rosato EF: Ten years experience with intravenous hyperalimentation and inflammatory bowel disease. *Ann Surg* 1978;187:523–529.
24. Driscoll RH, Rosenberg IH: Total parenteral nutrition in inflammatory bowel disease. *Med Clin North Am* 1978;62:185–201.
25. Holm E, Streibel JP, Moller P, Hartman M: Amino acid solutions for parenteral nutrition and for adjuvant treatment of encephalopathy in liver cirrhosis: Studies concerning 120 patients, in Walser M, Williamson R (eds): *Metabolism and Clinical Implications of Branched Chain and Ketoacids.* New York, Elsevier-North Holland, 1981, pp 513–518.
26. Elson CO, Layden RJ, Nemchausky BA, Rosenberg IL, Rosenberg IH: An evaluation of TPN in the management of inflammatory bowel disease. *Dig Dis Sci* 1980;25:42–48.
27. Dickinson RJ, Ashton MG, Axon ATE, et al: Controlled trial of intravenous hyperalimentation and total bowel rest as an adjunct to the routine therapy of acute colitis. *Gastrenterology* 1980;79:1199 (abstract).
28. Bos LP, Westerman IT: Total parenteral nutrition in Crohn's disease. *World J Surg* 1980;4:163–166.
29. Shiloni E, Freund HR: Total parenteral nutrition in Crohn's disease: is it primary or supportive mode of therapy? *Dis Colon Rectum* 1983;26:275–278.
30. Muller JM, Keller HW, Erasmi H, Pichlmaier H: Total parenteral nutrition as the sole therapy in Crohn's disease: A prospective study. *Br J Surg* 1983;70:40–43.
31. Martin LW, LeCoultre C, Schubert WK: Total colectomy and mucosal proctectomy with preservation of continence in ulcerative colitis. *Ann Surg* 1977;186:477–480.

32. Martin LW, LeCoutre C: Technical considerations in performing total colectomy and Soave endorectal anastomosis for ulcerative colitis. *J Pediatr Surg* 1978;13:762–770.
33. Martin LW, Fischer JE, Sayers HJ, Alexander F, Torres MA: Anal continence following Soave procedure: Analysis of results in 100 patients. *Ann Surg* 1986; 203:525–530.
34. Fischer JE: Nutritional assessment before surgery. *Am J Clin Nutr* 1982;35:1128–1131.
35. Rhoads JE, Alexander CE: Nutritional problems of surgical patients. *Ann NY Acad Sci* 1955;63:268–275.
36. Mullen JL, Buzby GP, Walman MT, Gertner MH, Hobbs CL, Rosato EF: Prediction of operative morbidity and mortality by preoperative nutritional assessment. *Surg Forum* 1979;30:80–82.
37. Buzby GP, Mullen JL, Matthews DC, et al: Prognostic nutritional index in gastrointestinal surgery. *Am J Surg* 1980;139:160–167.
38. Mullen JL, Buzby GP, Matthews DC, Small BF, Rosato EF: Reduction of operative morbidity and mortality by combined preoperative and postoperative nutritional support. *Ann Surg* 1980;192:604–612.
39. Ryan JA Jr, Taft D: A preoperative nutritional assessment does not predict morbidity and mortality in abdominal operations. *Surg Forum* 1980;31:96–98.
40. Higgens CS, Keighley MRB, Allan RN: Impact of preoperative weight loss and body composition changes on postoperative outcome in surgery for inflammatory bowel disease. *Gut* 1984;25:732–736.
41. Popp MB, Wagner SC, Brito OJ: Host and tumor responses to increasing levels of intravenous nutritional support. *Surgery* 1983;94:300–308.
42. Lee HA: Planning intravenous nutrition: Techniques and principles, in Lee HA (ed): *Parenteral Nutrition in Acute Metabolic Illness.* New York: Academic Press, 1974, pp. 307–331.
43. Holter A, Fischer JE: The effects of perioperative hyperalimentation on complications in patients with carcinoma and weight loss. *J Surg Res* 1977;23D:31–34.
44. Muller JM, Dienst C, Brenner V, Pichlmaier H: Preoperative parenteral feeding in patients with gastrointestinal carcinoma. *Lancet* 1982;1:68–71.
45. Yamada N, Koyama H, Hioki K, Yamada T, Yamamoto M: Effect of postoperative total parenteral nutrition (TPN) as an adjunct to gastrectomy for advanced gastric carcinoma. *Br J Surg* 1983;70:267–274.
46. Moghissi K, Hornshaw J, Teasdale PR, Dawes TA: Parenteral nutritional in carcinoma of the oesophagus treated by surgery: nitrogen balance and clinical studies. *Br J Surg* 1977;64:125–128.
47. Issell BF, Valdivieso M, Zaren HA, et al: Protection against chemotherapy toxicity by IV hyperalimentation. *Cancer Treat Rep* 1978;62:1139–1143.
48. Heatley RV, Williams RHP, Lewis MH: Preoperative intravenous feeding: A controlled trial. *Postgrad Med J* 1979;55:541–545.
49. Simms JM, Oliver E, Smith JAR: A study of total parenteral nutrition (TPN) in major gastric and esophageal resection for neoplasia. *J Parent Bnt Nutr* 1980;4:22 (abstract).
50. Lanzotti V, Copeland E, Bhuchar V, Wesley M, Corriere J, Dudrick S: A randomized trial of total parenteral nutrition (TPN) with chemotherapy for non-oat cell lung cancer (NOCLC). *Proc Am Assoc Cancer Res Am Soc Clin Oncol* 1980;21:377 (abstract).
51. Sako K, Lore JM, Kaufman S, et al: Parenteral hyperalimentation in surgical patients with head and neck cancer: A randomized study. *J Surg Oncol* 1981;16:391–402.
52. Valdivieso M, Bodey GP, Benjamin RS, et al: Role of intravenous hyperalimentation as an adjunct to intensive chemotherapy for small cell bronchogenic carcinoma. *Cancer Treat Rep* 1981;65(suppl 5):145–150.

53. Thompson BR, Julian TB, Stremple JF: Perioperative total parenteral nutrition in patients with gastrointestinal cancer. *J Surg Res* 1981;30:497–500.

54. Popp MB, Fisher RI, Wesley R, Aamodt R, Brennan MF: A prospective study of adjuvant parenteral nutrition in the treatment of advanced diffuse lymphoma: influence on survivial. *Surgery* 1981;90:195–203.

55. Nixon DW, Moffitt S, Lawson DH, et al: Total parenteral nutrition as an adjunct to chemotherapy of metastatic colorectal cancer. *Cancer Treat Rep* 1981;65 (suppl 5):121–128.

56. Serrou B, Cupissol D, Plagne R, Boutin P, Carcassone Y, Miche FB: Parenteral intravenous nutrition (PIVN) as an adjunct to chemotherapy in small cell anaplastic lung carcinoma. *Cancer Treat Rep* 1981;65:151–155.

57. Samuels ML, Selig DE, Ogden S, Grant C, Brown B: IV hyperalimentation and chemotherapy for state III testicular cancer: a randomized study. *Cancer Treat Rep* 1981;65:615–627.

58. Shamberger RC, Pizzo PA, Goodgame JR, et al. The effect of total parenteral nutrition on chemotherapy-induced myelosuppression: A randomized study. *Am J Med* 1983;74:40–48.

59. Shamberger RC, Brennan MF, Goodgame JT, et al: A prospective randomized study of adjuvant parenteral nutrition in the treatment of sarcomas: Results of metabolic and survival studies. *Surgery* 1984;96:1–13.

9

Traveler's Diarrhea
"Doctor, What Should I Take before I Leave Home?"

Jutta K. Preiksaitis

1. INTRODUCTION

Travel is often associated with new experiences. Unfortunately, a bout of debilitating diarrhea is often one of them. Although traveler's diarrhea may result in significant personal distress on a business trip, vacation, or honeymoon, it also has important economic, political, and military ramifications. The agents causing traveler's diarrhea in affluent travelers from the industrialized world visiting the tropics are the same agents that result in significant morbidity and mortality associated with infant diarrheal illness in developing countries. In this setting, traveler's diarrhea is a major public health problem.

2. EPIDEMIOLOGY

Over the years, the syndrome of traveler's diarrhea has been given a number of colorful and descriptive names—turista, Montezuma's revenge, Aztec two-step (Mexico), GI trots, Gyppy tummy, Spanish flux, Casablanca crud (Morocco), Aden gut (Yemen), Basra belly (Iraq), turkey

---

Jutta K. Preiksaitis ● University of Alberta, University Hospital, Edmonton, Alberta, Canada T6G 2C7.

trot, Hong Kong dog, Poona poohs, Malta dog, Rangoon runs (Burma), Tokyo trots, Trotsky's (USSR), Bombay runs, Ho Chi Minhs, emporiatic enteritis! The diagnosis of traveler's diarrhea can be made when a patient develops acute diarrhea (three or more loose, watery bowel movements per day) while abroad or shortly after arriving home. Symptoms associated with the diarrhea include abdominal pain or cramps, fever, nausea and vomiting, myalgias and arthralgias, headache, fatigue, chills, and anorexia. Bloody diarrhea is uncommon (less than 1% of diarrheal illness).[1-3] The symptoms experienced will be somewhat dependent on the agent causing the diarrhea.

The risk of acquiring traveler's diarrhea is dependent on both where you are from and where you are going. In a study based on interviews with 16,568 charter flight passengers returning to Europe from 13 destinations in various climatic regions, Steffen found that for travelers from highly industrialized nations, three grades of risk for traveler's diarrhea could be defined, depending on destination.[4] Low risk (<8%) was associated with travel to the United States, Canada, northern and central Europe, Australia, and New Zealand. Intermediate risk (8–20%) was found on most Caribbean islands, major resorts on the Northern Mediterranean and in the Pacific, Israel, Japan, and South Africa. High risk (>20%) was associated with travel to most developing countries in Africa, Asia, and Latin America.

Risk is also dependent on the traveler's country of origin. Visitors from a "low-risk" area traveling to a "high-risk" area appear to be at significantly higher risk of developing traveler's diarrhea than inhabitants of one high-risk area traveling to another high-risk area. When traveler's diarrhea was studied in visitors to a medical congress in Teheran (1968), only 8% of travelers from tropical countries became ill compared to 41% of those from countries with a more temperate climate.[5] Similar results were found in a study of microbiologists attending a meeting in Mexico City in 1970.[6] The attack rate for Americans, Canadians, and Northern Europeans was significantly higher than the combined attack rate for travelers from the Mediterranean, Far East, Africa, and Latin America. As illustrated by a study of Panamanian tourists in Mexico, among travelers whose country or origin is high risk visiting another high-risk area, members of upper socioeconomic classes appear to be at greater risk of developing traveler's diarrhea.[7] Travelers from a high-risk area to a low-risk area, however, are not at any greater risk of developing traveler's diarrhea than tourists traveling from one low-risk area to another low-risk area.[8]

The risk of acquiring traveler's diarrhea is also dependent on the duration of stay. In a study of crew members of the U.S.S. Belleau Wood visiting Mexico for two and a half days, 21% of subjects receiving no pro-phylaxis became infected.[9] In contrast, when U.S. students in Mexico were studied over a 3-week period, no cases of traveler's diarrhea were seen before the fourth day of the visit, but 61% of subjects not receiving prophylaxis had developed traveler's diarrhea by day 21. Between day 3 and 21 the risk was approximately 3.4% per day.[10] In a long-term study of U.S. students in Mexico, Brown et al.[11] found the greatest number of diarrheal episodes and most cases of diarrhea due to enterotoxigenic Escherichia coli (ETEC) occurred within the first 2 weeks after arrival in Mexico. Sporadic episodes of illness occurring after this time were usually associated with pathogens other than enterotoxigenic E. coli.

Infection with ETEC, usually the most common cause of traveler's diarrhea, has been related to exposure to contaminated food. Among U.S. students newly arrived in Mexico, Tjoa et. al.[12] found that the risk of acquiring traveler's diarrhea was significantly higher in students who ate in the school cafeteria, public restaurants, and street vendors compared to those who ate in private homes and apartments. Ericsson et al.[13] found differences in their data and Tjoa's regarding the risks of developing diar-rhea in students eating from street vendors. However, they state that only a small percentage of their students ate from vendors. Their conclusion is that there is an increased risk of developing diarrhea in people eating at restaurants, street vendors, and school cafeterias. A study of visitors attending a conference in Mexico City demonstrated an increased risk of infection with ETEC in those eating salads.[3] Vibrio parahemolyticus, a marine organism known to cause traveler's diarrhea, has been associated with the consumption of raw or only partially cooked contaminated seafood.[14]

Because a large dose of ETEC (10^8–10^{10} organisms) is required to cause illness in man, water is generally believed to be an unlikely source of infection, as gross contamination would be required to allow trans-mission of infection to man. Despite this theoretical consideration, at least three common-source community outbreaks of diarrhea due to ETEC have been associated with a contaminated water supply, one in an American national park and two in Tokyo.[15] The consumption of bottled beverages, however, does not guarantee protection of the traveler from water-transmitted enteric pathogens, as evidenced by an outbreak of typhoid fever in 1972 that was associated with a commercial bottled bev-erage.[16] A contaminated water supply also appears to be an important vehicle in the transmission of Giardia lamblia infection.[17]

Does dietary discretion prevent the traveler from acquiring diarrheal illness? The bulk of evidence suggests that traveler's diarrhea is difficult to elude. In two studies of travelers attending medical congresses in Mexico City, no association could be found between diarrheal illness and the consumption of tap water, iced drinks, salads, vegetables, or raw fruit.[3,6] In one study, those persons who took the greatest precautions had the highest attack rate.

3. ETIOLOGY

Although an infectious etiology for traveler's diarrhea has long been suspected, prior to the 1970s diarrheal illness associated with travel was often attributed to climatic changes, the effect of travel on circadian rhythm, psychological stress, or chilling of the abdomen by cold drinks or the cooling draft of a fan. However, in 1970, Rowe et al.,[18] in a study of British troops in Aden, first demonstrated the possible role of a strain of E. coli in producing traveler's diarrhea. A single serotype of E. coli, 0148:H28, was found in the stool of 19 of 33 soldiers with diarrheal illness. The pathogenicity of this serotype was subsequently demonstrated by the accidental infection of a laboratory worker. Later studies showed that pathogenicity of this and other strains of E. coli is related to the production of enterotoxins.

Subsequent studies have shown that ETEC is an important cause of traveler's diarrhea in many parts of the world including Mexico, Latin America, and Africa (Table 1).[3,7,18-24] In many studies ETEC has been isolated in 36–75% of travelers with diarrhea. Although ETEC appears to be worldwide in distribution, the likelihood that ETEC is the cause of an episode of diarrheal illness may be dependent on the destination of the traveler. Eccheverria et al., in a study of U.S. Army soldiers in South Korea, found that although 55% of the soldiers developed diarrhea, ETEC was never identified as the causative agent.[22] Relative immunity to infection with ETEC appears to exist in travelers whose country of origin is a high-risk area for traveler's diarrhea. This is illustrated by studies comparing the etiological agents causing diarrheal illness in Panamanian tourists and Latin American students to those causing illness in American tourists and students in Mexico.[7,25]

E. coli can also cause traveler's diarrhea by mechanisms other than toxin production. Enteroinvasive and enteroadherent E. coli are, however, quantitatively less important than ETEC (Table 1). Conventional bacterial pathogens such as Shigella and Salmonella are relatively infrequent causes of diarrhea in travelers. Shigella has been isolated from symptomatic individuals with frequencies varying from 5 to 22% and is usually the second most common cause of traveler's diarrhea next to

Table 1. Etiology of Traveler's Diarrhea[a]

Agent	Frequency (%)								
	Rowe[b]	Shore[c]	Gorbach[d]	Merson[e]	Sack[f]	Echeverria[g]	Guerrant[h]	Ryder[i]	Mathewson[j]
E. coli (ETEC)	54	36	72	45	75	0	56	4	57
E. coli (ETEC)	NT	0	0	4	NT	0	0	NT	NT
E. coli (EAEC)	NT	NT	NT	NT	NT	NT	NT	NT	9
Shigella	0	0	0	4	0	0	0	4	22
Salmonella	6	0	0	16	0	0	0	0	7
Campylobacter	NT	NT	NT	NT	NT	0	0	11	4
V. parahemolyticus	NT	NT	NT	2	0	0	0	NT	NT
Rotavirus (reovirus)	NT	NT	NT	4	0	7	NT	26	NT
Norwalk virus	NT	NT	NT	0	NT	0	NT	15	NT
Giardia	0	9	0	4	NT	2	NT	4	NT
Entaemoeba	0	0	6	0	NT	0	NT	4	NT
Unknown	40	54	22	37	25	90	44	37	19

[a]NT, not tested.
[b]Rowe et al. (1970)[18]—British troops to Aden.
[c]Shore et al. (1974)[19]—travelers to developing countries.
[d]Gorbach et al. (1975)[20]—U.S. students to Mexico.
[e]Merson et al. (1976)[3]—U.S. conventioneers to Mexico.
[f]Sack et al. (1977)[21]—Peace Corps workers in Kenya.
[g]Echeverria et al. (1979)[22]—U.S. troops in South Korea.
[h]Guerrant et al. (1980)[23]—U.S. students to Latin America.
[i]Ryder et al. (1981)[7]—Panamanian tourists in Mexico.
[j]Mathewson et al. (1983)[24]—U.S. students to Mexico.

ETEC. Gastroenteritis due to *Salmonella* species does occur in travelers, but more serious infections, such as typhoid fever, are rare.[4]

Over the past decade, infection with *Campylobacter* has been recognized as the most common bacterial cause of acute diarrhea in North America. Because bacteriological methods for isolation of this pathogen were not available until the mid-1970s, earlier studies of traveler's diarrhea did not include a search for this organism. More recent studies have demonstrated that *Campylobacter* species could be isolated from 4% of American students with diarrhea in Mexico[25] and 11% of Panamanian tourists who developed traveler's diarrhea in Mexico.[7] In a study of traveler's diarrhea in foreign visitors to Bangladesh, *Campylobacter jejuni* was isolated in 15% of cases, a frequency equal to that of the *Shigella* species.[26]

Vibrio parahemolyticus colonizes fish and shellfish and causes a diarrheal illness when these foods are eaten raw or partially cooked. This a common practice in Japan and the Far East. Outbreaks of diarrhea due to *V. parahemolyticus* have been described on cruise ships in the Caribbean.[27] In some areas of the world, *V. parahemolyticus* may play an important causative role in traveler's diarrhea. This was illustrated by a study in Bangkok, Thailand, where in 31% of all diarrheal episodes, *V. parahemolyticus* was identified as the pathogenic organism.[14]

Over the past decade, viruses, particularly the rotavirus (reoviruslike agents) and the parvoviruslike agents, have been implicated in the pathogenesis of acute nonbacterial gastroenteritis. These agents do not grow in tissue culture, and the diagnosis of infection is dependent on identification of the agent either by electron microscopy, by ELISA techniques, or by serological methods. The significance of viruses as a cause of traveler's diarrhea remains unclear. In a study of American students newly arrived in Mexico, rotaviruses were found in 26% of those with diarrhea, compared to 3% of controls without diarrhea. This suggests a causal relationship.[28] However, many of these students were also infected with bacterial pathogens, including ETEC. The significance of viruses in traveler's diarrhea may be dependent on the visitor's country of origin. Whereas ETEC appears to be the most significant pathogen in traveler's from a low-risk area going to Mexico, in one study of Panamanian tourists in Mexico, 41% of traveler's diarrhea was attributable to either rotavirus or Norwalk virus, a parvoviruslike agent.[7]

Parasitic infections are an uncommon cause of traveler's diarrhea. Although amebiasis is endemic in many high-risk areas for traveler's diarrhea, 1% or less of cases are due to infection with this organism. Infection with *G. lamblia* appears to be more common and may be underdiagnosed by stool examinaton for cysts alone. A duodenal–jejunal aspirate and/or small intestinal biopsy may be necessary to demonstrate the organism. *Giardia* infection should be an important consideration in patients consulting physicians after returning from travel. This is because symptoms from infection with giardiasis, unlike infection with bacterial and viral agents causing traveler's diarrhea, may persist for several months. Contaminated water supplies are most commonly implicated as the source of *Giardia* infection in travelers. Despite a search for the more recently recognized pathogens implicated as having a causal role in traveler's diarrhea, the cause of a significant proportion of cases remains unknown (Table 1). The efficacy of antimicrobial agents used as prophylaxis or treatment of traveler's diarrhea of "unknown" cause suggests that at least some of these cases are due to an as yet unidentified toxin producing or invasive coliform.

4. PATHOGENESIS OF DIARRHEA DUE TO E. COLI

Although *E. coli* is usually considered to be a normal commensal of the gastrointestinal tract, some strains cause acute diarrhea. These strains are grouped into three classes according to their pathogenic mechanisms: enteropathogenic (EPEC), enteroinvasive (EIEC), and enterotoxigenic (ETEC).[15]

Strains of EPEC have been associated with nosocomial outbreaks of neonatal enteritis in Europe and North America and community infections of infantile enteritis in developing countries. Organisms are identified as EPEC by using a slide agglutination test to determine the O serogroup of the *E. coli*. Although a "toxin" has long been suspected of playing a role in the pathogenesis of infection due to EPEC, most strains produce neither the heat-labile (LT) nor the heat-stable (ST) toxin characteristic of ETEC. Recently some serotypes identified as EPEC have been shown to produce a toxin that produces a cytotoxic effect on Vero cells. This toxin has been named Vero toxin (VT). VT-producing *E. coli* have been implicated in outbreaks of hemorrhagic colitis in the United States and Canada and have been associated with the hemolytic uremic syndrome in Canada.[29] Its possible role in traveler's diarrhea remains unclear.

The ability to colonize the epithelial mucosa of the small intestine appears to be important in the pathogensis of diarrhea due to EPEC. Some strains have colonization factors distinct from CFA/I and CFA/II of ETEC that can be measured by their ability to adhere to HEp-2 cells *in vitro*. *In vitro* studies using human fetal intestinal mucosa have suggested that inflammatory changes might result solely from the close attachment of the organisms to the intestinal mucosa.[30] These strains have been designated as enteroadherent (EAEC). In one study of traveler's diarrhea in U.S. students in Mexico, EAEC was the sole agent cultured from 6% of the cases.[24]

Some strains of *E. coli* are enteroinvasive (EIEC): i.e. they have the ability to penetrate the epithelial mucosa of the large bowel leading to inflammation and ulceration. This results in stools containing pus and/or blood. EIEC are an uncommon cause of traveler's diarrhea. In the laboratory these strains are identified using a Sereny test in which an ulcerative keratoconjunctivitis is produced by instilling living suspensions of the organism into the eye of the guinea pig.

Traveler's diarrhea is most often associated with infection with ETEC. These organisms are pathogenic because they produce either an LT or an ST toxin, or both. LT is a protein antigenically similar to cholera toxin. It consists of an A subunit, which is responsible for initiating the intracellular steps leading to fluid secretion, and five B subunits, which are necessary for binding of the enterotoxin to a receptor. LT and cholera toxin contain many homologous amino acid sequences. Like cholera toxin, LT acts through activation of adenylate cyclase, leading to increased levels of intracellular cyclic AMP and intestinal secretion. To demonstrate LT, an extract of the test strain is inoculated into a ligated ileal loop of an adult rabbit or other animal. LT is present if fluid secretion is induced. LT also produces cytotoxic changes induced by the accumulation of cyclic AMP in some cell lines *in vitro*. Cell lines commonly used to detect LT include Y-1 mouse adrenal cells and Chinese Hamster ovary cells. Although immunological techniques for detection of LT are available, they are not routinely used outside of research setting.

ST is a low-molecular-weight polypeptide that itself is only weakly antigenic. It is not antigenically related either to LT or to cholera toxin. It is believed to act through stimulation of guanylate cyclase. This leads to an increase in the cellular level of cyclic GMP, increasing fluid secretion and diarrhea. In the laboratory, ST is detected by injecting the *E. coli* extract into the milk-filled stomach of a newborn suckling mouse and then 4 hours later examining the small intestine for distention and weighing the small intestinal contents.

The test for LT and ST are laborious and usually not available outside of reference laboratories. Usually only 5–10 strains of *E. coli* per stool specimen are tested for toxin production. Therefore, unless the toxigenic strain has overgrown and is the predominant coliform in the stool, negative tests for toxin production do not totally exclude a toxigenic *E. coli* infection.

Both ST and LT are encoded on and transmitted by plasmids.[31] Plasmids are extrachromosomal genetic elements, usually present in bacteria as covalently closed circular DNA molecules. They are not essential for cell viability but are efficiently partitioned to daughter cells at the time of cell division. In addition, they can be efficiently transferred from cell to cell by simple contact (conjugation). Recent evidence suggests that at least some genetic sequences for ST are present on transposons. Transposons are plasmid elements that are highly mobile and can move readily from one DNA element of the cell to another. Since some antimicrobial resistance genes are also present on transposons, it would be possible to have *E. coli* that are both toxigenic (by virtue of their ability to produce ST) and resistant to a number of antibiotics—characteristics all mediated by the same plasmid.

Enterotoxin production alone is necessary but not a sufficient criterion for pathogenicity of an *E. coli* strain. The strain must also adhere to the mucosal epithelial cells of the small intestine. Pili are antigenic structures consisting of polymerized protein subunits. They are of regular size and shape and radiate from the bacterial cell. Attachment is mediated by an interaction of the pilus with specific receptors on the host mucosal cell. These pili are plasmid encoded and host specific. For example, one plasmid codes for a pilus K88 that is relatively specific for the epithelium of the small bowel of weanling piglets. This ETEC causes neonatal diarrhea in these animals. Another, pilus K99, is associated with colonization of the intestine of calves and lambs. Two analogous pili, CFA/I and CFA/II, have been described in man.[32-34] *In vitro,* these CFAs are detected by their ability to adhere to and subsequently hemagglutinate erythrocytes. Hemagglutination by ETEC-associated CFAs is not inhibited by mannose. CFA I causes agglutination of human group A red cells, whereas CFA II causes hemagglutination of bovine red cells. Receptors for enterotoxin are located on the luminal aspect of the membrane close to CFAs, thereby allowing toxin to be delivered to the membrane at high concentration. The enterotoxin receptor for ST is unknown, but that for LT is an oligosaccharide component of the GM_1 ganglioside.

In studies of human volunteers challenged with a wild-type strain which was LT+ ST+ CFA/I, or the same strain which through laboratory passage had become LT+ ST− CFA/I−, it was found that only those who received the wild strain developed watery diarrhea.[35,36] Colonization appears to be an important first step in pathogenicity. In a study of isolates of ETEC from U.S. students who developed traveler's diarrhea in Mexico, most, although not all, strains possessed CFAI or CFA II.[35,36] In the same study, Evans *et al.* also demonstrated that ETEC isolated from the stools of students without diarrhea are usually CFA negative.

Relative immunity to infection with ETEC appears to occur in populations. Evidence for this includes the decreased incidence of traveler's diarrhea in tourists from one high-risk area traveling to another[5,6] and the low incidence of diarrhea due to ETEC in Panamanian tourists in Mexico[7] and Latin American students in Mexico compared to their U.S. counterparts.[25] Diarrhea due to ETEC also becomes less common with more prolonged residence in a high-risk country.[11] The exact nature of this immunity is not clear, and a better understanding of it is important for possible vaccine development. The LT of ETEC is immunogenic, and antibody rises are detectable in infected individuals. However, studies in human volunteers have shown that although prior infection protects against homologous infection, prior infection does not protect against infection against a different strain of ETEC where the heat-labile enterotoxin was the only common antigen.[37] The role of local immunity, which may act by interference with colonization or inactivation of enterotoxin, remains unknown.

5. TREATMENT

It must be remembered that traveler's diarrhea is usually a mild, self-limited illness with a mean duration of 93 hrs. Many travelers will therefore take a "grin and bear it" attitude toward the illness. Nonetheless, a smaller number of patients will experience voluminous fluid losses and dehydration or severe systemic symptoms. In these patients treatment is indicated.

Adequate fluid replacement remains the mainstay of therapy for traveler's diarrhea.[38] Usually losses can be readily replaced orally by available fluids. In some cases oral hydration solutions are necessary. These are provided as UNICEF Oralyte anhydrous packages containing glucose, NaCl, $NaHCO_3$, and KCl. If Oralyte is not available, a homemade solution can be prepared by mixing 5 tsp glucose or 10 tsp of sucrose, ¾ tsp salt, ½ tsp baking soda, ¼ tsp KCl, with 1 liter of boiled drinking water. Depending on the level of dehydration, adults should take 250–500 ml/hour, and children over 2 years of age should take 125–250 ml/hr. If oral hydration cannot be maintained, arrangements for intravenous administration of fluids and electrolytes should be made. Coffee, tea, and some cola drinks should be avoided as the caffeine may inhibit phosphodiesterase activity in the intestine, thereby increasing intracellular levels of cyclic AMP further and aggravating the diarrhea.

The use of antidiarrheal drugs in traveler's diarrhea, as in other infectious diarrheas, remains controversial. The two synthetic narcotic analogs most commonly used, loperamide and diphenoxylate, exert their effect by inhibiting fluid secretion and reducing the propulsive activity of the intestine. Their use in inflammatory bowel disease and in pseudomembranous colitis may be associated with worsening of the symptoms of the disease and perhaps with induction of toxic megacolon. Diphenoxylate intake has also been associated with prolongation of fecal excretion of *Shigella*. In one study of the use of loperamide in American students with traveler's diarrhea visiting Latin America, the drug was found to be more effective than bismuth subsalicylate in relieving diarrhea.[39] Patients with bloody diarrhea and a temperature above 102°F were excluded from the study. Thus, the safety and efficacy of antidiarrheal drugs in mild to moderate traveler's diarrhea require further study.

Bismuth subsalicylate, or Pepto-Bismol, has been studied in the treatment of traveler's diarrhea. Although bismuth subsalicylate has been demonstrated to inhibit *E. coli* enterotoxin *in vitro* and *in vivo,* it probably acts through the inhibition of prostaglandin synthesis, with a subsequent reduction in fluid and electrolyte secretion. In a study by DuPont *et al.*[40] in which U.S. students who acquired traveler's diarrhea in Mexico were treated with 30–60 ml of bismuth subsalicylate every half-hour for eight doses, a significant decrease in stool frequency was noted in the treated versus the control group. Symptoms of nausea, vomiting, and abdominal cramps were also better in the treatment group, but only after patients with shigellosis were excluded from analysis.

Because traveler's diarrhea is caused by a number of bacterial agents, empiric antimicrobial therapy should have a sufficiently broad spectrum to be effective against most enteric pathogens. The results of prospective controlled trials studying several of these agents are summarized in Table 2. Although tetracycline has a broad spectrum of activity, the potential use of this agent is limited in some geographical areas because of a high incidence of tetracycline resistance in bacterial isolates. For example, 45% of ETEC strains from a study in Southeast Asia were tetracycline resistant.[41] Moreover, in a controlled study of tetracycline therapy in adults with diarrhea due to ETEC admitted to hospital in Bangladesh, only a slight improvement in symptoms was noted in patients with LT–ST disease. No effect was seen in ST disease when treated patients were compared to the placebo group.[42]

DuPont *et al.*[43] conducted a double-blind treatment study of traveler's diarrhea in U.S. students in Mexcio comparing the efficacy of trimethoprim/sulfamethoxazole (TMP/SMX) or trimethoprim (TMP) with a placebo. Both patients treated with TMP/SMX and TMP had a significant decrease in diarrhea by 24 hr after the initiation of therapy. The relief of nausea and abdominal cramps was more common in patients

Table 2. Prospective Controlled Studies of Treatment in Traveler's Diarrhea

Author	Population	Agent	Result
DuPont et al., 1977[40]	U.S. students in Mexico	Bismuth subsalicylate (Pepto-Bismol), 30 ml q½h × 8 doses or 60 ml q½h × 8 doses vs placebo	Significant decrease in stool frequency and associated symptoms in treatment group ($p < 0.05$)
Merson et al., 1980[42]	Adults admitted to hospital in Bangladesh	Tetracycline, 250–500 mg qid × 72 hr vs placebo	Slight effect in LT–ST disease, no effect in ST disease
DuPont et al., 1982[43]	U.S. students in Mexico	TMP/SMX (160 mg of TMP and 800 mg SMX) or TMP 200 mg b.i.d. vs placebo	Significant decrease in diarrhea by 24 hr TMP/SMX vs placebo, $p < 0.0002$, TMP, $p < 0.01$, beneficial effect on diarrhea due to ETEC, Shigella, and of unknown cause
Ericsson et al., 1983[44]	U.S. students in Mexico	Bicozamycin, 500 mg q.i.d. × 3 days vs placebo	Significant decrease in duration of diarrhea in treatment group, $p < 0.00009$, beneficial effect on diarrhea due to ETEC, Shigella, and of unknown cause

treated with the active drugs. The beneficial effect was seen not only in diarrhea due to ETEC, but also in diarrhea due to shigellosis and that not associated with a known enteropathogen. Side effects were minimal.

Bicozamycin is a poorly absorbed oral antibiotic with an antimicrobial spectrum that includes many aerobic gram-negative bacilli including most enteropathogens. Ericsson et al.[44] tested the efficacy of bicozamycin, 500 mg qid, for 3 days compared to placebo therapy in U.S. students in Mexico with traveler's diarrhea. The treatment group experienced a significant decrease in duration of diarrhea and relief of abdominal cramps when compared to the placebo group. As with TMP/SMX and TMP, bicozamycin was effective in the treatment of diarrhea due to ETEC, Shigella, and unknown pathogens. Side effects were limited to a rash in one patient. Although this drug shows promise as a therapeutic agent for enteric pathogens, it is an experimental drug and is not yet available commercially.

6. PROPHYLAXIS

Ideally, one would prefer to prevent rather than to have to treat traveler's diarrhea. Several approaches to the problem have been investigated.

Studies *in vitro* and *in vivo* have suggested that food products containing live lactobacilli might prevent ETEC from colonizing the gut and might produce local antitoxins. However, two placebo-controlled studies using lactobacilli as prophylaxis for traveler's diarrhea could demonstrate no beneficial effect.[45,46]

Bismuth subsalicylate has also been tested as a prophylactic agent. DuPont *et al.*[10] studied the relative efficacy of bismuth subsalicylate (Pepto-Bismol), 60 ml given four times daily for 21 days to U.S. students in Mexico, compared to a placebo preparation. The use of bismuth subsalicylate resulted in 68% protection against diarrheal illness. However, during the study period each student consumed more than 5 liters of Pepto-Bismol! Not only is compliance a problem, but unless one is willing to devote an extra suitcase to this product, under most circumstances the use of this agent for prophylaxis would not be practical.

Trials using antimicrobial agents for the prophylaxis of traveler's diarrhea were initiated even before the common etiological agents of traveler's diarrhea were identified. The results of these trials must be examined with caution. Not only was randomization often poor, but the protection offered by these agents was only 30–50%.[47] This represents a low degree of efficacy. A drug used for prophylaxis of what is usually a relatively mild illness should be safe. Clioquinol (iodochlorhydroxyquinoline, EnteroVioform) has been demonstrated to have some efficacy in the prevention of traveler's diarrhea when tested in British football players.[48,49] However, the serious neurological syndrome of subacute myeloptic neuropathy has been associated with the use of this drug.[50] Since it is often available "over the counter" in parts of the world where traveler's diarrhea is common, travelers should be warned about self-medication with this medication.

Antimicrobial agents that demonstrate the greatest promise when used as prophylaxis for traveler's diarrhea are doxycycline, TMP-SMX, and trimethoprim alone. The results of double-blind controlled studies using these agents are summarized in Table 3. In the initial studies, Sack and co-workers[51,52] examined the efficacy of doxycycline given in a dose of 100 mg daily as a prophylactic agent in Peace Corps workers in Kenya and Morocco. These were geographical areas in which at the time nearly all ETEC isolates were sensitive to doxycycline. In both these studies, doxycycline provided a high degree of protection against traveler's diarrhea when treatment and placebo groups were compared. In two later studies Echiverria and co-workers also studied Peace Corps workers, this time in the Honduras and Thailand.[53] In these geographical areas a significant proportion of ETEC were known to be doxycycyline resistant. Although 68% protection was observed using doxycyline prophylaxis in

Table 3. Prospective Controlled Studies of Prophylaxis with Doxycycline, Trimethoprim/Sulfamethoxazole, and Bismuth Subsalicylate in Traveler's Diarrhea

Author	Population	Agent	Result: Percent protection	Result: *p* value
Sack *et al.*, 1978[52]	Peace Corps workers in Kenya (antibiotic-sensitive area)	Doxycycline, 100 mg o.d. × 3 weeks	86	0.012
Sack *et al.*, 1979[51]	Peace Corps workers in Morocco (antibiotic-sensitive area)	Doxycycline, 100 mg o.d. × 3 weeks	83	<0.01
Sack, 1983[53]	Peace Corps workers in Honduras (antibiotic-resistant area)	Doxycycline, 100 mg o.d. × 3 weeks	68	<0.001
Sack, 1983[53]	Peace Corps workers in Thailand (antibiotic-resistant area)	Doxycycline, 100 mg. o.d. × 3 weeks	58	0.12
Freeman *et al.*, 1983[9]	Crew members of U.S.S. Belleau Wood visiting Mexico for 25 days	Doxycycline, 200 mg × 1 dose, then 100 mg o.d.	80	0.002
DuPont *et al.*, 1982[43]	U.S. students in Mexico	TMP/SMX (160 mg TMP/800 mg SMX), b.i.d. × 21 days	73	0.0001
DuPont *et al.*, 1983[55]	U.S. students in Mexico	TMP/SMX (160 mg TMP/800 mg SMX), o.d. × 14 days	95	<0.0001
		or: TMP, 200 mg o.d. × 14 days	52	<0.05
DuPont *et al.*, 1980[10]	U.S. students in Mexico	Bismuth subsalicylate suspension (17.5 mg/ml), 60 ml q.i.d. × 21 days	68	<0.0001

Honduras and 58% in Thailand, the protective effect was observed only against sensitive ETEC and against other as yet unrecognized doxycycline-sensitive bacteria. Although adverse effects were uncommon (< 1%), the number of subjects studied was small. During administration of doxycycline, there was rapid development of doxycycline resistance in normal fecal *E. coli*. This observation has important implications, in that antibiotic pressure through widespread use of prophylaxis may influence the emergence of resistant enteric pathogens. A more recent study of extremely short-term prophylaxis (3 days), in crew members of the U.S.S. Belleau Wood visiting Mexico, demonstrated the efficacy of doxycycline (80% protection) even when the period of exposure to potential pathogens is short.[9]

DuPont *et al.* have carried out two studies using TMP/SMX as prophylaxis for traveler's diarrhea in U.S. students in Mexico. In the first study, a double-strength tablet (160 mg TP, 800 mg SMX) was given twice daily for 3 weeks. This provided significant protection (73%). However, there was a large number of reported adverse events, primarily skin reactions.[54,55] In a second study, the dose of TMP/SMX was halved to one double-strength tablet daily, and another treatment group receiving trimethoprim alone, 200 mg o.d., was added.[55] A protection rate of 95% was observed in the group receiving TMP/SMX, and a more modest level of protection (52%) was seen in those persons receiving trimethoprim alone. Side effects were much fewer in this second study. In studies of TMP/SMX prophylaxis in granulocytopenic patients and in patients with recurrent urinary tract infection, a significant decrease in fecal enterobacteriaceae was observed, and colonization with resistant strains was unusual. In contrast, prophylaxis with TMP/SMX or trimethoprim alone for traveler's diarrhea was associated with no change in total fecal enterobacteriaceae and was associated with the development of high-level TMP and SMX resistance in virtually all these strains.[56]

Despite the apparent efficacy of doxycycline and TMP/SMX prophylaxis in traveler's diarrhea, the possible risks associated with their use should be considered. Although adverse reactions to these antimicrobial agents are usually mild and consist of a skin rash or photosensitivity, more severe reactions of marrow aplasia, Steven's–Johnson syndrome or antibiotic-associated colitis are possible. The use of prophylactic antibiotics may increase antibiotic resistance among diarrheal pathogens. Since antibiotic resistance and toxin production may be on the same plasmid, widespread antibiotic usage could lead to highly resistant ETEC. Although primarily a theoretical consideration, suppression of normal enteric flora by prophylactic antibiotics may predispose the traveler to infection with more serious pathogens such as cholera or typhoid fever. Finally, while taking prophylactic antibiotics, the traveler may avoid following sound preventative practices with respect to food and drink. Although this may not significantly alter the risk of acquiring traveler's diarrhea, it may predispose the person to more serious illnesses, such as typhoid fever or infectious hepatitis.

7. RECOMMENDATIONS FOR TRAVELERS

The bulk of evidence suggests that routine antibiotic prophylaxis should not be given to travelers. Possible exceptions to this guideline include persons on important business trips, military populations, individuals who are more susceptible to infection, or persons who are at greater risk of dehydration if they were to develop diarrhea. Because most bacteria are killed in the stomach when the gastric pH is 3 or less, patients who are achlorhydric or hypochlorhydric are much more susceptible to enteric infections such as cholera, salmonellosis, *Shigella,* and ETEC. Patients who have had gastric surgery, are receiving antacids or H_2-receptor antagonists, and possible cannabis users should be considered for prophylaxis for traveler's diarrhea. Those patients with renal, cardiac, or gastrointestinal disease who would poorly tolerate dehydration and electrolyte disturbances should also receive prophylaxis.

Depending on the known antibiotic sensitivity pattern of enteric pathogens found in the area of travel, the best prophylactic antibiotic regimen would be either TMP/SMX, one double-strength tablet daily, or doxycycline, 100 mg daily. Reasonable dietary precautions should be taken. Despite popular opinion, tap water is not usually a source of infection in traveler's diarrhea. Ice cubes, however, should be avoided since they may become contaminated by food handlers. Certain foods should also be avoided. These include raw vegetables, raw meat, raw fish and shellfish, food that has not been refrigerated, food that has been left out for several hours, and food purchased from street vendors. Food served "piping hot" should be safe.

If traveler's diarrhea does occur, the first objective should be to maintain hydration. In mild to moderate cases of traveler's diarrhea without fever, bismuth subsalicylate can be take (30 ml every 30 min for eight doses). If the diarrheal episode is intense or prolonged, TMP/SMX one double-strength tablet b.i.d., should be administered for 5 days. If symptoms do not respond to this therapy, medical attention should be sought.

REFERENCES

1. Kean BH: The diarrhea of travellers to Mexico. Summary of five-year study. *Ann Intern Med* 1963;59:605–614.
2. Gorbach SL, Hoskins DW: Travelers' diarrhea. *Disease-A-Month* 1980;27:1–44.
3. Merson MH, Morris GK, Sack DA, et al: Travelers' diarrhea in Mexico. A prospective study of physicians and family members attending a congress. *N Engl J Med* 1976;294:1299–1305.
4. Steffen R: Epidemiology of travellers' diarrhea. *Scand J Gastroenterol* 1983;18(suppl 84):5–17.
5. Kean BH: Turista in Teheran. Travellers' diarrhea at the Eighth International Congresses of tropical medicine and malaria. *Lancet* 1969;2:583–584.
6. Loewenstein MS, Balows A, Gangarosa EJ: Turista at an international congress in Mexico. *Lancet* 1970,1:529–531.
7. Ryder RW, Oquist CA, Greenberg H, et al: Travelers' diarrhea in Panamanian tourists in Mexico. *J Infect Dis* 1981;144:442–448.

8. Ryder RW, Wells JG, Gangarosa EJ: A study of travellers' diarrhea in foreign visitors to the United States. *J Infect Dis* 1977;136:605–607.

9. Freeman LD, Hooper DR, Lathen DF, Nelson DP, Harrison WO, Anderson DS: Brief prophylaxis with dexycycline for the prevention of travellers' diarrhea. *Gastroenterology* 1983;84:276–280.

10. DuPont HL, Sullivan P, Evans DG, et al: Prevention of traveler's diarrhea (emporiatric enteritis). Prophylactic administration of subsalicylate bismuth. *JAMA* 1980;243:237–241.

11. Brown MR, DuPont HL, Sullivan PS: Effect of duration of exposure on diarrhea due enterotoxigenic *Escherichia coli* in travelers from the United States to Mexico. *J Infect Dis* 1982;145:582.

12. Tjoa WS, DuPont HL, Sullivan P, et al: Location of food consumption and travelers diarrhea. *Am J Epidemiol* 1977;106:61–66.

13. Ericsson CD, Pickering LK, Sullivan P, DuPont HL: The role of location of food consumption in the prevention of travellers' diarrhea in Mexico. *Gastroenterology* 1980;79:812–816.

14. Sriratanaban A, Reinprayoon S: *Vibrio parahaemolyticus:* A major cause of traveller's diarrhea in Bangkok. *Am J Trop Med Hyg* 1982;31:128–130.

15. Rowe B: The role of *Escherichia coli* in gastroenteritis. *Clin Gastroenterol* 1979;8:625–644.

16. Lee JA: International conference on the diarrhea of travelers—New directions in research: A summary. *J Infect Dis* 1978;137:355–368.

17. Brandborg LL, Owen R, Fogel R, et al: Giardiasis and traveller's diarrhea. *Gastroenterology* 1980;78:1602–1614.

18. Rowe B, Taylor J, Bettelheim KA: An investigation of traveller's diarrhea. *Lancet* 1970;1:1–5.

19. Shore EG, Dean AG, Holik KJ, Davis BR: Enterotoxin-producing *Escherichia coli* and diarrheal disease in adult travellers: A prospective study. *J Infect Dis* 1974;129:577–582.

20. Gorbach SL, Kean BH, Evans DG, Bessudo D: Traveler's diarrhea and toxigenic *Escherichia coli. N Eng J Med* 1975;292:933–936.

21. Sack DA, Kaminsky DC, Sack RB, et al: Enterotoxigenic *Escherichia coli* diarrhea of travelers: a prospective study of American Peace Corps volunteers. *Johns Hopkins Med J* 1977;141:63–70.

22. Echeverria P, Ramirez G, Blacklow NR, Ksiazek T, Cukor G, Cross JH: Travelers' diarrhea among U.S. troops in South Korea. *J Infect Dis* 1979;139:215–219.

23. Guerrant RL, Rouse JD, Hughes JM, Rowe B: Turista among members of the Yale Glee Club in Latin America. *Am J Trop Med Hyg* 1980;29:895–900.

24. Mathewson JJ, DuPont HL, Morgan DR, Thorton SA, Ericsson CD: Enteroadherent *Escherichia coli* associated with travellers' diarrhea. *Lancet* 1983;1:1048.

25. DuPont HL, Olarte J, Evans DG, Pickering LK, Galindo E, Evans DJ: Comparative susceptibility of Latin American and United States students to enteric pathogens. *N Engl J Med* 1976;295:1520–1521.

26. Speelman P, Struelens MJ, Sanyal SC, Glass RI: Detection of *Campylobacter jejuni* and other potential pathogens in travellers' diarrhea in Bangladesh. *Scand J Gastroenterol* 1983;18(suppl 84):19–23.

27. Lawrence DN, Blake PA, Yashuk JC, Wells JG, Creech WG, Hughes JH: *Vibrio parahaemolyticus* gastroenteritis outbreaks aboard two cruise ships. *Am J Epidemiol* 1979;109:71–80.

28. Bolivar R, Conklin RH, Vollett JJ, Pickering LK, DuPont HL, Kohl S: Rotavirus in travellers' diarrhea: study of an adult student population in Mexico. *J Infect Dis* 1978;137:324–327.

29. Mechanisms in enteropathogenic *Escherischia coli* diarrhoea. *Lancet* 1983,1:1254.

30. Williams PH, Sedgwick MI, Evans N, Turner PJ, George RH, McNeish AS: Adherence of an enteropathogenic strain of *Escherichia coli* to human intestinal mucosa is mediated by a colicinogenic conjugative plasmid. *Infec Immun* 1978;22:393–402.

31. Falkow S, Portnoy DA: Bacterial plasmids—An overview. *Clin Invest Med* 1983;6:207–212.

32. Evans DG, Silver RP, Evans DJ, Chase DG, Gorbach SL: Plasmid-controlled colonization factor associated with virulence in *Escherichia coli* enterotoxigenic for humans. *Infec Immun* 1975;12:656–667.

33. Evans DG, Evans DJ, DuPont HL: Virulence factors of enterotoxigenic *Escherichia coli*. *J Infect Dis* 1977;136:S118–S123.

34. Evans DG, Evans DJ: New surface-associated heat-labile colonization factor antigen (CFA/II) produced by enterotoxigenic *Escherichia coli* of serogrousp 06 and 08. *Infect Immun* 1978;21:638–647.

35. Evans DG, Evans DJ: Colonization factor antigens of human-associated enterotoxigenic *Escherichia coli*, in Robbins JG, Hin JC, Sadoff JC (eds): Bacterial Vaccines, Vol IV. New York, Thieme-Stratton, 1982, pp 104–112.

36. Satterwhite TK, Evans DG, DuPont HL, Evans DJ: Role of *Escherichia coli* colonization factor antigen in acute diarrhoea. *Lancet* 1978;II:181–184.

37. Levine MM, Nalin DR, Hoover DL, Bergquist EJ, Hornick RB, Young CR: Immunity to enterotoxigenic *Escherichia coli*. *Infect Immun* 1979;23:729–736.

38. Nalin DR: Oral replacement of water and electrolytes losses due to travellers' diarrhea. *Scand J Gastroenterol* 1983;18(suppl 84):95–98.

39. Johnson PC, Ericsson CD, DuPont HL, et al: Comparison of loperamide to bismuth subsalicylate for the treatment of acute travellers' diarrhea. *Gastroenterology* 1986 (in press).

40. DuPont HL, Sullivan P, Pickering LK, Haynes G, Ackerman PB: Symptomatic treatment of diarrhea with bismuth subsalicylate among students attending a Mexican university. *Gastroenterology* 1977;73:715–718.

41. Echeverria P, Verhaert L, Ulyangco CV, et al: Antimicrobial resistance and enterotoxin production among isolates of *Escherichia coli* in the Far East. *Lancet* 2;1978:589–592.

42. Merson MH, Sack RB, Islam S, et al: Disease due to enterotoxigenic *Escherichia coli* in Bangladeshi adults, clinical aspects and a controlled trial of tetracycline. *J Infect Dis* 1980;141:702–711.

43. DuPont HL, Reves RR, Galindo E, Sullivan PS, Wood LV, Mendiola JG: Treatment of travellers' diarrhea with trimethorpim/sulfamethoxazole and with trimethoprim alone. *N Engl J Med* 1982;307:841–844.

44. Ericsson CD, DuPont HL, Sullivan P, Galindo E, Evans DG, Evans DJ: Bicozamycin, a poorly absorbable antibiotic, effectively treats travellers' diarrhea. *Ann Intern Med* 1983;98:20–25.

45. Clements ML, Levine MM, Black RE, et al: *Lactobacillus* prophylaxis for diarrhea due to enterotoxigenic *Escherichia coli*. *Antimicrob Agents Chemother* 1981;20:104–108.

46. deDios Pozo-Olano J, Warram JH, Gomez RG, Cavazos MG: Effect of a lactobacilli preparation on travellers' diarrhea. *Gastroenteorlogy* 1978;76:829–830.

47. Nye FJ: Travellers' diarrhea. *Clin Gastroenterol* 1970;8:767–781.

48. Richards DA: A controlled trial in travellers' diarrhea. *Practitioner* 1970;204:822–824.

49. Richards DA: Prophylactic value of clioquinol against travellers' diarrhea. *Lancet* 1971,1:44–45.

50. Oakley GP: The neurotoxicity of the halogenated hydroxyquinolines. *JAMA* 1973;225:395–397.
51. Sack RB, Froehlich JL, Zulich AW, et al: Prophylactic doxycyclinc for travellers' diarrhea. *Gastroenterology* 1979;76:1368–1373.
52. Sack RB, Kaminsky DC, Sack RB, et al: Prophylactic doxycycline for travellers' diarrhea. Results of a prospective double-blind study of Peace Corps volunteers in Kenya. *N Engl J Med* 1978;298:758–763.
53. Sack RB: Antimicrobial prophylaxis of travellers' diarrhea: A summary of studies using doxycycline or trimethoprim and sulphamethoxazole. *Scand J Gastroenterol* 1983;18(suppl 84):111–117.
54. DuPont HL, Evans DG, Rios N, Cabada FJ, Evans DJ, Dupont MW: Prevention of travellers' diarrhea with trimethoprim-sulfamethoxazole. *Rev Infect Dis* 1982;4:533–539.
55. DuPont HL, Galindo E, Evans DG, Cabada FJ, Sullivan P, Evans DJ: Prevention of travellers' diarrhea with trimethoprim-sulfamethoxazole and trimethoprim alone. *Gastroenterology* 1983;84:76–80.
56. Murray BE, Rensimer ER, DuPont HL: Emergency of high-level trimethoprim resistance in fecal *Escherichia coli* during oral administration of trimethoprim or trimethorprim-sulfamethoxazole. *N Engl J Med* 1982;306:130–135.

10

Sexually Transmitted Gastrointestinal Infections
An Update

Hillar Vellend

1. INTRODUCTION

In the past decade, sexually transmitted diseases have come to encompass not only the classical genital infections such as syphilis, gonorrhea, nonspecific urethritis, and herpes, but also anorectal infections caused by these microorganisms. There is also an increasing body of evidence that a number of specific gastrointestinal infections not commonly thought of as venereal, such as amebiasis, giardiasis, shigellosis, and campylobacteriosis, can, in fact, be acquired through specific sexual practices.[1-3]

2. EPIDEMIOLOGY

Sexually transmitted gastrointestinal infections (ST-GI) are predominantly, but not exclusively, seen in homosexual men. The major factors that have contributed to the high incidence of ST-GI in male homosexuals are the large number of different sexual partners (often anonymous) and certain specific sexual practices. Most cases are seen in the highly

Hillar Vellend • Departments of Medicine and Microbiology, Faculty of Medicine, University of Toronto, Toronto, Ontario, Canada M5G 2C4.

sexually active age group between 20 and 40. Additional factors that result in frequent transmission of these agents include the high prevalence of asymptomatic infection and failure to proscribe sexual activity during symptomatic infection. A specific microbiological diagnosis is made infrequently due to improper specimen collection and the limited availability of laboratory resources to detect *Treponema pallidum* on dark-field microscopy and for culturing microorganisms such as *Chlamydia trachomatis* and herpes simplex virus. Even when a specific diagnosis is made and effective treatment prescribed, sexual partners are often not evaluated or treated.

There are two major modes of acquisition of ST-GI. Most classical agents of anorectal infection such as *Neisseria gonorrhoeae*, *Treponema pallidum*, herpes simplex virus, and *Chlamydia trachomatis* are acquired by direct mucous membrane contact during receptive anal intercourse. On the other hand, enteric pathogens with a known low infecting inoculum, such as *Shigella*, *Entamoeba histolytica*, *Giardia lamblia*, and probably some *Campylobacter*-like organisms are acquired by direct fecal oral contact such as anilinctus or perhaps indirectly during oral–genital sexual activity.

3. MICROBIAL ETIOLOGY

Table 1 summarizes the medically important causes of ST-GI in North America. Although clearly important, sexually transmitted viral hepatitis will not be reviewed. Some causes will be described in more detail.

3.1. Anorectal Gonorrhea

Neisseria gonorrhoeae remains the single most common specific microbial cause of ST-GI.[4] Although anorectal involvement in women with uncomplicated genital gonorrhea is common (mean 44%), infection limited to the anorectum is much less frequent and is estimated to comprise no more than 4% of all gonococcal infections in women.[5] This infection is most commonly acquired by penoanal contact with or without anal intercourse. In men, anorectal gonorrhea is almost exclusively seen in homosexuals as a complication of rectal intercourse. Anorectal gonorrhea comprises 25–45% of all gonococcal infection in male homosexuals. Up to 1981, the incidence of pharyngeal and anorectal gonorrhea in men in the borough of Manhattan in New York City was approximately 500 per 100,000, almost as high as the total incidence of gonorrhea

Table 1. Sexually Transmitted Gastrointestinal Infection:
Specific Microbial Etiology

1. Bacterial
   a. *Neisseria gonorrhoeae*
   b. *Treponema pallidum*
   c. *Shigella* spp. *(flexneri)*
   d. *Campylobacter* spp. *(jejeuni)*
   e. *Salmonella* spp.
   f. *Clostridium difficile*
2. Viral
   a. Herpes simplex virus
   b. Papovavirus
3. Chlamydial
   a. *Chlamydia trachomatis* (LGV and non-LGV)
4. Parasitic
   a. *Entamoeba histolytica*
   b. *Giardia lemblia*

at all sites in women in new York City. However, by 1983, the incidence of pharyngeal and anorectal gonorrhea in men had fallen to about 200 per 100,000.[6] This abrupt decline is thought to be the result of modified sexual practices dictated by the fear of the acquired immunodeficiency syndrome (AIDS) in that city, which by 1983 had reported almost one-half of all cases of AIDS in the United States.

3.1.1. Symptoms

Anorectal gonococcal infection in male homosexuals is usually asymptomatic. From 20 to 70% of men who have *Neisseria gonorrhoeae* isolated from rectal swabs have either no symptoms or very mild symptoms. In a recent study of 194 homosexual men in Seattle,[4] the prevalence of anorectal gonococcal infection was not significantly different in a group of symptomatic men (31%) compared to a matched group of asymptomatic men (23%). The manifestations of symptomatic infection (i.e., disease) due to *N. gonorrhoeae* include a wide range of anorectal complaints such as rectal itching, discomfort (including dyspareunia), tenesmus, mucus on the stool, bleeding, discharge, diarrhea, and sometimes constipation.

3.1.2. Signs

Clinical signs, including endoscopic examination, predictably range from being absolutely normal to the finding of mucous discharge, purulent exudate, mucosal erythema, friability, and less commonly ulceration. Abnormal sigmoidoscopic findings are usually restricted to the distal 15 cm and typically involve multiple anal crypts.

3.1.3. Diagnosis

All these symptoms and signs are neither specific nor sensitive for the diagnosis of anorectal gonococcal infection. Diagnostic material should be obtained by swabbing the anorectal mucosa under direct visualization with a proctoscope or by "blindly" inserting a cotton-tipped swab about 2.5 cm into the anal canal and rotating the swab from side to side to maximize the absorption of mucous exudate into the swab. Stool is *not* an appropriate specimen. A stool-free swab should be promptly smeared and plated or placed in a suitable transport medium. A Gram's stain made directly from this type of specimen has a relatively low sensitivity (30–70%) but is particularly worthwhile to facilitate rapid diagnosis in a symtomatic individual. Culturing a specimen obtained by this "blind" technique appears to be as sensitive as one retrieved by direct observation of the anorectal mucosa.

3.1.4. Treatment

The recommended antibiotic regimens for anorectal gonorrhea include aqueous procaine penicillin G, 4.8 million units i.m., plus probenecid 1.0 g, or a single oral dose of ampicillin, 3.5 g with probenecid. The failure rate with either of these two treatment regimens is only about 5%. An effective alternative for the penicillin-allergic patient would be spectinomycin, 2–4 g i.m.[7] Two regimens that are useful for uncomplicated genital gonorrhea, tetracycline, 500 mg q.i.d. for 7 days, and amoxicillin, 3.0 g, plus probenecid, are associated with a 15% failure rate in anorectal gonorrhea and are therefore not recommended.[5] Why this should be the case is poorly understood but may be the result of the very large number of diverse bacteria that make up the normal fecal flora. Newer drugs such as cefoxitin and cefotaxime have been shown to be effective in clinical trials involving small numbers of subjects, but further experience needs to be accumulated before these antibiotics can be recommended.[8]

3.2. Herpes Simplex Virus Proctitis

Herpes simplex virus (HSV) is the most common cause of nongonococcal proctitis in sexually active homosexual men.[4] It is usually due to the type 2 virus and acquired by anal-receptive intercourse. In a recent study by Quinn *et al.*,[4] herpes simplex virus was isolated from 19% of symptomatic men compared to only 4% of asymptomatic controls. In fact, herpes simplex virus was the *only* specific microbe that was isolated significantly more frequently from symptomatic men compared to the asymptomatic controls.

3.2.1. Symptoms

Severe anorectal pain and tenesmus are virtually universal.[9] Other common complaints include anal discharge, constipation, anal pruritus, and hematochezia. The incubation period is usually less than 1 week, and the mean duration of symptoms is 21 days (range 7–44). About one-half of patients will experience some neurological symptoms which can be attributed to sacral radiculitis—most commonly difficulty in initiating micturition but also sacral paraesthesiae and posterior thigh pain.[9]

3.2.2. Signs

External perianal vesicular or ulcerative lesions are seen in up to two-thirds of patients. Anoscopic examination usually will demonstrate diffuse mucosal friability ("positive wipe test"), but discrete vesicular or ulcerative lesions may also be seen. The pathology is usually confined to the distal 10 cm. Fever and inguinal adenopathy are seen in about 50% of patients.

3.2.3. Diagnosis

A swab of an ulcerative lesions or abnormally friable anorectal mucosa should be immediately placed in viral transport medium, refrigerated at 4°C, and processed as promptly as possible. However, the symptoms and signs may be sufficiently characteristic of herpes simplex virus infection that the reliability of a clinical diagnosis is quite high. If a rectal biopsy is obtained, the finding of intranuclear inclusions and multinucleated giant cells correlate with HSV infection.

3.2.4. Treatment

To date, treatment of HSV proctitis has largely been symptomatic and supportive. Recent data suggest that oral acyclovir is effective in shortening the duration and symptoms of this infection (W. E. Stamm, personal communication).

3.2.5. Prognosis

There is little information on the natural history of HSV proctitis. Just as with genital HSV infection, recurrences may occur, but many clinicians have the impression that this may be less frequent and severe with HSV proctitis.

3.3. Chlamydia Trachomatis *Proctitis*

Chlamydia are obligate intracellular microorganisms that closely resemble bacteria. They undergo a developmental cycle in infected epithelial cells that results in an intracytoplasmic vesicle containing hundreds of individual microorganisms at various stages of development. Many different strains or serovars are responsible for the three major clinical syndromes caused by *Chlamydia:* trachoma (A, B, C); lymphogranuloma venereum (LGV) (L1, 2, 3); and the oculogenital strains (D–K).

The ability of LGV strains to produce severe anorectal infection has been known for almsot 50 years, although it is distinctly rare. More recently, *C. trachomatis* has been isolated from 10–15% of symptomatic men but also from up to 5% of asymptomatic controls.[10,11] *C. Trachomatis* proctitis can be separated into two distinct groups depending on the infecting serovars. Overall, about one-third are caused by the LGV type and two-thirds by the oculogenital (or non-LGV) serovars.

3.3.1. Symptoms

The LGV type produces an acute, severe, ulcerative proctitis that results in severe anorectal pain, discharge, tenesmus, hematochezia, and alterations in bowel function that may mimic Crohn's disease. On the other hand, the non-LGV strains usually produce asymptomatic infection or very mild disease.

3.3.2. Signs

The LGV strains usually produce diffuse mucosal friability with microulcerations. The non-LGV strains result in either no visible abnormality or focal erythema and friability.

3.3.3. Diagnosis

The LGV strains may produce granulomatous inflammation that is similar to that observed in Crohn's disease. Swabs of the involved rectal mucosa should be immediately placed in an antibiotic-containing transport medium suitable for *C. trachomatis*. It has been recommended that rectal specimens be sonicated prior to inoculation onto cycloheximide-treated McCoy cells to reduce contamination and improve the isolation rate.[12] A microimmunofluorescent antibody titer greater than or equal to 1:512 is strongly sugestive of infection due to the LGV type, but only seroconversion correlates well with infection due to the non-LGV type.

3.3.4. Treatment

Infected, particularly symptomatic, patients should be treated with tetracycline, 500 mg p.o. q.i.d. The duration of treatment should be 1–2 weeks for the non-LGV strains and 3 weeks for the LGV strains. This usually results in resolution of symptoms and negative cultures and fecal leukocytes after treatment.

3.4. Entamoeba Histolytica *Infection*

Harry Most, in his presidential address to the American Society for Tropical Medicine and Hygiene in 1968, first suggested the association between amebiasis and homosexuality.[13] Several subsequent studies have confirmed the high prevalence of both pathogenic and nonpathogenic intestinal protozoal infection in male homosexuals compared to heterosexual controls.[14] Oral–anal contact is the most likely mode of transmission. Keystone *et al.,* in a study from Toronto, demonstrated a 27% prevalence of *Entamoeba histolytica* infection in homosexual men compared to 1% in heterosexual controls.[14] The presence of symptoms could not be correlated with infection unless the infection was polymicrobial and included *Giardia lamblia*. Despite the high prevalence of potentially pathogenic *E. histolytica* in this population, no cases of amebic colitis or liver abscess have been documented. This suggests that these strains were relatively nonpathogenic.

In 1978, Sargeaunt devised a technique for characterizing pathogenic and nonpathogenic strains of *E. histolytica* on the basis of isoenzyme patterns called zymodemes. Patients with amebic disease were infected with strains II and XI. In a recent study of 52 strains isolated from homosexual men in Great Britain, all were nonpathogenic.[15] These findings have led to the growing consensus that asymptomatic cyst passers of *E. histolytica* need not necessarily be treated with drugs such as iodochlorhydroxyquin, metronidazole, diloxanide furoate, and diphetarsone.

3.5. Infections with Campylobacter-like Organisms

In a recent study from Seattle, Quinn et al.[16] reported the isolation of a heterogeneous group of Campylobacter-like organisms from 25 symptomatic and six asymptomatic homosexual men. No isolates were made from heterosexual controls. Infection was associated with oral–anal contact and was often accompanied by abdominal cramps, diarrhea, and hematochezia. Sigmoidoscopic examination usually demonstrated a proctocolitis with either focal or diffuse friability and occasional ulceration. Biopsies showed only nonspecific acute inflammatory changes. Direct plating of rectal swabs appears to be necessary to isolate these fastidious organisms, and special culture conditions are required.

4. EVALUATION OF THE PATIENT WITH SUSPECTED ST-GI

Very recently a comprehensive clinical and microbiological study of homosexual men with anorectal and intestinal infection was undertaken.[4] On the basis of this study, the authors have recommended the following approach.

1. A complete history and physical examination including at least anoscopy.
2. Initial laboratory investigations should include a Gram's stain, dark-field examination, and VDRL test. Swabs of rectal mucosa should be cultured for *N. gonorrhaeae* and *C. trachomatis*. The presence of leukocytes on a smear of the rectal mucosa is strongly suggestive of an infectious etiology.
3. Rapid diagnosis can be made for gonorrhea (gram stain), syphilis (dark field), and herpes simplex (clinical).
4. The clinical syndrome should be classified into one of the major groups (Table 2).
5. Additional microbiological investigations should be determined by the clinical syndrome.
6. Treatment should be optimized and directed toward specific microbial causes.
7. Careful clinical follow-up is mandatory.
8. Whenever possible, sexual partners should be evaluated and treated.
9. Empirical treatment should be avoided, but if it is necessary, a reasonable choice might be aqueous procaine penicillin G, 4.8

Table 2. Intestinal Infections in Homosexual Men

	Syndrome		
	Proctitis	Proctocolitis	Enteritis
Symptoms	Anorectal pain Rectal discharge Tenesmus Constipation	Combination	Diarrhea Abdominal pain Bloating Nausea
Anoscopy	Abnormal	Abnormal	Normal
Sigmoidoscopy	Normal beyond 15 cm	Abnormal beyond 15cm	Normal
Common microbial causes	*N. gonorrhoeae* Herpes simplex virus *C. trachomatis* *Treponema pallidum*	*Campylobacter* *Shigella* LGV ?*E. histolytica*	*Giardia lamblia*
Mode of acquisition	Receptive anal intercourse	Fecal–oral	Fecal–oral

million units i.m., plus probenecid, 1.0 g, followed by doxycycline, 100 mg p.o. b.i.d. for 10 days.

This group also emphasized the importance of polymicrobial infections in the symptomatic group where 22% had two or more pathogens compared to only 4% in the asymptomatic controls.

REFERENCES

1. Owen RL: Sexually transmitted enteric disease, in Remington JS, Swartz MN (eds): *Current Clinical Topics in Infectious Diseases—3*. New York, McGraw-Hill Book Co., 1982, pp 1–29.
2. Baker RW, Peppercorn MA: Gastrointestinal ailments in homosexual men. *Medicine* 1982;61:390–405.
3. Ma P, Armstrong D (eds): *The Acquired Immune Deficiency Syndrome and Infections of Homosexual Men*. New York, Yorke Medical Books, 1984.
4. Quinn TC, Stamm WE, Goodell SE, et al: The polymicrobial origin of intestinal infections in homosexual men. *N Engl J Med* 1983;109:576–582.
5. Klein EJ, Fisher LS, Chow AW, Guze LB: Anorectal gonococcal infection. *Ann Intern Med* 1977;86:340–346.
6. Department of Health and Human Services: Declining rates of rectal and pharyngeal gonorrhea among males—New York City. *Morb Mort Wkly Rep* 1984;33:295–297.
7. U.S. Department of Health and Human Services: Sexually transmitted diseases treatment guidelines 1982. *Morb Mort Wkly Rep* 1982;33S–60S.
8. Simpson ML, Khan MY, Siddiqui Y, et al: Treatment of gonorrhea: Comparison of cefotaxime and penicillin. *Antimicrob Agents Chemother* 1981;19:798–800.
9. Goddell SE, Quinn TC, Mkrtichian E, et al: Herpes simplex virus proctitis in homosexual men. *N Engl J Med* 1983;308:868–871.

10. Quinn TC, Goddell SE, Mkrtichian E, et al: *Chlamydia trachomatis* proctitis. *N Engl J Med* 1981;305:195–199.
11. Bolan RK, Sands M, Schachter J, et al: Lymphogranuloma venereum and acute ulcerative proctitis. *Am J Med* 1982;72:703–706.
12. Stamm WE: Proctitis due to Chlamydia trachomatis, in Ma P, Armstrong D (eds): *The Acquired Immune Deficiency Syndrome and Infections of Homosexual Men.* New York: Yorke Medical Books, 1984, pp. 40–47.
13. Most, H: Manhattan "A tropical isle." *Am J Trop Med Hyg* 1968;17:333–354.
14. Keystone JS, Keystone DL, Proctor EM: Intestinal parasitic infections in homosexual men: Prevalence, symptoms and factors in transmission. *Can Med Assoc J* 1980;123:512–514.
15. Sargeaunt PG, Oates JK, Maclennan I, et al: *Entamoeba histolytica* in male homosexuals. *Br J Vener Dis* 1983;59:193–195.
16. Quinn TC, Goodell SE, Fennell C, et al: Infections with *Campylobacter jejeuni* and *Campylobacter*-like organisms in homosexual men. *Ann Intern Med* 1984;101:181–192.

11

Medical Treatment of Variceal Bleeding

Jean-Pierre Villeneuve and Daphna Fenyves

1. INTRODUCTON

Acute variceal bleeding is a major complication of portal hypertension. It is the main cause of death in patients with cirrhosis.[63] Survival for cirrhotic patients following an episode of variceal hemorrhage is shown in Fig. 1.[64] Mortality is close to 50% at 3 months and 66% at 1 year after the initial variceal rupture. It should be pointed out that the survival slope is not linear. The risk of rebleeding and the risk of dying are much higher during the initial 3 months after the bleeding episode. This is followed by a long-term phase in which the risk of dying decreases. Survival is then primarily dependent on the severity of the underlying liver disease and largely independent of the bleeding episode. Commenting on this high early mortality, Conn stated that "the longer a patient survives, the better is the prognosis!"[16] Smith and Graham[64] demonstrated that early-phase mortality is the prime determinant of the long-term survival slope. Thus, any substantial improvement in long-term survival must rely on maneuvers that will improve survival for the early period.

Several forms of therapy have been devised and used to treat variceal hemorrhage in the hope of improving survival, but it is still difficult to determine whether any one treatment is clearly better than the others. Part of this confusion is due to the fact that several factors other than treatment can influence survival. The severity of liver failure is the key

Jean-Pierre Villeneuve and Daphna Fenyves ● Clinical Research Centre, Saint-Luc Hospital, Montreal, Quebec, Canada H2X 3J4.

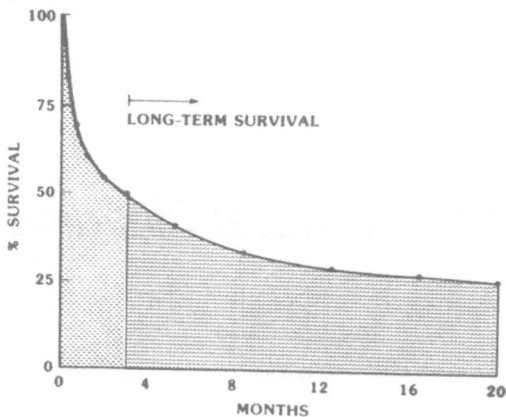

Figure 1. Life-table survival for 85 unselected variceal bleeders. From Smith and Graham[64] with permission of the authors and the editor of *Gastroenterology*.

determinant of survival in cirrhotics with acute variceal hemorrhage, irrespective of the treatment used (Table 1). The severity of the initial bleed and the occurrence of early rebleeding also influence mortality. Moreover, early rebleeding is related to the severity of liver failure. The more severe the liver disease, the higher the likelihood of early rebleeding.[1,51] Local expertise and enthusiasm for a given treatment at the hospital to which the patient is admitted are also likely to influence survival, but the importance of these factors is difficult to quantitate. In the presence of so many "confounding" variables, randomized controlled trials are the most dependable method to evaluate and compare treatment efficacy. Randomized trials provide reasonable assurance that these confounding variables will be equally distributed between two groups of patients, such that differences in outcome can be attributed to treatment effect. In this chapter, we shall review the available forms of medical therapy for variceal bleeding with particular emphasis on the results of randomized clinical trials. We shall first examine the measures used to stop the initial bleeding episode, namely, balloon tamponade, emergency scle-

Table 1. Estimated Natural History of
Variceal Bleeding in Cirrhosis of the Liver,
According to Child's Classification[a]

Child group	Survival		
	1 Month	1 Year	2 Years
A	>90%	76%	65%
B	70%	52%	39%
C	<55%	35%	23%

[a]Adapted from Schalm and Van Buren.[62]

2. EMERGENCY TREATMENT OF VARICEAL BLEEDING

Variceal rupture is a frequent cause of fulminant or severe persistent hemorrhage, which often precipitates liver failure. Nevertheless, in about half the patients, the bleeding stops spontaneously, at least temporarily. In these patients only general supportive measures are required.[2] In patients with massive or persistent bleeding, various hemostatic procedures are available.

2.1. Balloon Tamponade

The modified four-lumen Sengstaken-Blakemore tube is the most commonly used. Technical details concerning its use have been reviewed recently.[2] Two large prospective studies of gastroesophageal balloon tamponade in patients with *active* bleeding suggest a 90% efficacy for immediate hemostatsis, with a 14% rate of major complications and a 3% rate of lethal complications (Table 2). In a controlled trial comparing the Sengstaken–Blakemore tube and the Linton–Nachlas tube,[72] the Blakemore was found to be slightly more effective and better tolerated. A major problem of balloon tamponade is the high rebleeding rate (close to 50%) after removal of the tube. Therefore, balloon tamponade should be considered as an effective, but temporary, measure.

2.2. Emergency Schlerotherapy

Emergency endoscopic sclerotherapy is used to stop variceal bleeding with either intravariceal or paravariceal injection of sclerosing agents. Initial studies were carried out with rigid endoscopes under general anesthesia,[34,53,70] but more recently sclerotherapy with flexible endoscopes under light sedation has gained wider acceptance. Uncontrolled studies

Table 2. Hemostatic Procedures for Acute Variceal Bleeding[a]

	Balloon tamponade	Emergency sclerotherapy	Vasopressin	Somatostatin
Primary control of hemorrhage	90%	90%	57%	53%
Secondary rebleeding	52%	25%	50%	NA
Major complications	14%	10%	25%	0%
Short-term mortality	26%	33%	57%	47%

[a]References: Teres *et al.*,[72] Lewis *et al.*,[44] Chojkier *et al.*,[13] Kravetz *et al.*,[37] Hunt *et al.*,[30] Kjaergaard *et al.*,[35] Johnson *et al.*,[33] Stray *et al.*,[67] Takase *et al.*,[69] Soehendra *et al.*[66]

of emergency sclerotherapy with a flexible endoscope suggest a 90% efficacy for the immediate control of hemorrhage, a 25–30% rebleeding rate (within the first 2 weeks after the inital sclerotherapy), and a 10% rate of major complications (Table 2). These impressive results must be viewed with caution. The trials are uncontrolled, sclerotherapy was carried out in conjunction with tamponade in most instances, and it is difficult to determine the exact percentage of patients actively bleeding at the time of endoscopy.

Three controlled trials of emergency sclerotherapy have been published. Barsoum et al.[1] and Paquet and Feussner[55] compared endoscopic sclerotherapy to balloon tamponade. Both showed a beneficial effect of sclerotherapy on rebleeding rate and short-term mortality. The Copenhagen Esophageal Varices Sclerotherapy Project[18] compared sclerotherapy with tamponade to tamponade alone. They found no differences between the two groups in the severity and duration of the index bleed, short-term rebleeding, or short-term mortality, although long-term mortality was favorably influenced by the sclerotherapy. We have no satisfactory explanation for the discrepancy between these studies, although technical differences in the sclerotherapy methods and expertise of the endoscopists could play a role. For example, a controlled trial by Westaby et al.[76] suggests that sclerotherapy with an oversheath is slightly more effective than the free-hand technique for short-term control of bleeding. However, several other long-term sclerotherapy studies (to be discussed later) show a beneficial effect, despite the use of different sclerosing agents, sites of infection, and treatment schedules. The exact importance of technical variations as regards the efficacy of sclerotherapy remains unclear.[14]

Percutaneous transhepatic variceal obliteration has been proposed as an alternative method to control hemorrhage in actively bleeding patients.[45] Intraperitoneal bleeding, subcapsular hematoma, and portal vein thrombosis are serious complications of the technique. Two controlled trials[8,65] failed to show any advantage of the procedure for hemostatic effectiveness and short-term mortality.

2.3. Vasopressin

Vasopressin is a potent vasoconstrictor of the splanchnic circulation, but it has major effects on the heart and systemic circulation as well (Fig. 2). Vasopressin reduces hepatic blood flow and portal venous pressure.

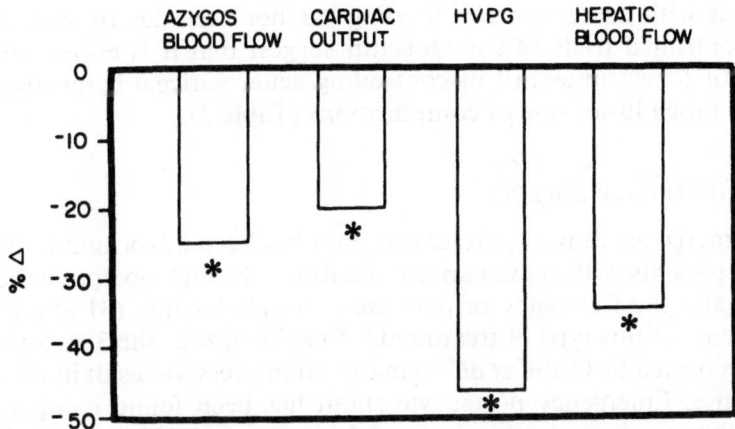

Figure 2. Hemodynamic effects of vasopressin 0.4 IU/min in patients with cirrhosis and portal hypertension. *, Significantly different from basal values. Adapted from Bosch et al.[5]

Recently Bosch et al.[5] have shown that vasopressin decreases azygos venous blood flow. Gastroesophageal collaterals, including esophageal varices, drain into the azygos venous system. This observation therefore suggests that blood flow through esophageal varices is reduced by vasopressin. Vasopressin also reduces cardiac output and coronary blood flow. Heart failure, acute infarction, and rhythm disturbances are serious complications of vasopressin administration.

Clinical trials of vasopressin suggest an efficacy of about 60% for primary hemostasis, with a 50% rebleeding rate following cessation of vasopressin infusion (Table 2). Major side effects, mostly of an ischemic nature, occur in 25% of patients. Controlled trials did not reveal a significant advantage for mesenteric versus intravenous infusion of the drug,[13,33] and even the efficacy of vasopressin over that of a placebo is questionable.

Various alternatives to vasopressin have been considered to avoid its side effects. Glypressin, a long-acting analog of vasopressin, has been reported to be more effective than vasopressin for the immediate control of bleeding while being associated with a lower toxicity[21]; however, the number of subjects in this controlled trial was small, and the response rate to vasopressin abysmal (9%).

Groszmann et al.[25] have shown that the addition of nitroglycerin reverses the detrimental effects of vasopressin while preserving its beneficial effects on the splanchnic bed. The efficacy of this combination in patients with acute variceal bleeding has not been determined. Finally, two controlled trials of somatostatin suggest that it is either equal[37] or superior to vasopressin[32] in controlling acute variceal hemorrhage, but with a much lower rate of complications (Table 2).

2.4. Emergency Surgery

Emergency central portacaval shunt has been advocated to treat cirrhotic patients with acute variceal bleeding. The high operative mortality (42%) and the frequency of postshunt encephalopathy (31%) are strong deterrents of this type of treatment.[52] In spite of this, the 38% 5-year survival reported by Orloff *et al.*[52] remains an impressive result in unselected cirrhotics. Emergency portacaval shunt has been found comparable to sclerotherapy in a randomized trial in patients with severe cirrhosis (Child class C).[12] There are no controlled studies in patients with less severe liver disease. In the absence of adequate data, one has to conclude that emergency portacaval shunt has never been given a fair trial.

Esophageal transection appears to be of limited value to improving survival,[11] but adequate studies are also lacking.

3. LONG-TERM PREVENTION OF VARICEAL REBLEEDING

Rebleeding is the hallmark of variceal hemorrhage. Among unselected patients treated conservatively, 40% will rebleed within 3 months and 75–80% after a year.[46,60,71] The mortality of a recurrent variceal hemorrhage varies between 25 and 35%.

Early rebleeding (within 1 or 2 weeks after the initial hemorrhage) is a particularly ominous event in patients with cirrhosis. Therefore, any treatment used to prevent recurrences should be instituted as early as possible after the index bleed. The choice between sclerotherapy, drugs (propranolol), or surgery is not an easy one.

3.1. Endoscopic Sclerotherapy

Seven controlled trials have compared endoscopic sclerotherapy and conservative medical management. In all trials, patients with both mild and severe liver disease were included (Child class A, B, and C). In most instances, sclerotherapy was carried out within 24 hr of the index bleed (Table 3). There were considerable variations in the sclerotherapy technique between investigators, but it is difficult to determine whether this influenced the results achieved. Two studies failed to show any improve-

Table 3. Randomized Controlled Studies of Endoscopic Sclerotherapy versus Conservative Medical Treatment in Patients with Cirrhosis and Variceal Bleeding

Reference	Interval: bleeding–randomization (days)	1 Year free of rebleeding (%)		1-Year survival (%)	
		Control	Sclerotherapy	Control	Sclerotherapy
MacDougall et al.[46]	1–5	25	57*	58	78*
Barsoum et al.[1]	1	26	68*	48	70*
Terblanche et al.[71]	1	21	35	50	54
Witzel and Wolbergs[79a]	NA[b]	NA	NA	39	65*
Copenhagen Sclerotherapy Project[18]	1	52	46	30	40*
Paquet and Fuessner[55]	1	NA	NA	35	80*
Korula et al.[36]	1–31	NA	NA	65	53

[a] Rebleeding and survival rates during the study period; explicit 1-year rates not given.
[b] NA, data not available in the article.
* Significantly different from the control group.

ment in survival, whereas the other five did (Table 3). Following sclerotherapy, patients remain at risk of rebleeding during the first 3–4 months until all varices are eradicated. Maximal benefit of the procedure on rebleeding and survival becomes more apparent after 6 months.[18,36,79] The severity of rebleeding, however, may be less in the sclerotherapy-treated patients. Therefore, long-term survival is a more pertinent end point than rebleeding in evaluating the value of sclerotherapy. Clearly, sclerotherapy does not worsen survival, and available evidence strongly suggests that it is an effective treatment for patients with variceal hemorrhage, that it can be used in almost all patients, and that it can be started soon after the index bleed.

3.2. Propranolol

Patients rebleeding from varices always have a significant degree of portal hypertension, as evidenced by a portal vein (or wedged hepatic vein) pressure gradient of at least 12 mm Hg.[23,75] Thus it seemed logical to postulate that a reduction of portal pressure could prevent variceal bleeding in cirrhotics. Vasopressin lowers portal pressure, but it can only be administered intravenously and is not suitable for long-term treatment. In 1980, Lebrec et al., showed that in patients with cirrhosis and portal hypertension, oral propranolol therapy reduced the portal pressure gradient by 25–35% and that this reduction was sustained on prolonged administration.[40,42]

However, more recent reports by other centers now suggest that the reduction of the portohepatic gradient after propranolol is unpredictable

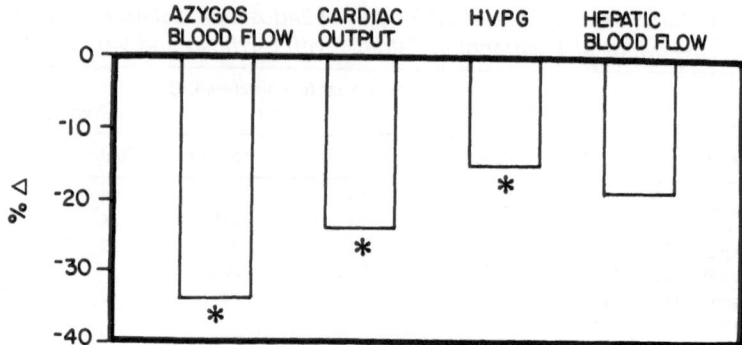

Figure 3. Hemodynamic effects of propranolol, 15 mg i.v., in patients with cirrhosis and portal hypertension. *, Significantly different from basal values. Adapted from Cales *et al.*[10]

(up to one-third of patients do not show a reduction) and most often of smaller magnitude (10–15%).[4,50,58]

It was initially postulated that this effect of propranolol was due to a reduction of cardiac output, with a secondary decrease of hepatic blood flow and portal pressure. However, the observation that cardioselective β blockers (atenolol, metoprolol) are less effective than propranolol in reducing portal pressure suggested an additional effect of propranolol.[29,77] Splanchnic vasoconstriction, due to the blockade of vasodilating β-2 adrenoreceptors by propranolol or to unopposed α-receptor stimulation, could result in a preferential reduction of portal blood flow. Bosch *et al.*[4] and Cales *et al.*[10] reported that azygos blood flow is reduced by propranolol to a greater extent than cardiac output or the portohepatic pressure gradient (Fig. 3), further suggesting that the effect of propranolol on portal and collateral blood flow may be more important than its effect on pressure per se.

Two placebo-controlled trials have been reported on the use of propranolol to prevent recurrent variceal bleeding in cirrhotic patients (Table 4). In both studies, treatment was begun 2–3 weeks after the initial bleeding episode. The results of the two studies are in sharp contrast. The French investigators[41,43] reported a significant effect of propranolol on both rebleeding rate and mortality, whereas the British study[7] did not demonstrate any benefit from propranolol. A variety of explanations have been proposed for the divergent results: different patient populations (more severe liver disease in the English study, more alcoholics in the French study), differences in patients' compliance, the inclusion of patients who had bled from portal hypertensive gastritis in the French

Table 4. Randomized Controlled Studies of Propranolol versus Conservative Medical Treatment in Patients with Cirrhosis and Variceal Bleeding

Reference	Interval: bleeding–randomization (days)	1 Year free of rebleeding (%)		1-Year survival (%)	
		Control	Propranolol	Control	Propanolol
Lebrec et al.[43]	24	42	87*	78	94
Burroughs et al.[7a]	11	56	54	77	85

[a]Survival during the 21-month study period; explicit 1-year survival not given.
*Significantly different from the control group.

study, and the possibility of a type II error in the English study (small number of patients).[15] Obviously, this controversy will only be resolved by further controlled trials which are now in progress. Whether it works or not, the use of propranolol has nevertheless been an important stimulus for research in the medical treatment of portal hypertension.

3.3. Other Drugs

Other β blockers have been reported to lower portal pressure such as nadolol and mepindolol, two nonselective blockers[24,57,78]; metoprolol and atenolol, β-1 selective blockers[9,29,77]; and ICI-11851, a β-2 selective blocker.[3,38] Preliminary results of a controlled trial with metoprolol suggest that it does not prevent rebleeding,[74] but long-term studies with other agents have not yet been reported.

Cimetidine was initially reported to decrease liver blood flow.[19] These results, however, were based on incorrect methodology, and subsequent studies have shown that cimetidine does not modify liver blood flow or portal pressure[6,27,28] and does not prevent recurrent variceal hemorrhage.[47]

Other candidates for the medical treatment of portal hypertension include prazosin[49] and long-acting nitrates,[26] but additional information is required before considering these drugs for clinical use.

3.4. Surgery

Four controlled trials of therapeutic central portacaval anastomosis have been published so far. Portacaval shunt is certainly effective, with a better than 90% success rate in preventing rebleeding, but also carries a 20–40% incidence of recurrent encephalopathy. Severe disabling encephalopathy is, however, rare. The three American studies showed a slight (but not statistically significant) improvement of survival in shunted patients as compared with conservative medical treatment,[31,59,60] but in the French study,[61] the shunt group had a less favorable survival. Distal splenorenal shunt is comparable to central shunt for the prevention of recurrent hemorrhage and long-term survival. In controlled trials, some investigators found a lower incidence of encephalopathy after distal shunts as compared with central shunts[39] while others did not.[17]

Esophageal transection with devascularization procedures, such as the Sugiura operation,[68] appear to be effective in preventing rebleeding. The 5-year survival rates of 51%[73] and 38%[22] reported by Japanese surgeons in cirrhotic patients are impressive, but whether such results can be reproduced in North American cirrhotic patients is still uncertain.

4. THERAPEUTIC STRATEGY

Clearly, all has not been said and done in the field of portal hypertension and variceal hemorrhage, and additional information (or confusion) is forthcoming. Meanwhile, what to do for patients with liver disease who present with variceal bleeding? It is important to remember that in such patients, the severity of the liver disease is the major determinant of survival, and it is unlikely that any treatment will alter the prognosis of subjects with severe cirrhosis. In addition, local expertise should be taken into account when selecting a treatment.

In our institution, balloon tamponade with the Sengstaken-Blakemore tube is the first choice for the immediate control of hemorrhage, when the bleeding does not stop spontaneously. Vasopressin is almost never used, and we find sclerotherapy with the free-hand technique quite difficult in the presence of active bleeding.

Rebleeding is the hallmark of variceal hemorrhage, and prevention of early recurrences should be the major goal of therapy. In patients with low-grade liver failure (Child class A or B), early sclerotherapy (within 12 hr of initial control of the bleeding) is a reasonable treatment and should be continued until varices are eradicated. If sclerotherapy fails, or if the patient bleeds from gastric varices or portal hypertensive gastritis, surgery should be considered. It is not known how emergency surgery would compare with early sclerotherapy. In patients with high-grade liver failure (Child class C) and variceal bleeding, it is unlikely that any long-term treatment will be effective. Injection sclerotherapy appears to be the simplest method to prevent rebleeding but will not improve the liver failure situation. Liver transplantation should be considered if the patient is a suitable candidate and survives the initial hemorrhage.

Finally, primary prophylaxis of variceal hemorrhage in patients with varices who have never bled will become a major focus of interest in the coming years. Two recent controlled trials suggest that prophylactic sclerotherapy improves survival,[54,80] and several prophylactic studies with β blockers are currently under way,[56] but it is still too early to make specific recommendations.

REFERENCES

1. Barsoum MS, Bolous FI, EL-Rooby AA, et al: Tamponade and injection sclerotherapy in the management of bleeding esophageal varices. Br J Surg 1982;69:76–78.
2. Bernuau J, Rueff B: Treatment of acute variceal bleeding. Clin Gastroenterol 1985;14:185–207.
3. Bihari D, Westaby D, Simson A, et al: Reductions in portal pressure by selective B_2-adrenoceptor blockade in patients with cirrhosis and portal hypertension. Br J Clin Pharmac 1984;17:753–757.
4. Bosch J, Mastai R, Kravetz D, et al: Effects of propranolol on azygos venous blood flow and hepatic and systemic hemodynamics in cirrhosis. Hepatology 1984;4:1200–1205.
5. Bosch J, Mastai R, Kravetz D, et al: Measurement of azygos venous blood flow in the evaluation of portal hypertension in patients with cirrhosis. Clinical and haemodynamic correlations in 100 patients. J Hepatol 1985;1:125–139.
6. Burroughs AK, Walt R, Dunk A, et al: Effect of cimetidine on portal hypertension in cirrhotic patients. Br Med J 1982;284:1159–1160.
7. Burroughs AK, Jenkins WJ, Sherlock S, et al: Controlled trial of propranolol for the prevention of recurrent variceal hemorrhage in patients with cirrhosis. N Engl J Med 1983;309:1539–1542.
8. Burroughs AK, Bass NM, Osborne RD, et al: Randomized controlled study of transhepatic obliteration of varices and eosophageal stapling transection in uncontrolled variceal hemorrhage. Liver 1983;3:383–384.
9. Butzow GH, Remmecke J, Brauer A: Metoprolol in portal hypertension: A controlled study. Klin Wochenschr 1982;60:1311–1314.
10. Cales P, Braillon A, Jiron I, et al: Superior portosystemic collateral circulation estimated by azygos blood flow in patients with cirrhosis. Lack of correlation with eosophageal varices and gastrointestinal bleeding. Effect of propranolol. J Hepatol 1984;1:37–46.
11. Cello JP, Cross R, Trunkey DD: Endoscopic sclerotherapy versus esophageal transection in Child's class C with variceal hemorrhage. Comparison with results of portacaval shunt: Preliminary report. Surgery 1982;91:333–338.
12. Cello JP, Crendell JH, Grass RA, et al: Endoscopic sclerotherapy versus portacaval shunt in patients with severe cirrhosis and variceal homorrhage. N Engl J Med 1984;311:1589–1594.
13. Chojkier M, Groszmann RJ, Atterbury CE, et al: A controlled comparison of continuous intra-arterial and intravenous infusions of vasopressin in hemorrhage from esophageal varices. Gastroenterology 1979;77:540–546.

14. Conn HO: Endoscopic sclerotherapy: an analysis of variants. *Hepatology* 1983;3:769–771.
15. Conn HO: Ideal treatment of portal hypertension in 1985. *Clin Gastroenterol* 1985;14:259–288.
16. Conn HO, Lindenmuth WW, May CV, et al: Prophylactic portacaval anastomosis. A tale of two studies. *Medicine (Baltimore)* 1972;51:27–40.
17. Conn HO, Resnick RH, Grace ND, et al: Distal splenorenal shunt vs portal systemic shunt: Current status of a controlled trial. *Hepatology* 1981;1:151–160.
18. Copenhagen Esophageal Varices Sclerotherapy Project: Sclerotherapy after first variceal hemorrhage in cirrhosis. A randomized multicenter trial. *N Engl J Med* 1984;311:1594–1600.
19. Feely J. Wilkinson GR, Wood AJJ: Reduction of liver blood flow and propranolol metabolism by cimetidine. *N Engl J Med* 1981;304:692–695.
20. Fogel MR, Knauer CM, Andres LL, et al: Continuous intravenous vasopressin in active upper gastrointestinal bleeding. A placebo-controlled trial. *Ann Intern Med* 1982;96:565–569.
21. Freeman JG, Cobden I, Lishman AH, et al: Controlled trial of terlipressin ("Glypressin") versus vasopressin in the early treatment of esophageal varices. *Lancet* 1982;2:66–68.
22. Futagawa S, Fukasawa M, Sanjo K, et al: Late results of esophageal transection with paraesophagogastric devascularization (Sugiura procedure) in the treatment of esophageal varices. *World J Surg* 1982;6:655.
23. Garcia-Tsao G., Groszmann RJ, Fischer RL, et al: Portal pressure, presence of gastroesophageal varices and variceal bleeding. *Hepatology* 1985;5:419–434.
24. Gatta A, Sacerdoti D, Merkel C, et al: Effects of nadolol treatment on renal and hepatic hemodynamics and function in cirrhotic patients with portal hypertension. *Am Heart J* 1984;108:1167–1172.
25. Groszmann RJ, Kravetz D, Bosch J, et al: Nitroglycerin improves the hemodynamic response to vasopressin in portal hypertension. *Hepatology* 1982;2:757–762.
26. Hallemans R, Naeije R, Mols P, et al: Treatment of portal hypertension with isosorbide dinitrate alone and in combination with vasopressin. *Crit Care Med* 1983;11:536–540.
27. Henderson JM, Ibrahim SZ, Millikan WJ, et al: Cimetidine does not reduce liver blood flow in cirrhosis. *Hepatology* 1983;3:919–922.
28. Herz R, Rossle M, Bonzel T, et al: Effect of cimetidine on the hepatic extraction of Indocyanine green, and portal pressure and the systemic circulation in patients with cirrhosis of the liver. *Klin Wochenschr* 1984;62:759–764.
29. Hillon P, Lebrec D, Munoz C, et al: Comparison of the effects of a cardioselective and a non selective beta-blocker on portal hypertension in patients with cirrhosis. *Hepatology* 1982;2:528–531.
30. Hunt PS, Korman MG, Hansky J, et al: An 8-year prospective experience with balloon tamponade in emergency control of bleeding esophageal varices. *Dig Dis Sci* 1982;27:413–416.
31. Jackson FC, Perrin EB, Felix WR, et al: A clinical investigation of the portacaval shunt: survival analysis of the therapeutic operation. *Ann Surg* 1971;174:672–701.
32. Jenkins SA, Baxter JN, Corbett W, et al: A prospective controlled trial comparing somatostatin and vasopressin in controlling acute variceal hemorrhage. *Br Med J* 1985;290:275–278.
33. Johnson WC, Widrich WC, Ansell JE, et al: Control of bleeding varices by vasopressin: a prospective randomized study. *Ann Surg* 1977;186:369–376.

34. Johnston GW, Rodgers HW: A review of 15 year's experience in the use of sclerotherapy in the control of acute hemorrhage from esophageal varices. *Br Surg* 1973;60:799–800.
35. Kjaergaard J, Fischer A, Miskowiak J, et al: Sclerotherapy of bleeding esophageal varices. *Scand J Gastroenterol* 1982;17:363–367.
36. Korula J, Balart LA, Radvan G, et al: A prospective, randomized controlled trial of chronic esophageal variceal sclerotherapy. *Hepatology* 1985;5:584–589.
37. Kravetz D, Bosch J, Teres J, et al: Comparison of intravenous somatostatin and vasopressin infusion in treatment of acute variceal hemorrhage. *Hepatology* 1984;4:442–446.
38. Kroeger RJ, Groszmann RJ; Effect of selective blockage of beta-2-adrenergic receptors on portal and systemic hemodynamics in a portal hypertensive rat model. *Gastroenterology* 1985;88:424–429.
39. Langer B, Taylor BR, Mackenzie DR, et al: Further report of a prospective randomized trial comparing distal splenorenal shunt with end-to-side portacaval shunt. An analysis of encephalopathy, survival and quality of life. *Gastroenterology* 1985;88:424–429.
40. Lebrec D, Nouel O, Corbic M, et al: Propranolol—A medical treatment for portal hypertension? *Lancet* 1980;1:180–182.
41. Lebrec D, Poynard T, Hillon P, et al: Propranolol for the prevention of recurrent gastrointestinal bleeding in patients with cirrhosis. A controlled study. *N Engl J Med* 1981;305:1371–1374.
42. Lebrec D, Hillon P, Munoz C, et al: The effect of propranolol on portal hypertension in patients with cirrrhosis. A hemodynamic study. *Hepatology* 1982;2:523–527.
43. Lebrec D, Poynard T, Bernuau J, et al: A randomized controlled study of propranolol for prevention of recurrent gastrointestinal bleeding in patients with cirrhosis: A final report. *Hepatology* 1984;4:355–358.
44. Lewis JW, Chunt RS, Allison JG: Injection sclerotherapy for control of acute variceal hemorrhage. *Am J Surg* 1981;142:592–595.
45. Lunderquist A, Vang J: Transhepatic catheterization and obliteration of the coronary vein in patients with portal hypertension and esophageal varices. *N Engl J Med* 1974;291:646–649.
46. MacDougall BRD, Westaby D, Theadossi A, et al: Increased long-term survival in variceal hemorrhage using injection sclerotherapy. *Lancet* 1982;1:124–127.
47. MacDougall BRD, Williams R: A controlled clinical trial of cimetidine in the recurrence of variceal hemorrhage: Implications about the pathogenesis of hemorrhage. *Hepatology* 1983;3:69–73.
48. Merigan TC, Plotkin GR, Davidson CS: The effect of intravenous pituitrin on hemorrhage from bleeding esophageal varices. A controlled evaluation. *N Engl J Med* 1962;266:134–135.
49. Mills DR, Rae AP, Farah DA, et al: Comparison of three adreno-receptor blocking agents in patients with cirrhosis and portal hypertension. *Gut* 1984;25:73–78.
50. Nakayama T, Ohnishi K, Saito M, et al: Effects of propranolol on portal vein pressure, portal blood flow, hepatic blood flow and cardiac output in patients with chronic liver disease. *Hepatology* 1983;3:812, (abstract).
51. Olsson R: The natural history of esophageal varices. A retrospective study of 244 cases with liver cirrhosis. *Digestion* 1972;6:65–74.
52. Orloff WJ, Bell RH, Hyde PV, et al: Long-term results of emergency portacaval shunts for bleeding esophageal varices in unselected patients with alcoholic cirrhosis. *Ann Surg* 1980;192:325–340.

53. Paquet KJ, Oberhammer E: Sclerotherapy of bleeding oesophageal varices by means of endoscopy. *Endoscopy* 1978;10:7–12.
54. Paquet KJ: Prophylactic endoscopic sclerosing treatment of the esophageal wall in varices. A prospective controlled randomized trial. *Endoscopy* 1982;14:4–5.
55. Paquet KJ, Feussner H: Endoscopic sclerosis and esophageal tamponade in acute hemorrhage from esophagogastric varices: A prospective controlled randomized trial. *Hepatology* 1985;5:580–583.
56. Pascal JF and a multicenter study group: Prophylactic treatment of variceal bleeding in cirrhotic patients with propranolol: A multicenter randomized study. *Hepatology* 1984;4:1092 (abstract).
57. Parker G, Ene MB, Daneshmend TK, et al: Do beta blockers differ in their effects on hepatic microsomal enzymes and liver blood flow? *J Clin Pharmacol* 1984;24:493–499.
58. Rector WG: Propranolol for portal hypertension. *Hepatology* 1982;2:678 (abstract).
59. Resnick RH, Iber FL, Ishihara AM, et al: A controlled study of the therapeutic portacaval shunt. *Gastroenterology* 1974;67:843–857.
60. Reynolds TB, Donovan AJ, Mikkelsen WP, et al: Results of a 12 year randomized trial of portacaval shunt in patients with alcoholic liver disease and bleeding varices. *Gastroenterology* 1981;80:1005–1011.
61. Rueff B, Prandi D, Degos F, et al: A controlled study of therapeutic portacaval shunt in alcoholic cirrhosis. *Lancet* 1976;1:655–659.
62. Schalm SW, Van Buren HR: Prevention of recurrent variceal bleeding: Nonsurgical procedures. *Clin Gastroenterol* 1985;14:209–232.
63. Sherlock S: Hematemesis in portal hypertension. *Br J Surg* 1964;51:746–749.
64. Smith JL, Graham DY: Variceal hemorrhage. A critical evaluation of survival analysis. *Gastroenterology* 1982;82:968–973.
65. Smith-Laing G, Scott J, Long RG, et al: Role of percutaneous transhepatic obliteration of varices in the management of hemorrhage from gastroesophageal varices. *Gastroenterology* 1981;80:1031–1036.
66. Soehendra N, de Heer K, Kempeneers I, et al: Sclerotherapy for esophageal varices: acute arrest of gastrointestinal hemorrhage or long-term therapy. *Endoscopy* 1983;15:125–129.
67. Stray N, Jacobsen CD, Rosseland A: Injection sclerotherapy of bleeding oesophageal and gastric varices using a flexible endoscope. *Acta Med Scand* 1982;311:125–129.
68. Sugiura M, Futagawa S: A new technique for treating esophageal varices. *J Thorac Cardiovasc Surg* 1973;66:677–685.
69. Takase Y, Ozadi A, Orri K, et al: Injection sclerotherapy of esophageal varices for patients undergoing emergency and elective surgery. *Surgery* 1982;92:474–479.
70. Terblanche J, Yakoob HI, Bornman PC, et al: Acute bleeding varices. A five year prospective evaluation of tamponade and sclerotherapy. *Ann Surg* 1981;194:521–528.
71. Terblanche J, Bornman PC, Kahn D, et al: Failure of repeated injection sclerotherapy to improve long-term survival after esophageal bleeding. *Lancet* 1983;11:1328–1332.
72. Teres J, Cecilia A, Bordas J, et al: Esophageal tamponade for bleeding varices. Controlled trial between the Sengstaken–Blakemore tube and the Linton-Nachlas tube. *Gastroenterology* 1978;75:566–569.
73. Umeyama K, Yoshikawa K, Yamashite T, et al: Transabdominal esophageal transection for esophageal varices: experience in 101 patients. *Br J Surg* 1983;70:419–422.
74. Uribe M, Ballesteros A, Strauss R, et al: Use of cardio-selective betablockers in portal hypertension: Relationship between bleeding varices and the portohepatic gradient. *Gastroenterology* 1983;84:1339.

75. Viallet A, Marleau D, Huet PM, et al: Hemodynamic evaluation of patients with intra-hepatic portal hypertension: Relationship between bleeding varices and the portohe-patic gradient. *Gastroenterology* 1975;69:1297–1300.
76. Westaby D, MacDougall BRD, Melia W, et al: A prospective randomized study of two sclerotherapy techniques for esophageal varices. *Hepatology* 1983;3:681–684.
77. Westaby D, Bihari DJ, Gimson AES, et al: Selective and non-selective beta-receptor blockade in the reduction of portal pressure in patients with cirrhosis and portal hyper-tension. *Gut* 1984;25:121–124.
78. Wink K: Acute and chronic effects of the beta-receptor blocker mepindolol on hemo-dynamics and the portal circulation. *Int J Clin Pharmacol Ther Toxicol* 1984;22:447–450.
79. Witzel L, Wolbergs E: Prospective Kontrollierte studie einer para and intravarikosen. Verodungstherapie bei osophagus varizen. *Schweiz Med Wochenschr* 1984;114:599–601.
80. Witzel L, Wolbergs E, Merki H: Prophylactic endoscopic sclerotherapy of esophageal varices. *Lancet* 1985;1:773–775.

12

Premalignancy of the Gastrointestinal Tract

Strategies for the Early Detection of Gastrointestinal Malignancy

Robert H. Riddell

1. INTRODUCTION

Premalignancy is a very broad term and needs further defining. Conceptually, the simplest definition is that premalignancy can be a condition, disease, or lesion; i.e., some factor increases the likelihood of a person developing a malignancy when compared with a control population without that factor. Examples of some of these factors can be as simple as age, for example, in colorectal carcinoma, or sex, as in the vast male predominance of adenocarcinoma complicating Barrett's esophagus or the presence of a ureterosigmoidostomy for large bowel cancer. Some diseases have a well-documented familial/hereditary component. Environmental factors may also be invoked, for example, the combination of alcohol and tobacco in the genesis of eosphageal squamous carcinoma.

A variety of benign *diseases* are known to predispose to gastrointestinal (GI) malignancy. For instance, in the stomach these include pernicious anemia and possibly the postgastrectomy stomach; in the periam-

Robert H. Riddell ● McMaster University Medical Centre, Hamilton, Ontario, Canada L8N 3Z5.

pullary region familial adenomatous polyposis coli can be associated with periampullary carcinomas; celiac sprue predisposes to the development of small intestinal lymphomas and carcinomas and possibly squamous carcinoma of the eosophagus; and in the large bowel inflammatory bowel disease, particularly ulcerative colitis, predisposes to adenocarcinoma of the colorectum.

The final level at which we may look at premalignancy is in premalignant *lesions*. These primarily are the adenomas wherever they occur in the GI tract but also dysplasia, the latter being particularly prevalent in diseases characterized by long-standing chronic inflammation.

Strategies for the early detection of GI malignancy involve a separate concept, namely, the early detection of invasive carcinoma as contrasted to the detection of noninvasive premalignant lesions discussed above. Currently, the pathological staging of these patients is purely a matter of chance; some will be relatively early and fortunately cured whereas similar patients may have disseminated disease and die rapidly. Implicit in the early detection of invasive carcinoma is the fact that early detection will result in an increased cure rate and not just increased survival times which might be the result of intrinsic biases such as lead time bias. Clinical strategies for early detection are surprisingly limited and will be discussed below. Nevertheless, it is important to decide whether one is searching primarily for premalignant as opposed to early invasive lesions, as the latter will occasionally prove to be advanced and will be associated with a definite mortality from disseminated carcinoma. This is much less likely when dealing with premalignant lesions as any invasive tumor found will be unexpected and therefore less likely to be advanced at the time of detection.

In this chapter I shall use the model of colorectal carcinoma as this embraces the spectrum of changes that may be found elsewhere in the GI tract.

2. PREMALIGNANT LESIONS

The main concept of looking for premalignant lesions can only be effective if at least the vast majority of invasive carcinomas arise from them. Thus, if the majority of carcinomas really did arise *de novo,* there would be little point in searching for preinvasive lesions. In the case of adenocarcinoma of the large intestine there is considerable evidence that most tumors probably have their origin in adenomas. What, then, is an adenoma?

Adenomas. An adenoma is a benign proliferation of neoplastic epithelium which can be readily identified by the presence of enlarged cells containing enlarged, usually hyperchromatic nuclei which produce a pseudostratified (picket fence) appearance, as illustrated in Fig. 1. Thus, any polypoid lesion in the GI tract that is composed of epithelium of this type is by definition an adenoma. Adenomas have a virtually identical morphology whether they occur in the large intestine, small intestine, or stomach. Furthermore, in the large bowel it is well documented that adenomas are more likely to have an associated invasive adenocarcinoma (i.e., infiltration into the submucosa), the likelihood being related to increasing size, increasing dysplasia, and the presence of a villus component.[1] Although this is useful information, it does not help in deciding whether an individual adenoma encountered clinically does or does not have an associated invasive carcinoma. Only resection of the polyp and histological examination of the specimen will determine this point. Nevertheless, one of the most interesting features of adenomas is that there needs to be a critical mass of about 5 mm of adenoma for invasion to occur. Beneath this figure invasion is excessively rare and can still be "written up."

A further study that strongly suggests that adenomas predispose to carcinoma is that of Gilbertson and Nelms[2] in which over 21,000 patients were examined over a 25-year period. All had sigmoidoscopy, and any polyps that were found were removed. In this population there were 27 initial cancers, but in the follow-up period, although between 85 and 100 cancers were expected, only five were encountered. One of these infiltrated into the muscularis propria, but the remaining four only reached the submucosa. It therefore appears that removal of incidental polyps, presumably including most adenomas, is effective in preventing subsequent rectal carcinoma. Nevertheless, even this study is not controlled and subject to a variety of biases.

As mentioned earlier, adenomas occurring in other parts of the GI tract are also predisposed to develop into invasive carcinoma. As with large-bowel adenomas we remain relatively ignorant about which adenomas tend to grow rather than remain stationary in size and which of those that grow ultimately become invasive. Furthermore, our knowledge of the time frames involved is sadly inadequate. From the management viewpoint it seems reasonable to assume that once a patient has developed an adenoma at any observable site, the premalignant potential of this organ has been demonstrated, and regular follow-up should be instituted. The means and interval between follow-up procedures will vary depending on local availability and should probably include routine air contrast barium studies or endoscopy every 2 or 3 years.

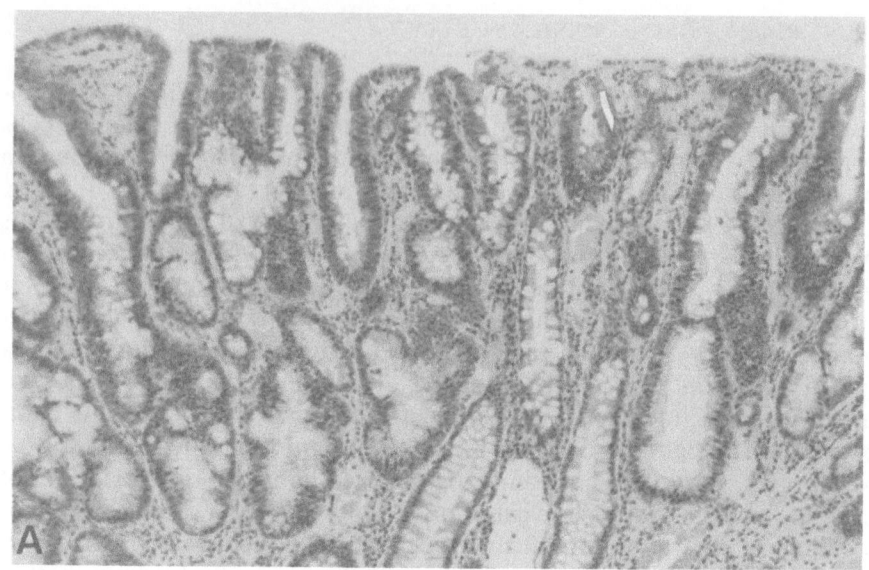

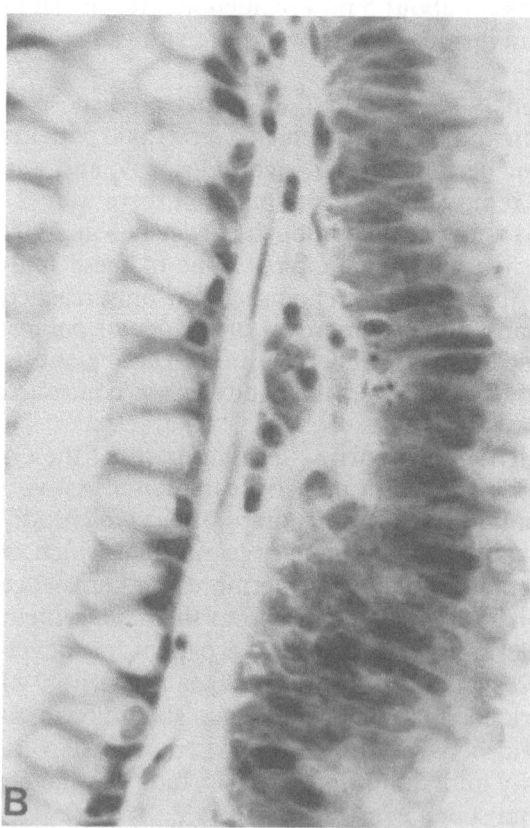

Figure 1. (A) Typical tubular adenoma in which the neoplastic glands, left and extreme right, can be contrasted with a few residual nonneoplastic glands just right of center. (B) Contrast between a normal gland (left) and a neoplastic (dysplastic) gland. The differences are apparent at a glance. In an appropriate clinical setting the abnormal gland would be "low-grade" dysplasia because the nuclei are largely retained in the basal half of the cells.

3. "FAMILIAL" LARGE-BOWEL CANCER

The familial diseases are best exemplified by the hereditary polyposis syndromes—familial adenomatous polyposis coli and, much less commonly, juvenile or Peutz-Jegher's polyposis. The familial nature of usual large-bowel carcinoma is surprisingly neglected, in view of the large impact that this might have on the number of patients presenting annually with advanced colorectal carcinoma.

The potential familial nature of "sporadic" colorectal carcinoma is exemplified by Lovett's study in which death certificates of relatives of patients with colorectal carcinoma were examined.[3] In this study it was found that 7–10% of parents of probands had died of the disease, and about 16% of their brothers and 18% of their sisters had also died of the disease. If one assumes that the overall mortality of this disease is about 50%, this would then imply that the prevalence figures of this disease are about double those stated. Practically, this means that perhaps one in three siblings of patients with large-bowel cancer might themselves develop the same disease. This sort of risk is surely such that regular surveillance of this group of patients should be seriously considered. Furthermore, it could even be argued that routine management and follow-up of patients with large-bowel carcinoma should include routine investigation of siblings and any living parents. It remains to be seen whether their offspring are at similarly high risk.

It should also be remembered that there are a variety of hereditary colon cancer syndromes which admittedly are all relatively uncommon but which tend to be characterized by the development of colon cancer, usually right-sided and at an earlier age than the general population, frequently while in the 40s. These include cancer family syndrome (hereditary adenocarcinomatosis in which carcinoma of the right colon occurs in association with gastric, uterine, ovarian, or breast carcinoma often in combination); hereditary gastrocolonic cancer with double primaries in either or both organs; hereditary colorectal cancer in which family members develop carcinoma (frequently at the same site in the colon); and Muir's (Torre's) syndrome, in which there is also an association with skin appendage tumors. It could, therefore, also be argued that the routine family history that is taken should include not only what relatives have died of, but careful enquiry as to whether they developed colorectal carcinoma.

Dysplasia. Dysplasia in the GI tract can be defined as an unequivocally neoplastic proliferation essentially equivalent to an adenoma; it usually occurs on the background of a long-standing inflammatory disease. It excludes all equivocal or regenerative lesions and may be the superficial part of an invasive carcinoma. The main differences between dysplasia and adenomas are that macroscopically adenomas can be regarded as well-circumscribed nodules of benign neoplastic tissue, whereas dysplasia is better regarded as a similar change in flat mucosa. In inflammatory conditions, however, a second difference becomes apparent. Adenomatous glands are readily distinguished from their adjacent "control," nonneoplastic crypts/glands (Fig.1B). In fact, in familial adenomatous polyposis coli even single crypts are easily distinguishable from their nonneoplastic counterparts. In inflammatory disorders such as Barrett's esophagus or inflammatory bowel disease, this change is part of a spectrum; any divisions within this spectrum are necessarily arbitrary and subjective. For this reason, biopsies taken to assess the presence of dysplasia can be categorized as negative, indefinite, and positive for dysplasia.[4] Those that are positive will look essentially like adenomas, those that are negative will resemble the normal mucosa, and the indefinite group is that part of the spectrum where one is uncertain whether progression from negative to positive is occurring, or whether changes are stable. Rebiopsy over several months and on several occasions may be necessary to establish the stability of these lesions or whether adjacent areas of unequivocal dysplasia are also present.

Changes that are negative for dysplasia include the whole gamut of regenerative changes that may be seen in these inflammatory conditions. Because this actively regenerating stage is characterized by enlarged vesicular nuclei with prominent eosinophilic nucleoli, confusion with neoplastic change can readily occur. Nevertheless, once these changes are recognized, such confusion is largely eliminated.[4]

The final point of this definition of dysplasia is that it may be the superficial part of an invasive carcinoma. It should be recognized that this may occur in the absence of *in situ* carcinoma. The original concept of the genesis of invasive carcinoma as going through different stages of dysplasia such as from mild to moderate to severe and finally to *in situ* carcinoma before becoming invasive has now given way to the concept that any dysplastic epithelium can give rise directly to infiltrating carcinoma without going through *in situ* phase. Indeed, it is imperative to recognize this, for if one chooses to follow low-grade dysplasia, it should be recognized that one is deliberately following a lesion that can directly give rise to invasive carcinoma and may therefore already have exerted that potential. Furthermore, these carcinomas may not be recognized clinically in patients with inflammatory disorders.

The distinction between a first "diagnostic" endoscopy and subsequent "surveillance" endoscopy is worth observing, particularly if dysplasia is found. This is likely to be much more serious when dysplasia is discovered on first rather than a subsequent endoscopy because in the former the length of time that dysplasia has been present is unknown and is probably more likely to be accompanied by an underlying invasive component.[5]

Although the classic descriptions of dysplasia are found in inflammatory bowel disease, it should be recognized that dysplasia in Barrett's esophagus is well documented but its significance is even more poorly documented than in inflammatory bowel disease. In both diseases we currently do not know the likelihood of an accompanying invasive carcinoma being present when either low-grade or high-grade dysplasia is found, an incidence that almost certainly rises if an endoscopic lesion has been detected and probably also rises further if found at the first endoscopy. However, Barrett's esophagus is unique in that of all the precancerous lesions occurring in the GI tract, this is the only one in which the precipitating disease (gastroesophageal reflux in this case) can be prevented by an antireflux operation. It is, therefore, interesting to speculate whether the removal of the underlying driving force can be accompanied by reversal of dysplastic or equivocal biopsies. Examples of regrowth squamous epithelium over typical Barrett's mucosa can certainly occur in this disease.[6]

4. STRATEGIES FOR EARLY DETECTION

Follow-up strategies or options are surprisingly straightforward and fall into one of five categories. These are

1. Do nothing.
2. Regular follow-up and biopsy.
3. Follow-up and biopsy at short intervals.
4. Removal of the driving force of the disease.
5. Excision of the diseased organ.

Doing nothing can be advocated in patients in poor health in whom further surgery would not be contemplated even if anything was found. Regular follow-up is carried out in patients without evidence of dysplasia. Early repeat biopsy (e.g., 1–3 months) is indicated in patients with suspicious or possibly dysplastic lesions for confirmation. Removal of the driving force could be contemplated in patients with Barrett's esophagus, possibly even those with low-grade dysplasia. Excision would include colectomy in ulcerative colitis or esophagectomy in Barrett's esophagus with dysplasia.

One of the most challenging aspects of GI disease today is when to change the mode of follow-up from one of these categories to another, particularly when this involves local surgery. Similarly, this is a juncture at which it is imperative to know whether one is dealing with cancer prevention, i.e., the detection of premalignant diseases or cases where early invasive cancer may be acceptable. The latter may only be acceptable if discovered early pathologically. Unfortunately, we are still not at the stage where this can be guaranteed.

Since the publication of the classification of dysplasia in inflammatory bowel disease the classification has been adapted with success at many hospitals.[7,8] Some newer techniques, including the use of mucins[9] or lectin binding, particularly with peanut lectin agglutinin[10] and other epithelial markers, now seem less specific than originally thought. However, it seems that measurement of DNA content using flow cytometry may be of value, particularly in predicting patients with ulcerative colitis with dysplasia or carcinoma.[11]

REFERENCES

1. Muto T, Bussey HJR, Morson BC: The evolution of cancer of the colon and rectum. *Cancer* 1975;36:2251–2270.
2. Gilbertson VA, Nelms JM: The prevention of invasive cancer of the rectum. *Cancer* 1978;41:1137–1139.
3. Lovett E. Family studies in cancer of the colon and rectum. *Br J Surg* 1976;63:13–18.
4. Riddell RH, Goldman H, Ransohoff DF, et al: Dysplasia inflammatory bowel disease. Standardized classification with provisional clinical applications. *Hum Pathol* 1983;14:931–968.
5. Fuson JA, Farmer RS, Hawk WA, Sullivan BH: Endoscopic surveillance for cancer in chronic ulcerative colitis. *Am J Gastroenterol* 1980;73:120–126.
6. Skinner DB, Walther BC, Riddell RH, et al: Barrett's esophagus. Comparison of benign and malignant cases. *Ann Surg* 1983;198:554–565.
7. Allen DC, Biggart JD, Pyper PC: Large bowel mucosal dysplasia and carcinoma in ulcerative colitis. *J Clin Pathol* 1985;38:30–43.
8. Rosenstock E, Farmer RG, Petras R, et al: Surveillance for colonic carcinoma in ulcerative colitis. *Gastroenterology* 1985;89:1342–1346.
9. Ehsanullah M, Morgan MN, Filipe MI, Gazzard B: Sialomucins in the assessment of dysplasia and cancer-risk patients with ulcerative colitis treated with colectomy and ileo-rectal anastomosis. *Histopathology* 1985;9:223–235.

10. Boland CR, Lance P, Levin B, et al: Abnormal goblet cell glycoconjugates in rectal biopsies associated with an increased risk of neoplasia in patients with ulcerative colitis: Early results of prospective study. *Gut* 1984;25:1364–1371.
11. Allen DC, Biggart JD, Orchin JC, Foster H: An immunoperoxidase study of epithelial marker antigens in ulcerative colitis with dysplasia and carcinoma. *J Clin Pathol* 1985;38:18–29.

13

Recent Advances in Gastrointestinal Radiology

Giles W. Stevenson

1. INTRODUCTION

The theme of this chapter is the need for closer integration between the various branches of clinical gastroenterology. To illustrate the theme I will review six aspects of gastrointestinal (GI) radiology.

2. HEARTBURN, CHEST PAIN, AND DYSPHAGIA

When patients are suspected of having gastroesophageal reflux disease, barium examination is the appropriate initial investigation.[1] When performed with care, it will demonstrate spontaneous reflux in about half the patients with reflux and, when used with the provocative water siphon test, will demonstrate reflux in almost all. Once reflux has been induced, the ability of the esophagus to clear refluxed acidic fluid can be documented, together with secondary motility disorders such as impairment of the primary wave or the presence of nonpropulsive contractions. Barium swallow can reliably demonstrate moderate or severe esophagitis,[2] and although the presence of a radiological hiatus hernia is of no value, the absence of an inducible hernia makes gastroesophageal reflux disease very unlikely. In most patients with reflux disease barium swallow is the only investigation required.

Giles W. Stevenson • McMaster University, Hamilton, Ontario, Canada L8N 3Z5.

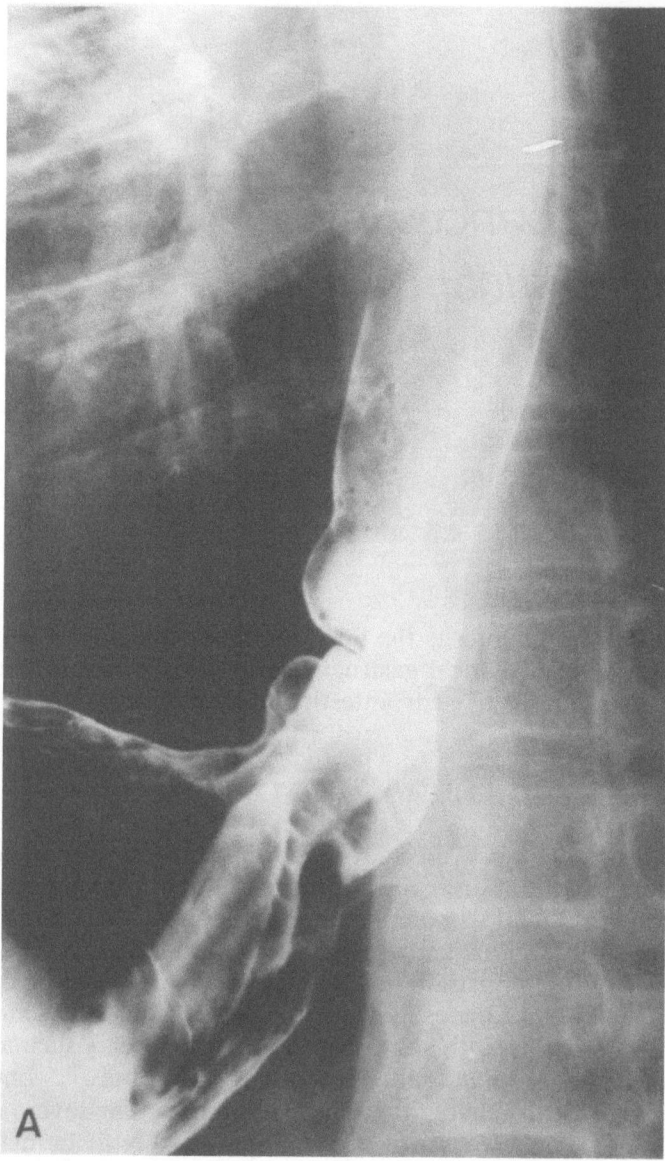

Figure 1. Prone oblique view showing the clarity with which rings can be demonstrated above a hiatus hernia (A), when this position is used to raise intraabdominal pressure and

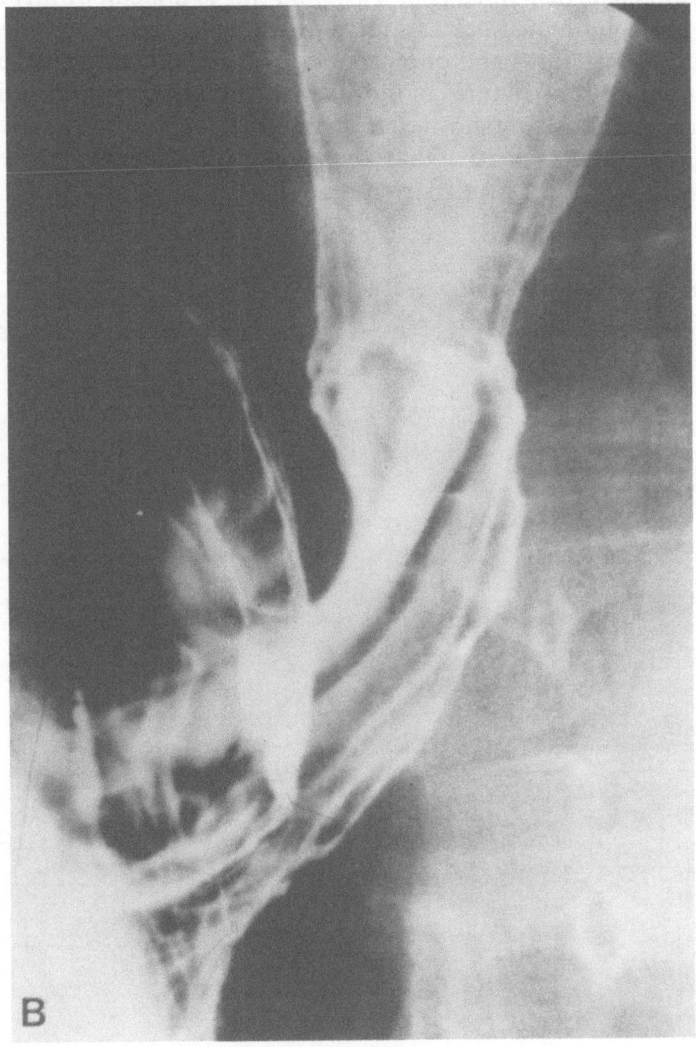

ensure distention. (B) The same projection demonstrating a hiatus hernia, esophagitis, and limited distensibility of the lower end of the esophagus.

Several studies have documented the inadequacies of the conventional barium swallow in excluding stricture in patients with dysphagia. A prone oblique view is an important technique to show the lower end of the esophagus distended (Fig. 1). When this is difficult or inconclusive, the use of a solid bolus such as a marshmallow provides a reliable method of excluding strictures and of reproducing the symptoms of dysphagia in patients with mild strictures of motility disturbances. A prospective comparison with endoscopy showed the marshmallow barium swallow (Fig. 2) to be slightly more sensitive than the pediatric endoscope, particularly in the detection of mild peptic strictures.[3]

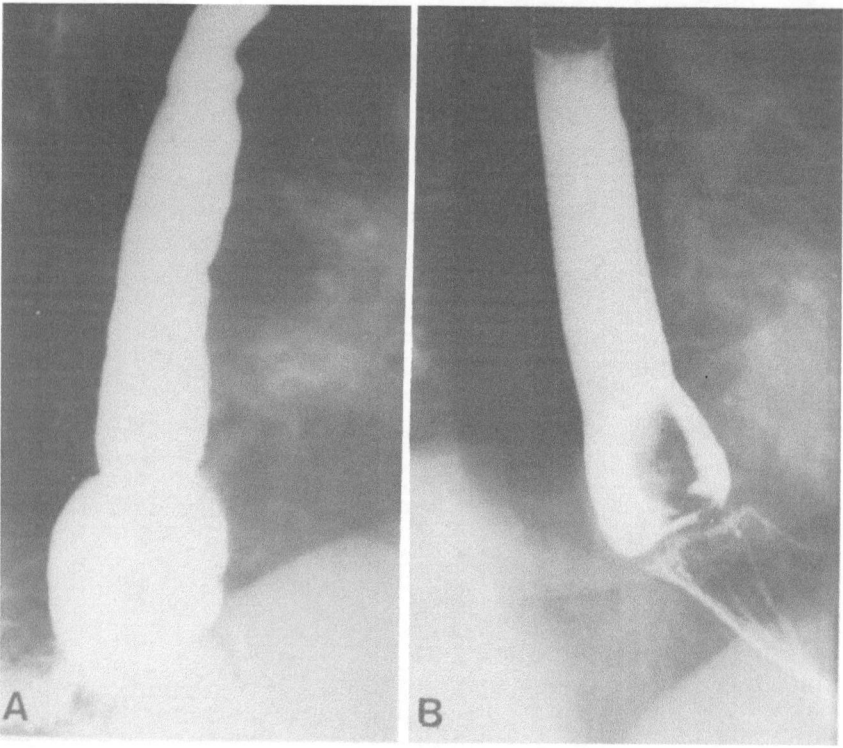

Figure 2. Fifty-seven-year-old man with intermittent dysphagia. Supine film while swallowing barium suggests hiatus hernia but does not reveal stricture (A). Half of a large marshmallow has impacted in his gastroesophageal junction ring, supported a column of barium, and also reproduced his dysphagia (B). When the routine films are negative, the marshmallow is a useful method to avoid overlooking a mild stricture.

A substantial minority of patients with atypical chest pain, in whom a cardiac cause has been excluded, will have pain due to esophageal disease.[4] Of these, most have reflux disease and a small proportion have a primary motility disorder. Manometry may be required to sort out these problems, although the finding of abnormal motility does not mean that it is the cause of the patient's symptoms. Provocative drugs such as ergonovine, bethanecol, or edrophonium may help to reproduce both the symptoms and the abnormal motility at the same time. Motility laboratories are not yet widely available, and a carefully performed barium swallow with video recording, induction of reflux and clearance assessment, use of a marshmallow as a provocative test, and possibly the use of Tensilon (edrophonium chloride) as a provocative agent will enable a diagnosis to be made radiologically in many of these patients. Barium fluoroscopy is unable to diagnose nutcracker esophagus since in these patients all that will be observed is an apparently normal, effective primary peristaltic wave which may be revealed by manometry to be of very high pressure and prolonged duration. If barium swallow is to remain competitive and useful in the endoscopic and manometric era, it requires meticulous technique, extensive use of video recording, assessment of esophageal motility and clearance, and the use of provocative agents.

3. DYSPEPSIA

Most patients referred to gastroenterologists with dyspepsia have already had previous investigations including barium x rays, and it is appropriate that in these difficult patients endoscopy should be used as the primary investigation. However, the majority of patients with dyspepsia are seen by family physicians and treated symptomatically. Many are referred for imaging of the upper GI tract without reference to gastroenterologists and will have barium meals because that is what is available to family physicians. The question arises whether these patients should be having endoscopy?

Dyspeptic patients can be divided into four groups: fit, healthy individuals with no previous ulcer history; physically impaired or immobile patients with no previous history of gastric disease; patients with known previous gastric or duodenal ulceration; and patients with previous gastric or duodenal surgery. In the first group high-quality barium meals can be performed with an accuracy up to 95% of that achieved by endoscopy.[5] If high-quality radiology is available, and costs half of what endoscopy

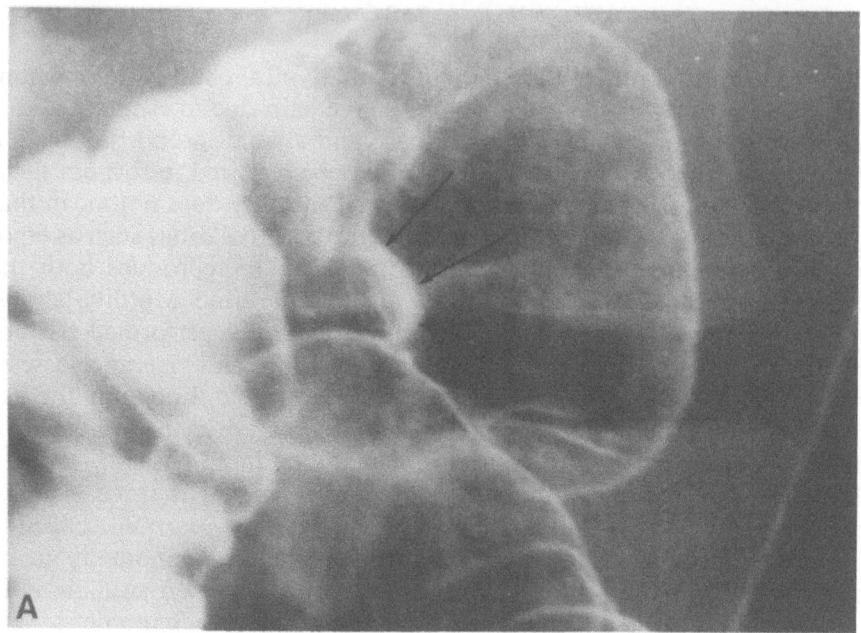

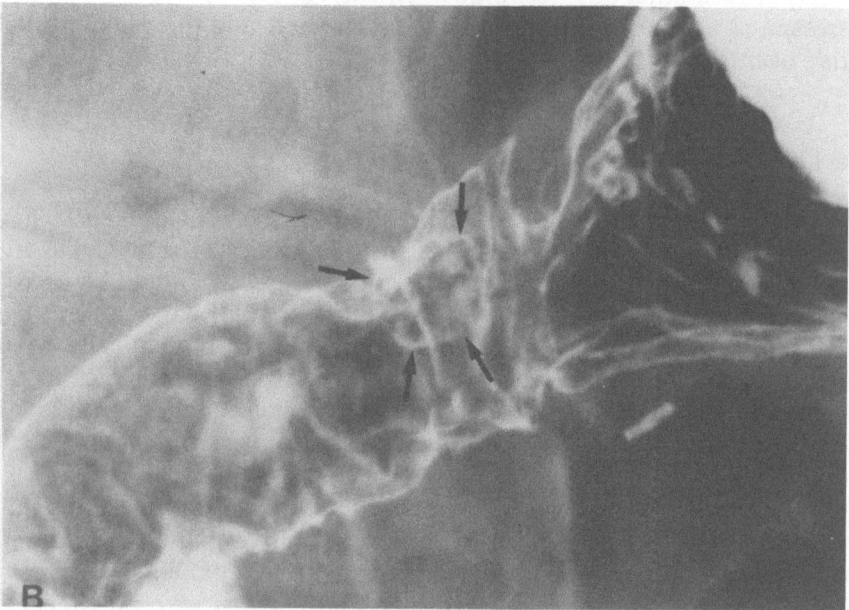

Figure 3. Two patients with duodenal ulceration. The first (A) has a linear ulcer diagnosed on this film with moderate confidence and confirmed endoscopically. Many ulcers become linear as they heal, but the moderate confidence expressed on these findings was clinically inadequate for the referring physician. The patient was 22 years old, was being seen for the first time, and an unequivocal diagnosis was required. The second patient (B and C) had

does, it should arguably be the investigation of choice (Fig. 3). However, studies have shown that in some settings many patients prefer endoscopy to barium meal, and, therefore, if costs are similar, it would be reasonable to offer endoscopy as a first-line investigation. For patients who are immobile and in whom poor-quality barium meals will be performed, and in patients with duodenal ulcer disease in the past[6] or previous gastric

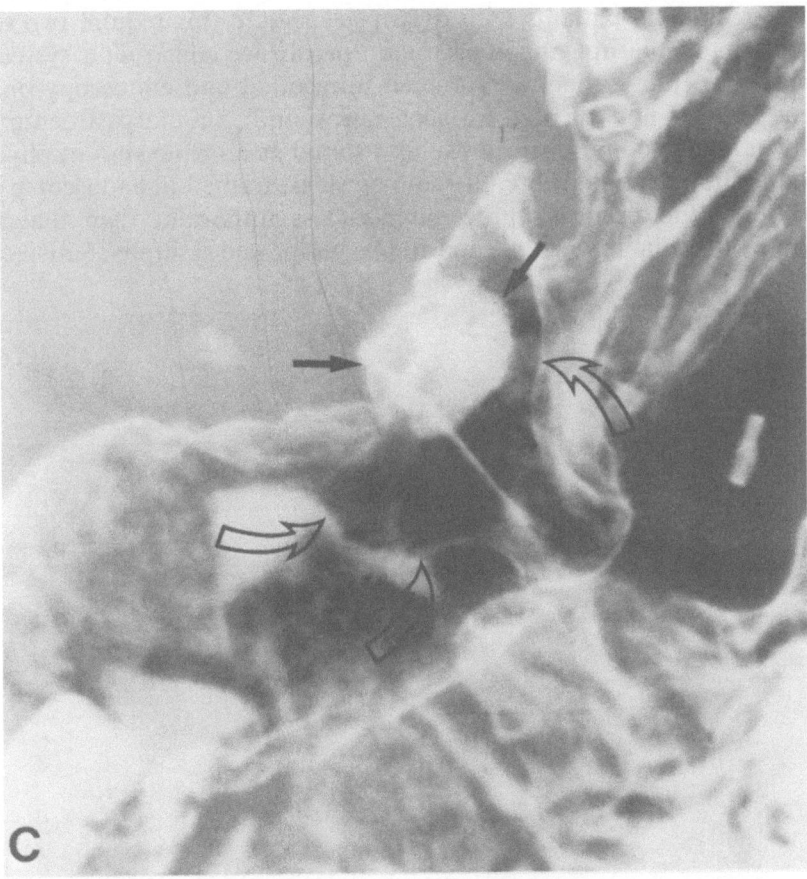

had an antrectomy and presented with further abdominal pain. Although endoscopy would be the more appropriate investigation, in this instance the films revealed a duodenal ulcer with a clarity that permits complete confidence in the diagnosis. The ulcer (arrows) can be seen as a ring shadow (A), and also barium filled (B) with surrounding edema (open arrows).

survery,[7] the evidence clearly shows that barium radiology is not very accurate and endoscopy should be used.

How does a radiology department to whom these patients are referred obtain endoscopic examination rather than perform inappropriate barium studies? There is a need for an integrated GI service,[8] for rapid and flexible rescheduling.

In some patients with dyspepsia, the cause is found in the biliary tract rather than in the stomach or duodenum. A case can therefore be made for using ultrasound of the gallbladder as one of the two primary investigations in patients with dyspepsia. Should this require two separate visits to the imaging department, or can we construct a system in which dyspeptic patients are offered ultrasound and endoscopy on the same visit? Who will perform such ultrasound? Should gastroenterologists in a large clinic learn to use ultrasound as an extension of physical examination? Should more GI radiologists be trained in endoscopic procedures? Who performs procedures is less important than that they should be available when needed and be performed skillfully. Satisfactory

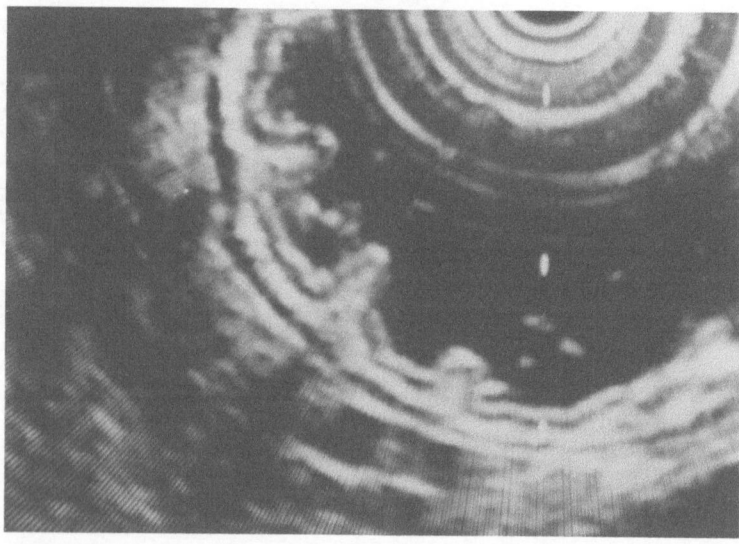

Figure 4. Endoscopic ultrasound image of the gastric wall using a 7.5-MHz mechanically rotating transducer. Several layers of alternating high and low echogenicity can be seen. These represent acoustic interfaces that correspond roughly but not exactly with the histological layers. A broad area of high echogenicity, for example, appears to include both the submucosa and the superficial part of the muscularis propria.

answers to these questions may require some adjustment to conventional boundaries of subspecialization.

3.1. Endoscopic Ultrasound

This procedure has been developing over the last few years and is now showing promise of clinical usefulness.[9] It gives magnificent views of the heart and, from the GI point of view, can show mediastinal and esophageal wall disease clearly and show very small liver lesions and pancreatic abnormalities, especially pancreatic endocrine tumors. It provides detail of gastric and esophageal wall invasion that is not obtainable by any other form of imaging (Fig. 4). The equipment is expensive and requires physicians who are endoscopists and who are prepared to devote the time to become expert at ultrasound interpretation, and therefore the procedure will only come slowly into clinical use.

4. CHOLELITHIASIS AND JAUNDICE

Gallbladder ultrasound has been shown to have an accuracy equal to, or slightly better than, oral cholecystogram for the detection of gallstones and is now the investigation of choice. However, oral cholecystography (with tomograms if opacification is poor) does have a sensitivity of around 95%. There is, therefore, still a place for the oral cholecystogram when ultrasound is technically difficult, or when the ultrasound report is at variance with the likely clinical diagnosis.

Three recent radiological studies raise interesting questions about the future management of cholelithiasis. A report by Niederau et al. described bile duct diameters in 830 blood donors.[10] The mean diameters were 2.8 mm for those with normal biliary systems, 4.8 mm for those with stones in the gallbladder, and 6.2 mm for those with previous cholecystectomy. The finding of slightly increased bile duct diameters in the presence of gallbladder stones is most easily explained by the assumption that when patients are forming small gallstones, they are being passed through the sphincter in large numbers every time the gallbladder contracts and reduces its volume. It may well be that the symptoms of biliary dyspepsia are principally due to the passage of these small concretions through the spincter of Oddi. The second report is one from London showing that when patients with stones in the gallbladder have an endoscopic sphincterotomy for duct stone, 50% of such patients have emptied their gallbladders of stones within 6 months. Third, there are now several reports indicating that following such spincterotomy the likelihood of cholectystectomy being required later is low, between 5 and 12% by 3–5 years.[11] Moreover, at least half of these operations were performed within the first month after spincterotomy, suggesting that the original problem was probably the gallbladder, rather than the duct stone. These three pieces of evidence together raise the possibility that endoscopic spincterotomy might be an appropriate treatment for cholelithiasis (Fig. 5).

The role of ultrasound in the investigation of jaundice has recently been questioned. Connon has suggested that because an ultrasound report of a nondilated biliary duct cannot always be relied on, direct cholangiography should be the initial investigation in patients with jaundice.[12] Standards of ultrasound do vary, and a normal ultrasound report

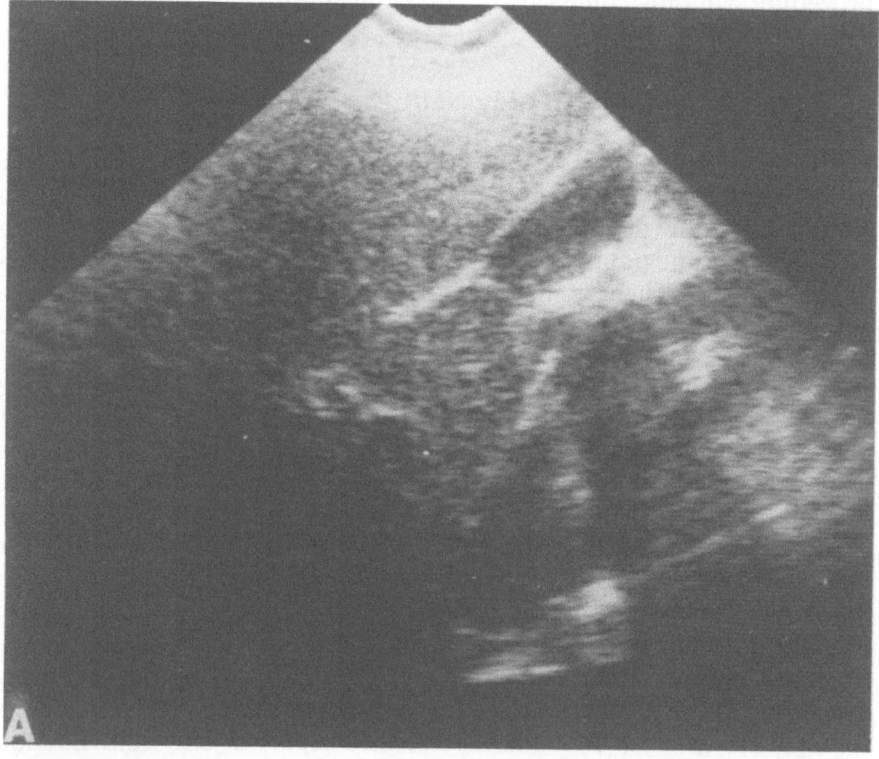

Figure 5. Ultrasound images from a female patient, aged 24, who developed severe pancreatitis 3 months postpartum. On transfer to a teaching hospital 4 weeks later she had a pancreatic abscess and ultrasound showed stones in the gallbladder (A). She was treated by percutaneous abscess drainage and by endoscopic sphincterotomy (which produced a gush

in the presence of suspicious blood chemistry should not delay direct cholangiography. However, the main reason for performing ultrasound examination is to help direct the most appropriate form of direct imaging. If ultrasound shows a large mass in the porta hepatis with very high obstruction, percutaneous cholangiography may be appropriate (Fig. 6). If ultrsound shows numerous hepatic metastases, liver biopsy may be more useful. If ultrasound shows a low obstruction or the presence of stones, endoscopic retrograde pancreatography (ERCP) with possible spincterotomy or stenting may be indicated. Thus, ultrasound does retain a useful initial role in patients with jaundice.

Most gastroenterologists still peform liver biopsy blindly. This seems a little odd to radiologists who are accustomed to using ultrasound or

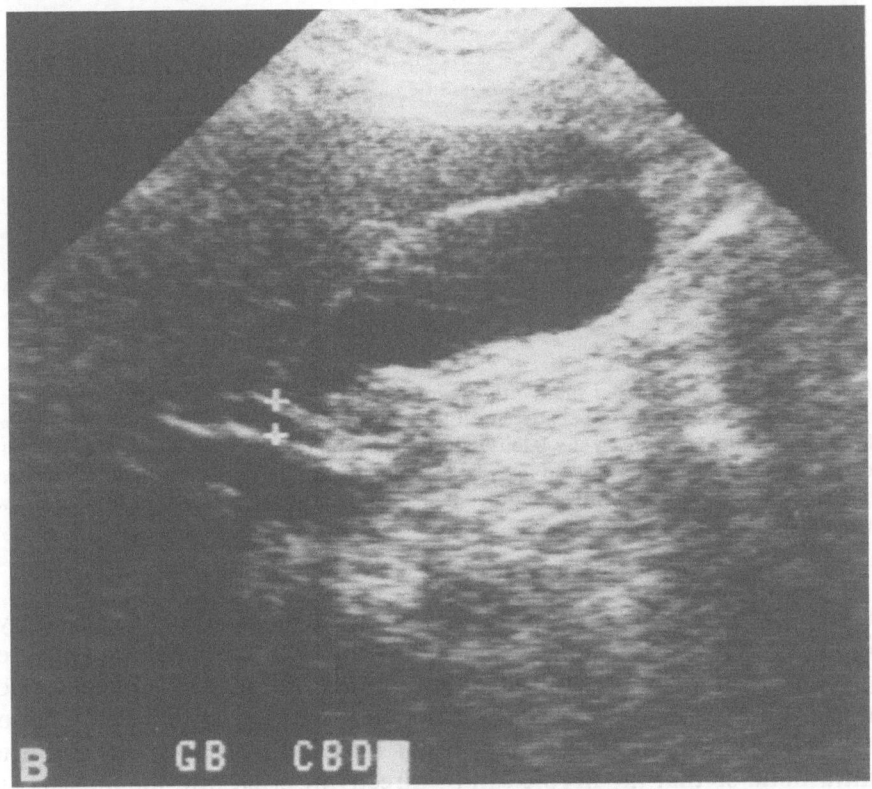

of pus and gravel from the bile duct). Elective cholecystectomy was scheduled, but follow-up preliminary ultrasound study 6 months after discharge from hospital showed that the gallbladder was free of stones (B). She remains well 1 year later.

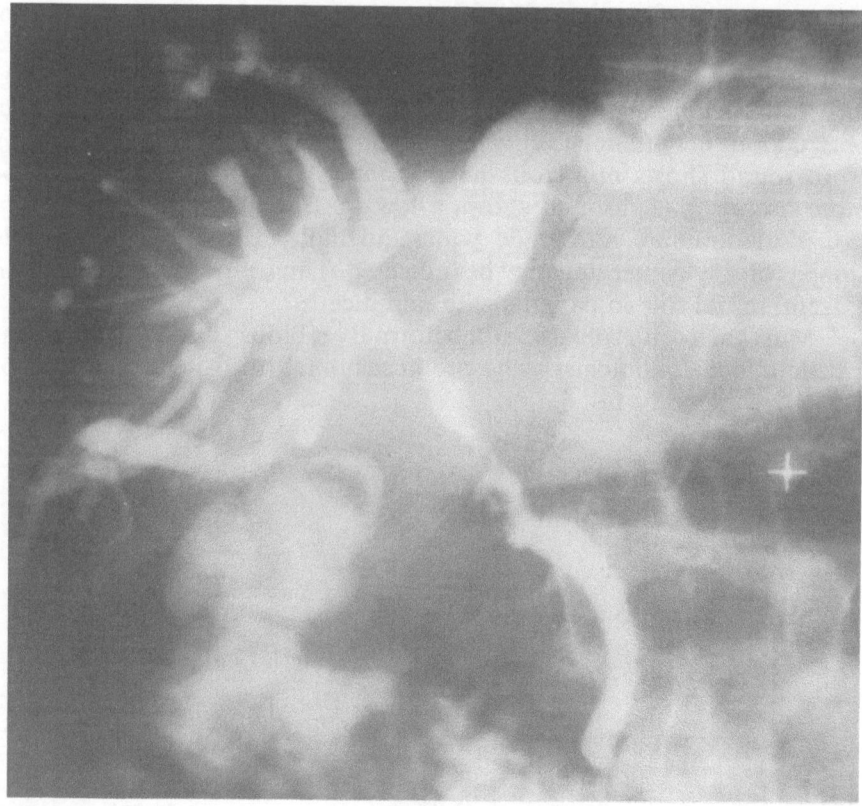

Figure 6. Sixty-four-year-old man with progressive jaundice and weight loss. Ultrasound showed a mass in the porta hepatis, and ERCP was unhelpful in that it showed only the lower end of the stricture in the bile duct. Transhepatic cholangiography showed the full extent of the malignant lesion and allowed insertion of a drainage catheter which provided effective palliation for 4 months. Endoscopic palliation is at present best for lesions below the bifurcation.

computerized tomography (CT) for guiding their needles. When biopsy is performed for diffuse liver disease, it may be reasonable not to use guidance, although even in that situation why risk putting a large needle through a major branch of the portal vein when it is not necessary to do so? When peforming a liver biopsy for metastatic disease, why not use ultrasound so that the needle can be directly inserted into the metastasis instead of putting it in blindly and passing it between the three lesions present in the right lobe of the liver? Depending on the degree of impaired coagulation, a wise gastroenterologist would not do a liver biopsy in patients with defective clotting. The transjugular approach under fluoro-scopic control offers a safer alternative approach.[13] Many radiologists plug the liver track with a Gelfoam plug after transhepatic procedures, but this practice has not yet found much acceptance among gastroenterologists.

5. DIARRHEA AND INFLAMMATORY BOWEL DISEASE

Double-contast barium enema is established as the technique of choice for radiology of the colon. The best method of imaging the small bowel is not clear. Small-bowel enema is extolled as being much more accurate than the small-bowel meal or barium follow-through, but the evidence for this is poor. Moreover, small-bowel enema is more expensive, much more uncomfortable for the patient, involves a greater radiation dose, and takes much more physician time. There is no good evidence that the slightly better detail is useful in diagnosing Crohn's disease. The carefully performed small-bowel meal done as a specific small-bowel examination is probably just as good,[14] with the possible exceptions of looking for minor stenoses (in which case a rapid flow rate is helpful), and looking for small tumors in patients who have been bleeding. Although refinements in technique are needed for the small-bowel meal to improve the rather poor images that we often produce, it seems doubtful that routine enteroclysis is the answer.

A common radiological problem is the difficult terminal ileum in which radiologists cannot be certain whether slight nodularity represents disease or is a variant of normality, particularly in teen-agers and young adults (Figs. 7 and 8). In these patients direct colonoscopic inspection of the terminal ileum is invaluable, and permits biopsy and fluid collection.[15,16]

Barium enema usually provides adequate imaging of the colon in patients with inflammatory bowel disease. Double-contrast enema will reveal active ulcerative colitis and Crohn's disease with almost the same reliability as colonoscopy, and although endoscopy shows a greater extent of colitis than is detectable on barium enema, there is no evidence that this is clinically important. Barium enema appearances are, however, almost never specific to particular diseases, and biopsy and culture will frequently be required. Barium enema appearances of Crohn's disease may be mimicked by amebiasis, herpes infection, and occasionally ischemia. The appearances of ulcerative colitis may be seen in numerous infections, particularly *Campylobacter,* and pseudomembranous colitis may give similar appearances. Thus, barium enema is excellent for detecting an abnormality but less good at making specific diagnoses.[17]

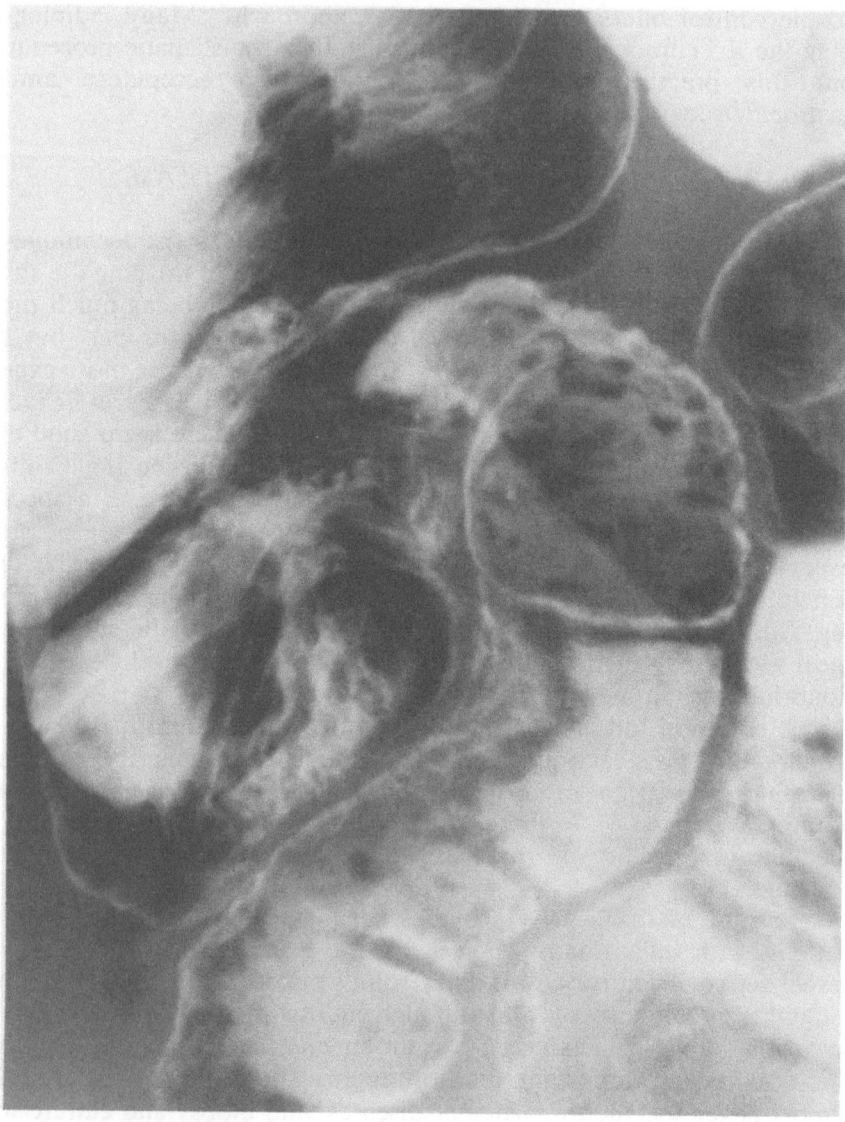

Figure 7. Normal lymphoid tissue in the terminal ileum of a 17-year-old male patient. No colonoscopy is required here, but in a patient aged 50 this amount of lymphoid tissue would pose a diagnostic problem.

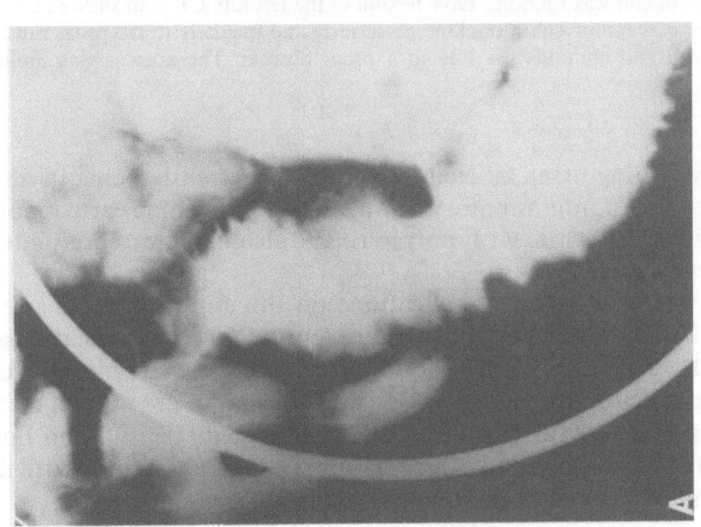

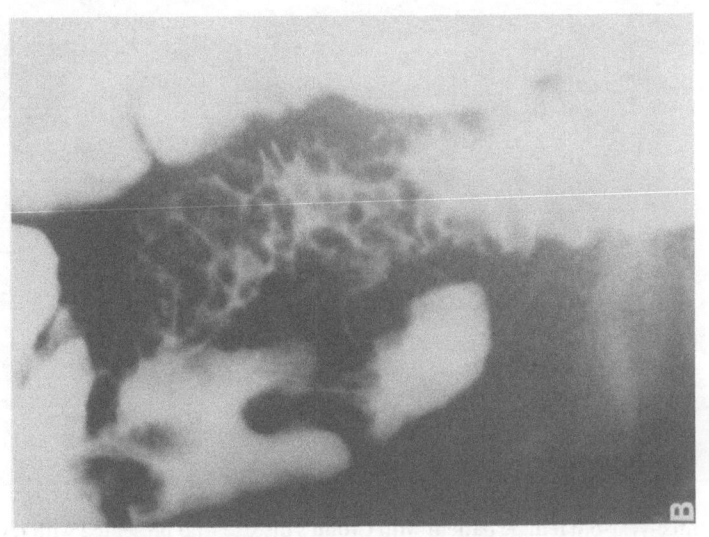

Figure 8. Thickened folds and nodularity in a 15-year-old boy. No ulceration is visible, and *Yersinia* infection was suggested as the likely diagnosis with Crohn's disease a less likely possibility. The radiological appearances are not specific. The diagnosis was confirmed when *Yersinia* was cultured from the stool, but otherwise colonoscopy and ileal biopsy would have been helpful.

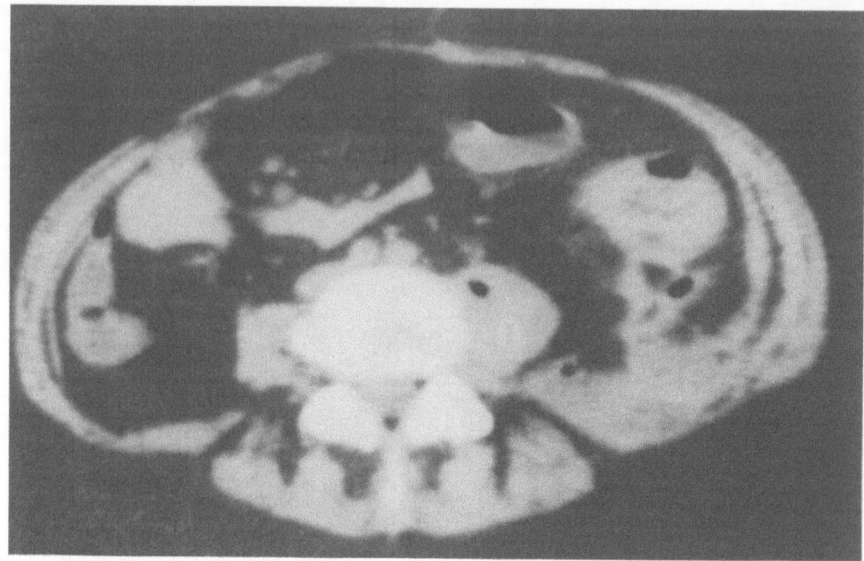

Figure 9. Forty-three-year-old female patient with Crohn's disease who presented with fever and abdominal pain and was found to have flexion of the left hip. CT scan showed a mass around the upper descending colon tracking posteriorly and medially to the psoas muscle, which is expanded and contains gas due to a psoas abscess. The abscess was drained percutaneously.

Indium scanning using labeled leukocytes is currently being investigated for detection of inflammatory bowel disease, and some early reports are encouraging.[18] Labeling with porphyrins is also being explored but is not yet clinically useful.[19]

There have been several publications on the appearances of ultrasound and CT scanning in patients with inflammatory bowel disease, particularly Crohn's disease.[20,21] The different appearances are now recognized, but the precise indications for each examination are not yet clear. In general, they are useful when abscess is suspected (Fig. 9), and both may be helpful in guiding percutaneous drainage of abscess in patients with inflammatory bowel disease.

6. ANORECTAL DYSFUNCTION

Evacuation proctography is becoming popular for investigation of this problem. A barium paste is introduced into the rectum and the patient is examined fluoroscopically with video recording and spot films, in the lateral projection, while sitting on a commode. Pelvic floor movement is assessed with the patient at rest, squeezing, straining, and evacuating. Adequacy of the anal sphincter, ability of the levator ani to lift and descend, and ability of the puborectalis sling to relax and contract appropriately can all be assessed. During evacuation intrarectal intussusception can be observed (Fig. 10) together with the formation of a rectocoele or external prolapse. There are not many reports available yet, but it looks as though the examination, which is simple to perform, may turn out to be useful in planning therapy in some of these patients.[22,23]

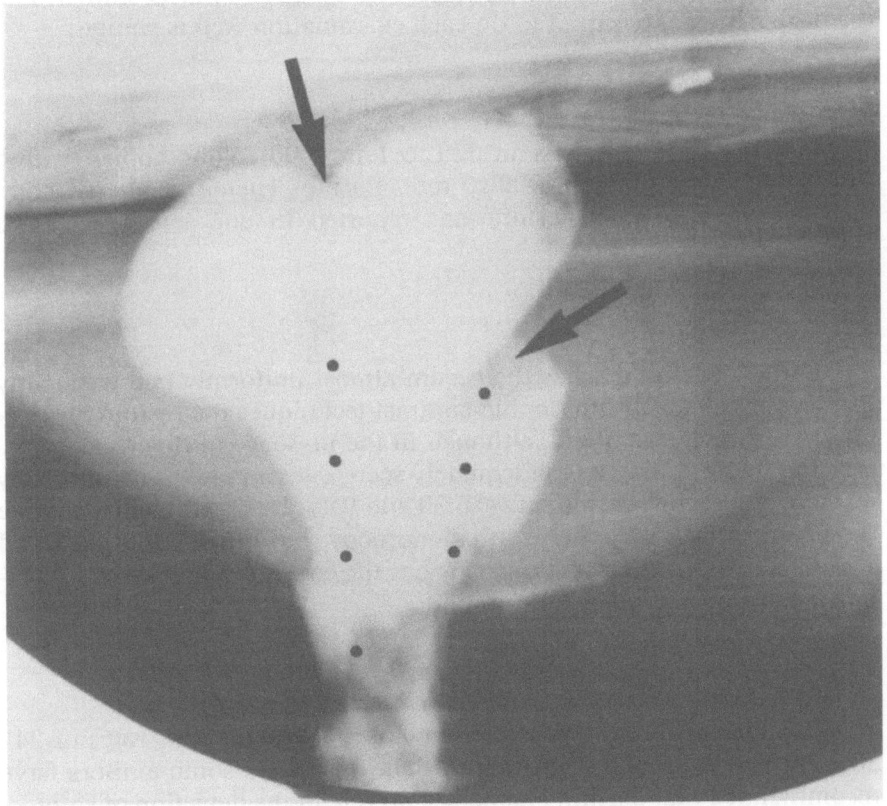

Figure 10. Evacuating proctography film taken during evacuation of barium paste. The patient complained of obstructed defecation with intermittent inability to empty the rectum. The film shows that rectoanal intussusception is occurring with the prolapsed mucosa (arrows) preventing further emptying.

7. COLORECTAL NEOPLASIA

The principal diagnostic controversy here is whether barium enema or colonoscopy should be used for primary investigation. Standards of barium enema and colonoscopy vary widely. When deciding which examination should be used, four factors should be taken into account—cost, safety, completeness, and reliability.

7.1. Cost

Colonoscopy costs from 2 to 10 times as much as barium enema. The cost difference is illogical since the purchase and maintenance costs of the endoscopic equipment are less, physician time required is similar, and the degree of skill required to do each examination well is similar.

7.2. Safety

Perforation occurs in 1 in 500 to 1 in 1000 colonoscopies, with a substantial subsequent mortality rate. Barium enema is almost completely safe, with four perforations reported in one series of 23,500 examinations.

7.3. Completeness

Barium enema reaches the cecum almost uniformly and frequently the terminal ileum. With double-contrast techniques the rectum and sigmoid are clearly examined, although in the presence of diverticular disease the sigmoid may be inadequately seen. Success rate of colonoscopy reaching the cecum varies between 30 and 95%. It is possible to examine the ileum in 90% of patients at colonoscopy, but this is attempted and achieved in few centers. Colonscopy has the enormous advantage of permitting biopsy and collection of fluid.

7.4. Reliability

Barium enema may often miss colorectal carcinoma—rates of 24–30% are not unusual.[24,25] With such high miss rates some authors have recommended that barium enema has no role in the detection of colorectal carcinoma.[25] Other studies, however, show that colorectal carcinoma can be detected with a sensitivity of 94%, by double-contrast barium enemas, and that most of the misses were due to perceptive errors.[26] Thus, in this series 99% of colorectal carcinomas were visible on the x-ray films.

This is a satisfactory detection rate unequaled by many other diagnostic methods.

At its best, barium enema is not quite as sensitive as colonscopy for the detection of polyps, and although good comparative figures are hard to obtain, one study from St. Mark's indicated that polyps 7 mm and larger were missed in 14% of patients by barium enema and in 8% by colonoscopy.[27]

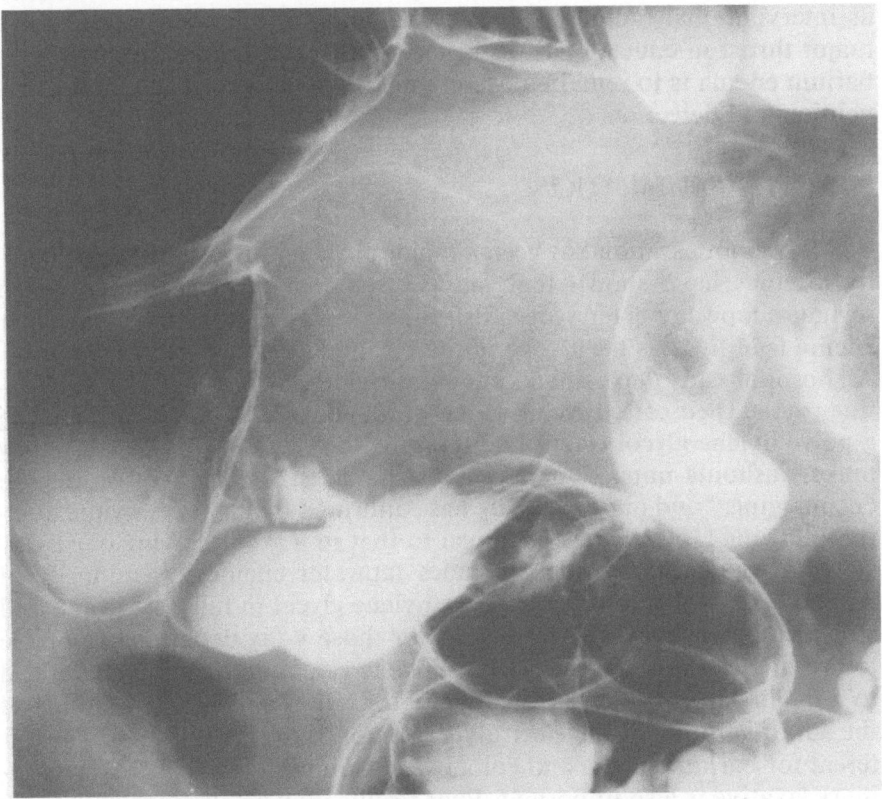

Figure 11. Eighty-four-year-old female patient presenting with rectal bleeding. Barium enema reported as normal due to perceptive error. The cecum, usually the widest part of the right colon, is relatively opaque indicating either that it contains a mass or that it is compressed. There is also a concave border to the cecal barium puddle confirming the presence of a mass, either intrinsic or extrinsic. At surgery a large metastatic deposit from the pancreas was adherent to and invading the cecum. Most errors with double-contrast enemas are perceptive mistakes, and physicians should always read these films themselves in addition to the radiological review.

7.5. Reasons for Errors

Perceptive mistakes are by far the greatest problem, occasionally exacerbated by poor technique, with failed bowel preparation being one of the major technical factors (Fig. 11). The avoidance of perceptive error requires provision of x-ray reading facilities that encourage mental and visual concentration, with appropriate illumination, and perhaps the introduction of double reading of all barium enema examinations. Many radiologists are uncomfortable with modern double-contrast techniques, and most technical training at present is devoted to new modalities such as interventional radiology, ultrasound, and CT. There is a need for a major thrust in educational workshops on double-contrast techniques if barium enema is to remain a useful method of colorectal carcinoma prevention and detection.

8. BOWEL PREPARATION

Bowel preparation has been a major problem in barium enema quality. Studies have shown that only bowel preparation methods which include a tapwater enema are satisfactory,[28] and the provision of tapwater enema facilities has been beyond the resources of many radiology units. All hospital x-ray departments should provide washout facilities as a routine part of their care. Having said that, the new bowel preparation using a polyethylene glycol electrolyte mixture shows great promise and may make washouts unnecessary for most patients. Preliminary results are encouraging,[29] and our own study has confirmed that barium enema quality following Golytely was identical to that in a group having our 2-day standard preparation which includes tapwater enemas. A minority of patients are unable to tolerate polyethylene glycol in full dosage and will still require washouts. Nevertheless, for those x-ray departments unable to provide washout facilities, polyethylene glycol preparation could lead to a major improvement in the quality of bowel enemas. The timing of the administration of the electrolyte solution is critical and has to be different for barium enema and colonoscopy, and the timing of the preliminary laxative is also important. Poor results may be obtained with these solutions without attention to such details. A few patients are unable to complete the preparation and have to be identified by radiology staff so that they can have bowel washouts before their barium enema.

9. STRATEGY OF LARGE-BOWEL INVESTIGATION

With these facts on cost, safety, completeness, and reliability, we are in a position to construct a strategy for investigation of the large bowel, separating patients into groups depending on whether they are over or under 40 years old, and whether or not they have rectal bleeding.

9.1. Category 1

Patients under 40 who are not bleeding are a fit mobile group in whom good-quality barium enemas can be obtained and polyps are relatively unlikely. They should have barium enema because it is cheaper, safer, more complete, and sufficiently accurate.

9.2. Category 2

Patients over 40 who are not bleeding are more likely to have polyps and more likely to have diverticular disease. Barium enema is relatively weaker in the sigmoid colon in this group. A case can, therefore, be made for performing flexible sigmoidoscopy as well as barium enema. However, if flexible sigmoidoscopy shows a polyp at 50 cm, there is little point in doing a barium enema since the patient will need colonoscopy for removal of that polyp and any others that may be present further round.

These patients should, therefore, have flexible sigmoidoscopy first. Since the results will be better if the bowel is clean, it should be performed not in the clinic but after full bowel preparation immediately before the barium enema and for convenience on the x-ray table. If flexible sigmoidoscopy is negative, the patient should go straight on to barium enema. However, if sigmoidoscopy shows polyps (likely in 8–12%), the patient should be moved next door so that colonoscopy can be performed instead.

9.3. Category 3

In patients under the age of 40 with rectal bleeding, flexible sigmoidoscopy and anoscopy may be used to guide further investigation. If these examinations are negative, investigation should cease unless bleeding persists. If initial endoscopic examination shows hemorrhoids, they should be treated. If inflammatory bowel disease is shown, barium enema is usually going to be useful to confirm extent and to examine the small bowel. If polyps are found, colonoscopy will be required.

9.4. Category 4

There are no good prospective studies looking at the effect of colonoscopy and barium enema on management of patients over the age of 40 with rectal bleeding. Retrospective studies, usually performed on patients who have had negative barium enemas and who have continued to bleed, suggest that colonoscopy may have a yield of neoplasia in up to 25% of such patients.[30,31] This suggests that colonoscopy is the investigation of choice in patients over 40 with rectal bleeding. This remains to be proved, but it is the logical inference to be drawn from the literature such as it is. Prospective studies are required comparing colonoscopy with flexible sigmoidoscopy and barium enema in patients with rectal bleeding.

In summary, barium enema does retain a useful role in patients with colorectal neoplasia but only if it is performed to a high standard. Colonoscopy is also variable in quality. Flexible sigmoidoscopy could have a pivotal role in directing the most efficient use of the other two investigations. The implementation of a strategy such as the one outlined here would require very close cooperation between gastroenterology and radiology departments.

10. FUTURE TRENDS

The future of GI radiology lies in integration. In the upper GI tract many patients now coming for a barium meal should be having endoscopy, and some patients who are coming for endoscopy for esophageal problems should be having barium radiology. The ability to move patients from one to the other is helpful. In the investigation of dyspepsia ultrasound examination should be available at the same time as endoscopy or barium studies. For the colon, flexible sigmoidoscopy should guide whether a barium enema or colonoscopy is needed so that both must be available on a rapid-service basis. Ultrasound should be available for some, if not all, liver biopsies. Immediate percutaneous transhepatic cholangiography may be required for failed ERCP.

Both radiology and endoscopy have started to become integral parts of modern therapeutics and have emerged from their limited diagnostic beginnings. The selection of the best therapy often involves consideration of drug, endoscopic, radiological, and surgical approaches, and this is forcing surgeons, gastroenterologists, and radiologists to start working as integrated teams.

These trends require a GI imaging unit that includes endoscopy rooms, barium fluoroscopy rooms with video-recording facilities, laser, ultrasound, and perhaps, if it lives up to its initial promise, endoscopic ultrasound. In some hospitals this will lead to the diminishing of traditional barriers with gastroenterologists, surgeons, and radiologists all performing some endoscopic procedures. Some gastroenterologists or surgeons may learn to use ultrasound and some ultrasound radiologists may learn to use endoscopy in order to further develop endoscopic ultrasound. More surgeons will learn diagnostic and therapeutic biliary endoscopy as part of their surgical biliary practice. The worst possible scenario sees the separate development of units of surgical endoscopy, medical endoscopy, and radiologic endoscopy with gastroenterologists buying fluoroscopy equipment for ERCPs and tube placements, and perhaps surgeons buying real-time ultrasound for occasional examination of the upper abdomen on their patients in the emergency room. The challenge of the next few years is going to be in the harmonious development of integrated units of diagnostic and therapeutic GI imaging.

REFERENCES

1. Ott DJ, Dodds WJ, Wu WC: Current status of radiology in evaluating gastroesophageal reflux disease. *J Clin Gastroenterol* 1982;4:365–375. 1982.
2. Ott DJ, Wu WC, Gelfand DW: Reflux esophagitis revisited: Prospective analysis of radiologic accuracy. *Gastrointest Radiol* 1981;6:1–7.
3. Somers S, Stevenson GW, Thompson G: Comparison of endoscopy and barium swallow with marshmallow in dysphagia. *J Can Assoc Radiol* 1986 (in press).
4. Benjamin SJ, Castell DO: Esophageal causes of chest pain, pp. 85–98. in Castell DO, Johnson LF (eds): *Esophageal Function in Health and Disease.* New York: Elsevier Biomedical 1983.
5. Laufer I: Assessment of the accuracy of double contrast gastrointestinal radiology. *Gastroenterology* 1976;71:874–878.
6. Holdsworth CD, Bardhan KD, Balmforth CV, et al: Upper gastrointestinal endoscopy: its effects on patient management. *Bri Med J* 1979;1:775–777. 1979.
7. Max MH, West B, Knutson CO: Evaluation of postoperative gastroduodenal symptoms: Endoscopy or upper gastrointestinal roentgenography? *Surgery* 1979;86:578–582.
8. De Luca VA: The G.I. unit as a centralized interdepartmental hospital division. *J Clin Gastroenterol* 1980;2:219–220.
9. Cotton PB, Shorvon PJ, Lees WR: Endoscopic ultrasonography, a new look from within. *Br Med J* 1985;290:1373.
10. Niederau C, Muller J, Sonnenberg A, et al: Extrahepatic bile ducts in healthy subjects, in patients with cholethiasis, and in postcholecystectomy patients: A prospective ultrasonic study. *J Clin Ultrasound* 1983;11:23–27.
11. Safrany L, Cotton PB: Endoscopic management of cholelithiasis. *Surg Clin North Am* 1982;62:825–836.
12. Connon JJ: Direct cholangiography: its diagnostic and therapeutic role. *Can Med Assoc J* 1984;130:264–268.
13. Gamble P, Colapinto RF, Stronell RD, et al: Transjugular liver biopsy: A review of 461 biopsies. *Radiology* 1985;157:589–593.
14. Ott DJ, Chen YM, Gelfand DW, et al: Detailed peroral small bowel examination versus enteroclysis. *Radiology* 1985;155:29–34.
15. Coremans G, Rutgeerts P, Geboes K, et al: The value of ileoscopy with biopsy in the diagnosis of intestinal Crohn's disease. *Gastrointest Endosc* 1984;30:167–172.

16. Ileoscopy—If forsaken will it be forgotten. *Gastrointest Endosc* 1984;30:213–214 (editorial).
17. Gardiner R, Stevenson GW: The colitides. *Radiol Clin North Am* 1982;20(4)797–818.
18. Sverymuttu SH, Peters AM, Humphrey HJ, et al: 111 Indium scanning in small bowel Crohn's disease. *Gastrointest Radiol* 1983;8:157–161.
19. Biarnason I, Zanilli G, Smith I, et al: Intestinal imaging: Comparison of 111 Indium labelled leucocytes and 99 m Tc porphyrin. *Gut* 1985;5:553.
20. Kaftori JK, Pery M, Kleinhaus U: Ultrasonography in Crohn's disease. *Gastrointest Radiol* 1984;9:137–148.
21. Goldberg HI, Gore RM, Margulis AR, et al: Computed tomography in the evaluation of Crohn's disease. *Am J Roentgenol* 1983;140:277–282.
22. Mahieu P, Pringot J, Bodart P: Defecography: Description of a new procedure and results in normal patients. *Gastrointest Radiol* 1984;9:247–251.
23. Ekberg O, Nylander G, Ford FT: Defecography. *Radiology* 1985;155:45–48.
24. Stevenson GW, Robertson A, Hecker R: Barium enema in the diagnosis of colonic carcinoma. *Aust Clin Rev* 1984;13:13–17.
25. Gilbertsen VA, Williams SE, Schuman L, McHugh R: Colonoscopy in the detection of carcinoma of the intestine. *Surg Gynecol Obstet* 1979;149:877–878.
26. Kelvin FM, Gardiner R, Vas W, Stevenson GW: Colorectal carcinoma missed on double contrast barium enema study: A problem in perception. *Am J Roentgenol* 1981;137:307–313.
27. Williams CV, Macrae FA, Bartram CI: A prospective study of diagnostic methods in adenoma follow up. *Endoscopy* 1982;14:74–78.
28. Present AJ, Jansson B, Burhenne HJ: Evaluation of twelve colon cleansing regimens with single contrast barium enema. *Am J Roentgenol* 1982;139:855–860.
29. Chan CH, Diner WC, Fontenot E, et al: Randomized single blind clinical trial of a rapid colonic lavage solution (Golytely) vs. standard preparation for barium enema and colonoscopy. *Gastrointest Radiol* 1985;10(4):378–382.
30. Swarbrick ET, Hunt RH, Fevre DI, et al: Colonoscopy for unexplained rectal bleeding. *Gut* 1976;17:823 (abstract).
31. Hunt RH: Rectal bleeding, in: Hunt RH, Waye JD (eds): *Colonoscopy.* London: Chapman and Mall, 1981, pp. 267–288.

14

Gastrointestinal Disorders of the Elderly
A General Approach, Examples, and Caveats

Lawrence J. Brandt

1. INTRODUCTION

Study of the physiology of aging is in its infancy, and it has only recently been recognized that the aged subject is a unique individual who reacts to disease processes differently than he or she did in earlier years.[1] In this short account, one can only present a general approach to those gastrointestinal disorders associated with aging illustrated with some clinical examples. The latter have been chosen from a group of disorders which present with symptoms common to the young as well as the old and for which a pathophysiological basis has been elucidated. I have attempted to highlight several points of clinical relevance and to offer some guidelines to patient management. Each clinical section is introduced by a brief outline of senescent physiological alterations as they pertain to the organ or disorder under discussion. First, a few comments to illustrate a general approach to gastrointestinal disorders in the elderly that I have found particularly valuable:

1. Certain disorders are chiefly found in senescence, such as presbyesophagus, atrophic gastritis, diverticulosis, and mesenteric vascular ischemia.

Lawrence J. Brandt ● Montefiore Hospital and Medical Center, Bronx, New York 10467.

2. For any given symptom, the differential diagnosis may be very different in an elderly patient. What is routinely diagnosed as heartburn in a 30-year-old may reflect esophageal candidiasis in an octogenarian. Severe rectal bleeding may suggest Crohn's disease in a 20-year-old, whereas vascular ectasias or diverticulosis is of greater concern in patients beyond age 65.

3. The same disease process may be markedly different at extreme ends of the age spectrum. Celiac sprue in a youngster typically manifests with foul-smelling diarrhea or growth retardation, whereas in an elderly patient, osteoporosis and hip fracture may be the sole expression of intestinal malabsorption.

4. What appears to be the same disease process in disparate age groups may reflect totally different etiologies. Examples include the achalasialike presentation of gastric carcinoma and the "atypical" behavior of ulcerative colitis in the elderly.

5. Complications that occur only after many decades of disease are more usually seen in the elderly. The neoplastic complications of celiac sprue and postgastrectomy carcinoma are illustrative.

2. ESOPHAGUS

What alterations in esophageal motility are due to the aging process itself? Most important is the realization that age-related changes in esophageal function and disease seem to lie in the degree rather than in the nature of the motility changes.[2,3] Whether an entity warranting the term "presbyesophagus"[4] truly exists is controversial. It appears that with aging

1. The incidence of normal peristalsis and a complete lower esophageal sphincter response after swallowing is reduced.

2. The incidence of failure of the lower esophageal sphincter to relax after swallowing is increased.

3. Resting esophageal pressures are higher, and the incidence of tertiary contractions after swallowing is increased.

4. Esophageal emptying and postdeglutitive clearance is delayed. Esophageal dilatation may result.

5. Peristaltic contractions appear to be relatively weaker and their velocity slower, especially in the upper esophagus.

Esophageal disorders usually present with dysphagia and/or chest pain. Less commonly wheezing, lung abscess, or recurrent pneumonia suggest pulmonary disease. Dysphagia is not a diagnosis, only a symptom, and its causes in the elderly differ somewhat from those in a younger age population (Table 1). Chest pain due to an esophageal disorder is often confused with angina pectoris and usually is caused by a motility disorder—most often a "nutcracker" esophagus or diffuse esophageal spasm.

Because it may present with anginal-type chest pain which is indistinguishable from that of coronary artery disease and which may be relieved by nitroglycerin,[5–8] *symptomatic diffuse esophageal spasm* is a vexing clinical problem. The predominant symptoms of esophageal spasm are chest pain and dysphagia, which may present independently of one another, but most often are associated. The pain of diffuse spasm can be quite variable. It may be mild or severe, dull, sharp, colicky, squeezing, intermittent, or persistent. It is usually felt substernally. In some patients radiation of the pain into the neck, back, or down the upper extremities may raise concern that the problem is one of cardiac rather than esophageal disease. The pain of diffuse esophageal spasm may come on suddenly, and often it is associated with eating or precipitated by a

Table 1. Dysphagia in the Elderly

Oropharyngeal dysphagia
  Malignancy
  Central nervous system disease (Parkinson's disease, cerebrovascular accident)
  Peripheral nervous system disease (diabetes mellitus)
  Motor end-plate disease
  Myopathy (hypothyroidism)
  Mechanical
    Intrinsic (carcinoma, stricture)
    Extrinsic (cervical spine disease)
  Postoperative (laryngectomy, tracheostomy)
  Medication induced (antibiotics, quinidine)
Midesophageal dysphagia
  Malignancy—primary, contiguous
  Motility disorder—("nutcracker" esophagus, esophageal spasm)
  Stricture—(Barrett's)
  Infectious—(*Candida,* herpes)
Distal esophageal dysphagia
  Malignancy—gastric > esophageal
  Reflux—esophagitis, stricture
  Webs, rings, diverticula
  Hernia—paraesophageal

---

tense, emotionally charged situation. Occasionally, pain is provoked by ice-cold liquids, which is especially interesting because ingestion of cold liquids significantly depresses the amplitude and frequency of esophageal peristalsis in normal persons. Furthermore, the pain accompanying rapid ingestion of cold liquids is associated with a complete absence of motor activity in the body of the esophagus.

Dysphagia is usually not as prominent a symptom as chest pain in patients with esophageal spasm, and it is usually felt as a diffuse substernal sensation. Syncope on swallowing has also been described in patients with esophageal spasm and has been shown to be associated with cardiac arrhythmias suggesting a vagal reflex.

The diagnosis of esophageal spasm is usually made by barium esophagography, cinefluorography, and esophageal manometry. Barium esophagography may reveal a normal esophagus or a distortion of the esophageal contour. A variety of colorful synonyms has been coined to describe the impressive abnormalities of the barium column including curling, beading, corkscrew esophagus, rosary bead esophagus, knuckle duster, pseudodiverticulosis, and tertiary waves. Some patients with diffuse esophageal spasm have a normal barium esophagram, whereas many elderly individuals shown profound roentgenological abnormalities but without dysphagia, chest pain, or manometric abnormalities.

The contraction waves following a swallow in esophageal spasm are typically high in amplitude, increased in duration, repetitive, and simultaneous—particularly throughout the lower two-thirds of the esophagus. Occasionally, a sustained "tetanic" contraction is seen which may be associated with chest pain. Peristaltic waves of high amplitude characterize the nutcracker esophagus. If a patient is suspected of having diffuse esophageal spasm, and the manometric examination is normal at the time of study, symptoms and characteristic manometric findings of spasm may be elicited by administration of cholinergic agents, pentagastrin, or even ergonovine. The latter drug may also induce coronary artery spasm and therefore should not be used during routine clinical manometry.

The pain arising in the esophagus may be clinically indistinguishable from the pain of angina pectoris or myocardial infarction. In recent years coronary angiography has been increasingly used to determine the presence of coronary artery disease and to investigate the etiology of chest pain. Brand and colleagues studied a group of 58 patients with anginalike chest pain who were referred for esophageal manometry.[5] Forty-three of these had no evidence of coronary artery disease, and of this group one-third were found to have esophageal motility disorders that accounted for the chest pain. Most common was an increased amplitude of the force of contraction, which on occasion bore a direct relationship to the intensity of the patient's chest pain. Diffuse spasm, which is commonly believed to be the most frequently occurring motility disorder during attacks of anginalike chest pain, was observed in only 20% of the abnormal tracings in Brand's series. Esophageal spasm also occurs in response to gastroesophageal reflux, and therefore most patients with chest pain who are having esophageal manometric studies should also have a simultaneous acid infusion (Bernstein) test and an esophageal pH study performed to clarify whether acid reflux plays a role in the production of the chest pain. This information is crucial to the successful management of the patient because the therapy for acid peptic disease of the esophagus is quite different from that of a primary motility disorder. It was of interest that in Brand's study[5] fully one-third of the group with proven coronary artery disease and anginalike pain had intermittent dysphagia and heartburn. Furthermore, one-fourth of these subjects had chest pain and half had abnormal motility tests during the manometric study. In the subset of patients with documented coronary artery disease and an esophageal motility disorder, esophageal manometry is particularly useful in differentiating which intrathoracic organ is responsible for the patient's symptom.

The keystone in the medical treatment of esophageal hypermotility disturbances is the use of smooth muscle relaxants such as nitroglycerin or long-acting nitrites[8] or calcium-channel-blocking agents.[9,10] Diffuse esophageal spasm can be effectively managed with long-acting nitrites over a prolonged period in the absence of reflux. However, if esophageal spasm is associated with reflux, the use of nitrites is unpredictable and less effective. Thus, all patients with diffuse esophageal spasm should not necessarily receive the same treatment, and a complete esophageal evaluation, including manometry and pH testing, may be necessary to establish appropriate therapy.

Calcium-channel-blocking agents block the movement of calcium and other ions across cell membranes and thereby interfere with the genesis of the action potential and subsequent muscle contraction. Nifedipine[9] and verapamil[10] have been shown to affect esophageal peristalsis and lower esophageal sphincter pressure. In one study of six patients with diffuse esophageal spasm, nifedipine was demonstrated to improve symptoms and reduce the amplitudes of peristaltic waves and the amplitude and frequency of nonperistaltic contractions.[9] Obviously, the exact role these new agents will play in the management of muscular disorders of the gastrointestinal tract is yet to be determined, but preliminary results of their use are interesting and clinical trials are awaited.

For selected patients with well-documented esophageal spasm and severe symptoms that do not respond to currently available medical therapy, a long esophagomyotomy may be advisable.[11] Although surgical therapy usually results in improvement of symptoms, such is not always the case. In view of the strides being made in our understanding of the physiology of normal and abnormal muscular function, and the recent advances in the pharmacotherapy of muscular disorders, it seems prudent to avoid surgery except for those patients with severe or debilitating symptoms that do not respond to intensive medical therapy.

3. STOMACH

It is generally accepted that gastric secretion diminishes with advancing age and that relative hypochlorhydria is more common than absolute anacidity. But the early methods used to establish this are not presently considered sensitive enough to evaluate gastric secretory function.[12-14] In the elderly, pentagastrin is preferable to histamine or Histalog because of its fewer adverse effects. The latter, in a dosage sufficient for maximal parietal cell stimulation, may produce severe and potentially hazardous side effects, including flushing, hypotension, nausea, and cramps.

In an effort to understand why acid secretion is reduced in the elderly, the histological appearance of the aged stomach has been studied and correlated with gastric secretion. Two such extensively studied age-related disorders associated with diminished acid secretion are *atrophic gastritis* and *gastric atrophy*. In atrophic gastritis there is a variable amount of inflammation accompanied by equally variable degree of atrophy. Atrophic gastritis tends to be progressive and may result in gastric atrophy, whereas gastric atrophy is a more diffuse disorder characterized by a reduction in the number of chief and parietal cells in the mucosa of the gastric body and fundus with atrophy of the deeper antral mucosal glands. There is an increased frequency of such atrophic changes with advancing age and a close correlation between gastric secretory function and the histological appearance of the gastric mucosa.[15] With development of atrophic gastritis or gastric atrophy, the ability to secrete acid is progressively reduced.

Atrophic gastritis has been classified into two types.[16] Type A is characterized by antiparietal cell antibody in the serum and is a diffuse process with relative antral sparing. Acid secretion is markedly reduced with resultant hypergastrinemia, and eventually vitamin B_{12} absorption is impaired resulting in pernicious anemia. Type B lacks serum antiparietal cell antibody and is a more focal antral process with less reduction of acid secretion, normal gastrin levels, and only rarely malabsorption of vitamin B_{12}.

Atrophic gastritis and gastric atrophy are usually asymptomatic, but dyspepsia, abdominal pain, distention, nausea, and vomiting may develop. Intermittent diarrhea has been noted in approximately 10% of achlorhydric patients ("gastrogenous diarrhea") and justifies a search for parasitic infestation or bacterial overgrowth. Iron deficiency anemia is also seen in atrophic gastritis. Gastric ulcer occurs with increased frequency, and the incidence of cancer in atrophic gastritis is similar to that in pernicious anemia, approximating 10% in patients observed for up to 20 years.[17] An etiological role for intestinal metaplasia has been postulated for some gastric cancers, and occasionally a clear transition is seen between metaplastic and neoplastic epithelia.

Having discussed disorders characterized by reduced acid secretion, let us turn our attention to one associated with relative hyperchlorhydria, namely *peptic ulcer disease*. The number of elderly patients hospitalized with peptic disease, especially with duodenal ulcer, is increasing. Ulcer disease in the elderly frequently exhibits a virulent course with more complications and a higher mortality than in the young.[18] Duodenal ulcer occurs two to three times more frequently than gastric ulcer, but the latter is responsible for two of every three ulcer-related deaths. The incidence of ulcer-related deaths seems unchanged in those older than 60 years, and the death rate increases with advancing age.

A history of exposure to drugs capable of precipitating ulcer disease is common in elderly patients. Anticoagulants and drugs used in the treatment of arthritic disorders, including corticosteroids and the nonsteroidal antiinflammatory agents (e.g., aspirin, indomethacin, phenylbutazone), are especially notorious.

The presentation late in life tends to be rather acute, often with bleeding or perforation. Conversely, it is not uncommon for symptoms to be more variable and subtle than in younger years, especially with gastric ulcers. So-called "geriatric" ulcers high in the cardia may cause misleading symptoms such as dysphagia mimicking esophageal neoplasm or substernal pain mistaken for angina. Chronic blood loss is more common with gastric than duodenal ulcers. The resultant anemia may lead to cardiac or cerebral symptoms, which can further confuse the clinical picture and suggest a malignancy.

Ulcer-related complications increase with advancing age. In one representative series, the complication rate rose progressively from 31% in patients 30–64 years old to 76% in those 75–79 years of age.[19] *Bleeding* is the most common complication and accounts for one-half to two-thirds of all fatalities.[19] In a surgical series reporting patients with exsanguinating hemorrhage, the age distribution peaked during the seventh decade with 40% of patients being over 65 years of age.[20] Endoscopic therapy with heater probes, bipolar electrocoagulation, or lasers is playing an increasing, but as yet unproven, role in the management of upper gastrointestinal tract hemorrhage and may be lifesaving in unstable patients. Angiography with the intraarterial administration of embolic agents is another alternative nonsurgical therapeutic modality. Bleeding that is persistent, massive, or unresponsive to management by endoscopic or angiographic techniques, especially from a gastric source, should prompt surgical intervention. It is unclear which operation is the preferred procedure. Surgical therapy should not be withheld or delayed solely because of advanced age.

Perforation is the second most frequent complication. Signs and symptoms may differ from the classic picture of acute severe pain and rapidly developing boardlike abdominal rigidity seen in younger patients. The less dramatic or subtle presentation associated with atypical signs and symptoms often leads to delay in diagnosis and a higher mortality.[21]

Gastric outlet *obstruction* complicates ulcer disease in 10–15% of patients over 60 years and is seen almost exclusively in those with a long history of peptic disease.[21] Since gastric carcinoma not infrequently causes antropyloric obstruction in the advanced years, coexistence of a malignant lesion must be excluded. The initial therapy of gastric outlet obstruction includes correction of fluid and electrolyte balance and nasogastric intubation to decompress the stomach. In selected cases, stenosis of the pylorus may be treated endoscopically, using dilating balloon catheters.

Intractability is an uncommon problem in elderly patients with peptic disease and rarely necessitates surgical intervention. Intractable pain usually indicates a superimposed complication or the presence of a particularly severe form of ulcer disease, e.g., giant duodenal ulcer or giant gastric ulcer.

3.1. Giant Duodenal Ulcer

When an ulcer exceeds 2 cm in diameter or involves most of the surface area of the bulb, it often behaves so differently from the smaller, more usual ulcer that it should be considered a separate entity. Giant duodenal ulcer presents most frequently in the seventh decade. It occurs predominantly in males, many of whom have no preceding history of ulcer disease. Abdominal pain is the most frequent symptom and often radiates to the back or right upper quadrant mimicking pancreatic or gallbladder disease. It is variably relieved by antacids and may be worsened by eating. Significant weight loss often accompanies the pain and may raise the suspicion of malignancy. Gastrointestinal bleeding occurs in most patients, and serum albumin levels are usually below normal, probably because of protein loss from the ulcer bed. The diagnosis is usually established by radiology, though these large ulcers may be mistaken for the duodenal bulb. Giant duodenal ulcers are frequently complicated by bleeding, penetration, pyloroduodenal obstruction, perforation, and inflammatory masses. Surgical therapy has been considered preferable, but in an individual who is stable and without pressing need for emergency surgery, a course of medical therapy including H2 blockers is reasonable. Twenty-five years ago giant duodenal ulcers were uniformly fatal, but a recent report consisting of medically and surgically treated patients demonstrated a giant ulcer-related mortality rate of only 8%.[22]

3.2. Giant Gastric Ulcer

A giant gastric ulcer is one with a diameter of 3 cm or more. It occurs more commonly in males, with a peak incidence at age 60–70 in men and 70–80 in women. Pain is not a major complaint, but only about 10% of patients are totally pain-free. In about 20% the pain is atypical with radiation to the chest, periumbilical region, or lower abdomen.[23] Hemorrhage is the most common complication, and many of these ulcers penetrate the stomach wall resulting in hemorrhage from the splenic or left gastric arteries. Perforation and obstruction are less frequently encountered. Giant gastric ulcers are much more likely to be benign than malignant. Nonetheless, achlorhydria is presumptive evidence that the ulcer is malignant. In the absence of hemorrhage or perforation, an intensive program of medical therapy with H2 blockers is warranted.

Medical therapy is a double-edged sword in the elderly, and its risks must be carefully weighed. Rigorous administration of antacids is associated with an increased salt load often sufficient to upset the delicate balance in patients with renal disease or congestive heart failure. Further problems of antacids include change in bowel habits and drug interactions. The aluminum hydroxide compounds have been shown to adsorb several drugs, e.g., digoxin and quinidine, and to interfere with their absorption. Side effects of the H2 blocker cimetidine that are of particular concern in the elderly include mental obtundation or confusion, sinus node dysfunction, and drug interactions. Ranitidine may be safer. Anticholinergic agents may precipitate gastric stasis, intestinal atony, obstructive uropathy, and acute glaucoma.

4. SMALL INTESTINE

The weight of the human intestine decreases after the fifth decade of life, and the jejunal villi of elderly subjects may be broader and shorter with a greater population of leaf-shaped and convoluted forms than is found in normal young controls. Barium studies of the small intestine occasionally reflect those morphological changes and show a coarser mucosal pattern in patients over 60. It is probable that such senescent changes result from diminished cell turnover and that there is an "ineffectual enteropoiesis" in the aged gut.[24] Age-related changes demonstrated in animals include increased mucosal fibrosis, glandular atrophy, a decrease in intestinal lymphocytes, Peyer's patches, lymphoid follicles, and a generalized basophilia. The functional and immunological consequences of these alterations are only now beginning to be investigated.

Absorption and Malabsorption

The functional capacity of the small intestine decreases with aging. The diminished ability to absorb carbohydrates with aging is subtle and not accompanied by clinical evidence of undernutrition. The validity of D-xylose testing to document intestinal malabsorption in the elderly is controversial. This is because low urinary values are often obtained in the absence of malabsorption. Such false-positive results are usually attributed to impaired renal function and the diminished ability of the aged kidney to excrete the sugar load. Hence, the ratio of urinary D-xylose excretion after oral and intravenous D-xylose was shown not to change with age.[25] However, not all investigators agree that the apparently diminished monosaccharide absorption actually reflects reduced renal function. In older population groups, Webster and Leeming used the combined results of oral and intravenous xylose tests to demonstrate that one-fourth of patients older than 63 years of age absorbed D-xylose from the small bowel less efficiently than did younger subjects.[26] In only 10% of these elderly subjects, however, was the physiological impairment as severe as that of patients with celiac disease or tropical sprue. Determination of the serum levels of D-xylose in addition to the urinary excretion does not substantially help resolve the question, because diminished urinary excretion also retards clearance of the sugar from the circulation. Thus, the issue of whether absorption of this monosaccharide is altered with age remains unsettled. It is nonetheless important to ensure a fasting state when performing a D-xylose test in the elderly as the presence of food may diminish absorption of the sugar. The exaggerated decrease in

D-xylose excretion with eating forms the basis of the "provocative" D-xylose test for chronic intestinal ischemia.

The effect of aging on carbohydrate absorption has recently been studied using breath hydrogen analysis following a standard 100-g carbohydrate meal.[27] Evidence of intestinal carbohydrate malabsorption was observed in one-third of subjects over 65 years of age but in no control subjects less than 65. Furthermore, testing of subjects with meals containing 25–200 g of carbohydrate demonstrated a progressive reduction in absorptive capacity with advancing age. Young controls absorbed up to 200 g of carbohydrate in a meal, whereas only one-third of elderly subjects had negative breath tests, i.e., no evidence of carbohydrate malabsorption, when meals containing up to 200 g of carbohydrate were consumed.

There does not seem to be a consistent decrease in disaccharide (e.g., lactose) tolerance with advancing age. Diminution in mucosal lactase content and resultant lactose maldigestion has been offered as an explanation of symptoms—gaseous dyspepsia, bloating, and diarrhea—experienced by some elderly patients labeled as having "functional" bowel disease.

Multiple studies have demonstrated that the pattern of fat absorption in the elderly differs from that seen in the young. In one report, for example, the serum level of chylomicrons after an oral fat load was less than that in younger subjects. Moreover, the addition of lipase to the original fat load abolished the observed differences between the age groups, suggesting an element of pancreatic dysfunction.[28] Indeed, impaired pancreatic function has been demonstrated in the elderly but in most patients is not evident clinically. Suggestive evidence has been presented showing reduced absorption of both radioactive triolein and oleic acid in patients older than 60 years of age, suggesting the coexistence of both digestive and absorptive abnormalities in the aged.[29] Some studies have actually shown cholesterol absorption to increase with advancing age,[30] which, if true, could conceivably help to explain in part the development of atherosclerosis.

Vitamin deficiencies in the elderly generally reflect diminished intake or disease states. The concept of "physiological avitaminosis" should be discarded. However, the aged gut seems to absorb calcium and vitamin D poorly despite an apparently greater need for these nutrients. The diets of elderly people are frequently deficient in calcium, and the adaptive response of the intestine to increase absorptive capacity with low intake is blunted. Perhaps this contributes to the progressive loss of bone with advancing age. When iron deficiency occurs, gastrointestinal blood loss must be excluded, although some factors that may adversely influence iron absorption in the elderly include hypochlorhydria and an increased ingestion of cereal grains from which iron is poorly absorbed.

The differential diagnosis of *malabsorption* syndrome in the elderly encompasses a large number of disorders (Table 2). Some entities cause symptoms by interfering with the intraluminal digestion of nutrients (pancreatic insufficiency); others alter the mucosa (celiac sprue); and still others interfere with intestinal blood flow (irradiation). Elderly individuals may also suffer from systemic disorders which directly involve the intestine (amyloidosis) or affect it as an innocent bystander (congestive heart failure).

An example of a malabsorptive disorder that can occur in the elderly is *celiac sprue*. In one large series,[31] approximately 7% of cases presented during the seventh decade of life, and in another, celiac disease was the most common cause of steatorrhea in patients older than 50 years of

Table 2. Causes of Maldigestion and
Malabsorption in the Elderly

Maldigestion
  Pancreatic insufficiency
  Zollinger–Ellison syndrome
  Postgastrectomy
Malabsorption
  Bacterial overgrowth
    Structural disorders
      Jejunal diverticulosis
      Stricture
    Motility disorders
      Diabetes, neuromuscular disease
  Short-bowel syndrome
  Hepatocellular–biliary tract disease, e.g., cholestasis
  Celiac sprue
  Crohn's disease
  Malignancy
    Lymphoma, melanoma, retroperitoneal disease
  Vascular disorders
    Radiation
    Chronic mesenteric ischemia
  Drug-induced, e.g., colchicine
  Systemic disorders
    Congestive heart failure
    Endocrine diseases
    Mastocytosis, carcinoid
    Dysgammaglobulinemia, amyloidosis
    Skin diseases (diffuse)

age.[32] As in childhood, diarrhea, steatorrhea, weight loss, and the sequelae of malabsorption constitute the features of this disorder. However, a substantial proportion of patients in later life do not present with any symptoms referable to the digestive tract whatsoever, but with insidious anemia or metabolic bone disease. Individuals having intestinal symptoms for the first time in later life may be demonstrating the onset of the clinical disease but may also show physical evidence such as healed rickets or short stature, reflecting many years of subclinical disease activity. When the disease does present acutely during adulthood, a precipitating event is often identifiable. For example, the patient may have a bout of antibiotic-associated diarrhea or "traveler's diarrhea" which fails to resolve and progresses to "typical" celiac disease. Occasional cases present in an acute form after abdominal surgery (especially vagotomy and partial gastrectomy) for peptic ulcer disease.

In elderly patients the possibility of celiac disease should be kept in mind, especially in the presence of cachexia, anemia (iron, vitamin B_{12}, or folate malabsorption), osteomalacia (calcium and vitamin D malabsorption), edema (gastrointestinal protein loss), bleeding diatheses, often manifesting after administration of aspirin, nonsteroidal antiinflammatory agents, or Coumadin (vitamin E deficiency), and neurological disorders (peripheral neuropathy, myeloradiculopathy, depression, psychiatric disturbances).

After many years of celiac disease (which may be in remission for decades), several complications emerge, which, because they develop only after a long interval, are more common in the elderly. These include osteomalacia, malignancy (lymphoma and carcinoma), multiple intestinal ulcers, and, rarely, amyloidosis.[33]

5. COLON

A now commonly diagnosed disorder that illustrates how descriptions of new entities can influence and alter prevailing concepts of disease is ischemic colitis. Described in 1963,[34] it is now recognized to be the most common cause of noninfectious colitis in patients older than 50 years of age. Furthermore, its misdiagnosis as ulcerative colitis probably explains why inflammatory bowel disease in the elderly was said to behave in an atypical fashion, exhibiting many of the features now recognized as characteristic of colonic ischemia, i.e., the frequency of rectal sparing and segmental colonic involvement, the high incidence of spontaneous resolution, the lack of response to conventional therapy, and the high incidence of stricture formation.[35-37]

5.1. Ischemic Colitis

During the past decade, it has become increasingly clear that the spectrum of colitis in the elderly varies from that in the young. In contrast to ulcerative colitis, which is more common in the younger population, ischemic colitis is the most prevalent noninfectious cause of colitis after the age of 50 years. Nonetheless, because such organisms as *Shigella, Campylobacter, Clostridium difficile,* and *Entamoeba histolytica* can clinically mimic both ischemic colitis and ulcerative colitis, the possibility of an infectious etiology must always be excluded before beginning therapy.

Despite the growing appreciation of ischemic colitis as a distinct entity, this condition is often still misdiagnosed as ulcerative colitis. Indeed, in a recent study involving 81 elderly patients with the onset of colitic symptoms after the age of 50 years, ischemic disease was diagnosed retrospectively in 75%. In 30% of patients, an index diagnosis of ulcerative colitis at the time of hospital discharge had been incorrect.[36]

The term ischemic colitis is not suitable for all episodes of colonic ischemia but rather applies only to those specific forms of transient and chronic ischemic damage characterized by inflammation. In our experience with more than 300 cases of colonic ischemia, such a colitis occurred in approximately 40% of affected patients, one-third of which were chronic. It is the chronic form of colonic ischemia that is so commonly mistaken for ulcerative colitis in the elderly.

In general, patients with colonic ischemia do not appear seriously ill. Most patients present with the sudden onset of bloody diarrhea or bright-red blood per rectum. Diarrhea alone is uncommon. Blood loss is usually not hemodynamically significant, and only 10% of patients are anemic at the time of hospitalization. Patients often complain of mild crampy, left-sided abdominal pain, although this pain is not a prominent complaint and is usually overshadowed by the bleeding. Careful questioning can usually elicit the sequence of initial pain followed by bleeding within 24 hr. Other symptoms such as nausea and vomiting are uncommon. Abdominal distention may be seen in 20% of affected patients, half of whom will have had a period of constipation prior to the onset of rectal bleeding. Physical examination typically detects mild left-sided, lower-abdominal tenderness. Signs of peritoneal irritation are uncommon and, when they do occur, usually indicate irreversible ischemic damage. Fever and leukocytosis may be present and also reflect severe colonic injury.

A plain film of the abdomen in patients with ischemic colitis most often shows a nonspecific gas pattern. Ileus is seen in about 30% of cases. Thumbprinting is apparent in less than 10% of examinations. This thumbprinting is caused by submucosal hemorrhage or edema and is the radiological hallmark of ischemia.

Rigid sigmoidoscopy can be helpful if performed soon after the onset of symptoms, but this procedure is of value in only 10–20% of cases, i.e., when the segment of involved bowel is within 25 cm from the anal verge. Even then, the mucosal abnormalities associated with ischemic colitis are nonspecific. Segmental distribution of mucosal abnormalities and submucosal hemorrhage are highly suggestive of colonic ischemia. Flexible sigmoidoscopy or colonoscopy may be performed in order to more fully evaluate the colon, but these diagnostic techniques carry a risk of iatrogenic complications. Air insufflation and the resultant increase in intraluminal colonic pressure diminish mucosal blood flow and may intensify an ischemic injury. Experimentally, distention of the bowel and increases in intraluminal pressure to more than 30 mm Hg result in step-by-step decreases in intestinal flood flow and the shunting of blood away from the mucosa.[38] During routine colonscopy, Kozarek and his colleagues[39] demonstrated that intraluminal pressures ranged up to 57 mm Hg when the endoscope tip was free in the bowel and were further increased by external abdominal pressure, a change in the patient's position, or Valsalva maneuver. Utmost caution must be exercised to use the least amount of air necessary to enable adequate inspection of the mucosa and passage of the instrument. If typical findings of ischemia are seen in the left colon, examination of the remainder of the bowel is unnecessary.

Because the mucosal abnormalities found in most colitides are similar, endoscopic mucosal biopsies taken from abnormal areas of the bowel are usually not specific for ischemia. Biopsies taken from areas that appear grossly normal are more helpful in the differential diagnosis. If such biopsies demonstrate inflammation, ulcerative colitis is likely, whereas if the specimen is microscopically normal, an ischemic etiology for the colitis is probable. Biopsies are diagnostic only if histological changes specific for ischemia, e.g., mucosal infarction or hemosiderin-containing macrophages, are apparent.

A barium enema performed within 48 hr of the onset of symptoms should demonstrate findings strongly suggestive of the diagnosis of colonic ischemia. Thumbprints that disappear spontaneously on serial studies performed over several weeks are a major criterion for a radiological diagnosis of colonic ischemia. Thumbprints represent submucosal hemorrhages and hence are present only in the acute stages of colonic ischemia. Barium enema repeated 1 week after the initial study will show either a return to normal or replacement of the thumbprints with a segmental colitis pattern as the overlying mucosa becomes necrotic. The ischemic nature of the ischemic process may not be appreciated if the initial barium enema is delayed until these later stages. Diner and colleagues[40] measured intraluminal pressure in the distal colon during barium enema examination with and without air contrast studies. Mean pressures ranged from 20 mm Hg to 33 mm Hg during the examination, with no significant difference observed between the two techniques, and all pressures recorded were lower than those sustained with straight-leg raising or the Valsalva maneuver. Because these pressures are lower than those demonstrated during colonoscopy, barium enema examination should theoretically interfere less with colonic blood flow and therefore be safer than colonoscopy in evaluating a patient with ischemic colitis. Colonoscopy, however, offers the advantage of enabling visualization of fine mucosal vascular abnormalities, e.g., erythema, and also of permitting biopsy.

Because acute abnormalities in the vascular tree are seldom present, angiography is *not* usually helpful in the evaluation of patients with ischemic colitis. Most likely, the initial ischemic episode occurs before the onset of symptoms and in vessels beyond the resolution of current angiographic technique.

The clinical course of patients with colonic ischemia varies. Complete resolution is seen in 40–50% of cases, colitis persists in approximately 20%, gangrene and perforation develop in about 20%, and stricture formation occurs in about 15%. Second episodes of ischemia are unusual and are seen in less than 5% of affected patients. In patients with reversible ischemic lesions, symptoms and signs rapidly subside within 24–48 hr, and complete healing usually occurs within 1–2 weeks. More severe ischemia may require 1–6 months to heal completely. Patients with such prolonged disease may be clinically well even in the presence of persistent roentgenological abnormalities.

Irreversible lesions may become obvious in hours if gangrene or perforation occurs or may follow a protracted course if chronic colitis or stricture develops. Chronic colitis usually causes persistent bloody diarrhea and weight loss. In most of these patients persistent symptoms necessitate colonic resection. In others, the colitis may eventually heal, but submucosal fibrosis occurring during the healing process may result in stricture formation. Such strictures are reported in up to 30% of patients with ischemic colitis and may produce increasing bowel obstruction which ultimately necessitates surgical therapy. Such obstruction usually follows a period of apparent well-being.

Chronic irreversible ischemic damage may be difficult to diagnose if the patient was not seen during the acute ischemic episode (Table 3). Barium enema studies usually show either a segmental ulcerative-colitis pat-

Table 3. Differential Evaluation of Ischemic Colitis and Ulcerative Colitis in the Elderly

	Ischemic colitis	Ulcerative colitis
Sigmoidoscopy	Abnormal rectum (5%) Segmental disease	Abnormal rectum in 100% Diffuse involvement beginning at the anal verge and extending proximally in a continuous fashion
Initial barium enema	Submucosal hemorrhage Thumbprinting	Diffuse colitis beginning in the rectum
	Segmental colitis Obstructing lesion distal to segment of colitis (20%)	Universal colitis Pseudopolyps
Subsequent barium enema (2 weeks later)	Rapid resolution or progression to a segmental colitis pattern stricture	No change
Gross pathology	Segmental distribution of disease	Continuous involvement, including the rectum
	Infarction or gangrene Submucosal hemorrhage	Pseudopolyps
Microscopic pathology	Mucosal necrosis Submucosal granulation tissue Submucosal fibrosis Submucosal hemosiderin-laden macrophages	Mucosal inflammation

tern or a stricture that may resemble a constricting carcinoma.[41] The *de novo* occurrence of segmental colitis or the presence of a colonic stricture in an elderly patient should be considered ischemic until such other diagnostic possibilities as infectious colitis, Crohn's disease, and colonic carcinoma have been excluded.

Colonic ischemia is associated with a distal, potentially obstructive lesion in 20% of cases.[37] Carcinoma accounts for 50% of these lesions, whereas the other 50% includes diverticulitis, fecal impaction, and stricture. An obstructive lesion in the distal colon should be strongly suspected in any patient with ischemic colitis who reports a history of constipation or in whom abdominal distention is found on physical examination. Even when the clinical manifestation of colonic ischemia consists solely of bloody diarrhea without any clinical suggestion of obstruction, the possibility of an associated potentially obstructive distal lesion should be excluded.

Treatment of ischemic colitis is primarily supportive if the clinical evaluation does not suggest intestinal gangrene or perforation. If the colon is distended, it should be decompressed. Antibiotics are recommended if the patient has abdominal pain or tenderness, fever, or leukocytosis. Systemic corticosteroids are not indicated in the treatment of colonic ischemia and theoretically may increase the risk of intestinal perforation or secondary infection. No good evidence exists to suggest that patients with chronic ischemic colitis respond to long-term treatment with sulfasalazine, as do patients with idiopathic ulcerative colitis. Rectal administration of corticosteroids may be successful in treating distal ischemic colitis.

If deterioration during the clinical course is suggested by increasing abdominal signs, fever, and leukocytosis, emergency surgery may be necessary. Surgical treatment may also be indicated for persistent diarrhea and bleeding and consists of local resection of the involved area and primary anastamosis.

5.2. Ulcerative Colitis

Ulcerative colitis is said to have a bimodal age distribution, with a peak incidence in the third and fourth decades and a second, smaller peak in the sixth and seventh decades. Many of the studies describing this second peak were published before the initial description of ischemic colitis by Boley and his colleagues in 1963.[34] Our recent experiences have taught us that many of the elderly patients who were diagnosed in the past as having ulcerative colitis would be diagnosed today as having ischemic colitis. A retrospective study of the records of patients older than 50 years of age who were admitted to Montefiore Medical Center during a 10-year interval showed that the initial discharge diagnosis in 50% of those we retrospectively considered to have ischemic colitis was inflammatory bowel disease, mostly ulcerative colitis.[36] This observation may well explain why ulcerative colitis appears to occur with a second peak and why numerous articles written prior to the recognition of ischemic colitis as a distinct entity reported that ulcerative colitis behaved differently in the elderly than in the young. Moreover, the so-called atypical features described in elderly patients with ulcerative colitis are now recognized as characteristic of ischemic colitis, namely, the segmental distribution of the disease, the less frequent involvement of the rectum, the high incidence of spontaneous resolution, and the frequent progression to a fibrotic stenosis with the delayed manifestation of colonic obstruction.

Nevertheless, bona fide ulcerative colitis does occur in the elderly. Recent studies evaluating hundreds of patients with ulcerative colitis have shown that 12–20% of cases occur after the age of 60 years.[42,43] In our study, we found that 14% of the 81 patients with colitis whose symptoms began after the age of 50 years had clinical, roentgenological, and pathological evidence of ulcerative colitis.

Although numerous series have described characteristic features of ulcerative colitis in the elderly, it is unclear whether these differences are attributable to a truly distinct disease process or represent the interaction of aging with the same disease process seen in younger patients. The situation is further confused because many of these older reports include elderly patients whose disease began when they were younger than 50 years of age as well as those in whom the disorder developed after age 50. Eighty percent of our elderly patients presented with the same features as do younger patients, namely, bloody diarrhea or bright-red blood per rectum. Moreover, symptoms of ulcerative colitis were gradual rather than sudden in onset in 75% of the cases. At the initial evaluation, 25% of elderly patients with new-onset ulcerative colitis had a fever ($>100°F$), 50% had leukocytosis (white blood cell count $> 10,000$ mm^3), and 30% had a low serum albumin concentration (<3 g/dl). In addition, approximately 20% of the patients presented with extraintestinal manifestations of ulcerative colitis, including arthritis, iritis, and pyoderma gangrenosum.

All too often ulcerative colitis in the elderly is unsuspected, and the diagnosis delayed or missed. The most common erroneous initial diagnoses are colonic carcinoma and diverticular disease. Diethelm et al.[44] noted that the correct diagnosis was made at the time of the initial evaluation in only 2 of 10 elderly patients with ulcerative colitis. In the study by Toghill and Benton,[42] 25% of 19 patients with ulcerative colitis whose symptoms began after the age of 65 years underwent surgery or died before the correct diagnosis was established. When an elderly patient presents with bloody diarrhea or bright-red blood per rectum, the possibility that colitis is responsible for the symptoms should be strongly considered, and sigmoidoscopy should be performed as part of the initial physical examination. Sigmoidoscopy demonstrates an abnormal mucosa in all untreated patients with ulcerative colitis and is an especially important examination because the barium enema may be negative early in the course of disease.

A characteristic of ulcerative colitis in the elderly is the increased severity of disease. Elderly patients more often present with total colonic involvement than do younger patients. In various studies, the incidence of universal colonic involvement documented during the first attack of ulcerative colitis was 33–45% in elderly subjects,[35,42] as compared with 14–25% in younger patients.[43] The course of the disease is also more aggressive in the elderly. In one study,[42] 9 of 19 patients with ulcerative colitis seen after the age of 65 years had colonic perforation or toxic megacolon, and six of these patients died within the first few months after the initial attack. In our study,[35] 6 of the 11 patients with ulcerative colitis whose symptoms appeared after age 50 had a complicated course with recurrent bleeding or toxic megacolon not responsive to medical treatment. This increased virulence with advancing age is further manifested by a progressively higher mortality rate during the initial attack. In one study, the mortality associated with the first attack was 5.9% for patients younger than 30 years of age, 10.1% for patients between the ages of 30 and 59 years, and 16.3% for patients older than 60 years of age.

The mainstays of medical therapy for ulcerative colitis in the elderly include sulfasalazine and systemic and topical corticosteroids, just as in the young. Indications for steroid usage are more stringent in the elderly because as a group they are more susceptible to develop complications of long-term corticosteroid use including osteoporosis, fractures, salt and water retention, hypertension, and possibly infection.

REFERENCES

1. Brandt LJ: *Gastrointestinal Disorders of the Elderly*. New York, Raven Press, 1984.
2. Kahn TA, Shragge BW, Chrispin JS, Lind JF: Esophageal motility in the elderly. *Am J Dig Dis* 1977;22:1049–1054.
3. Bhanthumnavin K, Schuster M: Aging and gastrointestinal function, in Finch C, Hayflick L (eds): *Handbook of the Biology of Aging*. New York, Van Nostrand Reinhold, 1977, p. 209.
4. Soergel KH, Zboralski F, Amberg JF: Presbyesophagus: Esophageal motility in nonagenarians. *J Clin Invest* 1964;43:1472–1479.
5. Brand DL, Martin D, Pope II CE: Esophageal manometrics in patients with angina-like chest pain. *Dig Dis* 1977;22:300–304.
6. Ferguson SC, Kodges K, Hersh T, Jinich H: Esophageal manometry in patients with chest pain and normal coronary arteriogram. *Am J Gastroenterol* 1981;75:124–127.
7. Kline M, Chesne R, Sturdevant RAL, McCallum HW: Esophageal disease in patients with angina-like chest pain. *Am J Gastroenterol* 1981;75:116–123.
8. Swamy N: Esophageal spasm: Clinical and manometric response to nitroglycerin and long-acting nitrates. *Gastroenterology* 1977;72:23–27.
9. Blackwell JH, Holt S, Heading RC: Effect of nifedipine on oesophageal motility and gastric emptying. *Digestion* 1981;21:50–56.
10. Richter JE, Sinar DR, Cordova CM, Castell DO: Verapamil—A potent inhibitor of esophageal contractions in the baboon. *Gastroenterology* 1982;2:882–886.
11. Ellis FH Jr, Olsen AM, Schlegel JF, Code CF: Surgical treatment of esophageal hypermotility disturbances. *JAMA* 1964;188:862–866.
12. Baron JH: An assessment of the augmented histamine test in the diagnosis of peptic ulcer. *Gut* 1963;4:243–253.
13. Blackman, AH, Lambert DL, Thayer WR, Martin HF: Computed normal values for peak acid output based on age, sex and body weight. *Am J Dig Dis* 1970;15:783–789.

14. Grossman MI, Kirsner JB, Gillespie IE: Basal and Histalog-stimulated gastric secretion in control subjects and in patients with peptic ulcer or gastric ulcer. *Gastroenterology* 1963;45:14–26.

15. Bock OAA, Richards WCD, Witts LJ: The relationship between acid secretion after augmented histamine stimulation and the histology of the gastric mucosa. *Gut* 1963;4:112–114.

16. Strickland RG, Mackay IR: A reappraisal of the nature of chronic atrophic gastritis. *Dig Dis Sci* 1973;18:426–440.

17. Walker IR, Strickland RG, Ungar B, Mackay IR: Simple atrophic gastritis and gastric carcinoma. *Gut* 1971;12:906–911.

18. Narayanan M, Steinheber FU: The changing face of peptic ulcer in the elderly. *Med Clin North Am* 1976;60:1159–1172.

19. Leverat M, Pasquier J, Lambert R, Tissot A: Peptic ulcer in patients over 60: Experience in 287 cases. *Am J Dig Dis* 1966;11:279–285.

20. Brooks JR, Eraklis AJ: Factors affecting the mortality from peptic ulcer: the bleeding ulcer and ulcer in the aged. *N Engl J Med* 1964;271:803–809.

21. Stafford CE, Joergenson EJ, Muray GC: Complications of peptic ulcer in the aged. *Calif Med* 1956;84:92–94.

22. Eisenberg RL, Margulis AR, Moss AA: Giant duodenal ulcer. *Gut* 1978;11:592–599.

23. Strange SL: Giant innocent gastric ulcer in the elderly. *Gerontol Clin* 1963;5:171–189.

24. Holt PR, Pascal RR, Kotler DP: Ineffectual enteropoiesis in aging rat gut. *Gastroenterology* 1982;82:1086 (abstract).

25. Kendall MJ: The influence of age on the xylose absorption test. *Gut* 1970;11:498–501.

26. Webster SGP, Leeming JT: Assessment of small bowel function in the elderly using a modified xylose tolerance test. *Gut* 1975;16:109–113.

27. Feibusch JM, Holt PR: Impaired absorptive capacity for carbohydrate in the aging human. *Dig Dis Sci* 1982;27:1095–1100.

28. Becker GH, Meyer J, Necheles H: Fat absorption in young and old age. *Gastroenterology* 1950;14:80–92.

29. Citi S, Salvani L: The intestinal absorption of ^{131}I-labelled olein and triolein, of ^{58}CO, vitamin B and ^{59}Fe, in aged subjects. *J Gerontol* 1961;12:123–126.

30. Hollander D, Morgan D: Increase in cholesterol intestinal absorption with aging in the rat. *Exp Gerontol* 1979;14:201–204.

31. Cooke WT, Asquith P (eds): *Clinics in Gastroenterology*, Vol 3. Philadelphia, WB Saunders, 1974.

32. Prince HL, Gazzard BG, Dawson AM: Steatorrhoea in the elderly. *Br Med J* 1977;1:1582.

33. Harris OD, Cooke WT, Thompson H, Waterhouse JAH: Malignancy in adult coeliac disease and idiopathic steatorrhoea. *Am J Med* 1967;42:899–921.

34. Boley SJ, Schwartz S, Lash J, Sternhill V: Reversible vascular occlusion of the colon. *Surg Gynecol Obstet* 1963;116:53–60.

35. Fischer Z, Brandt LJ: Differentiation of ischemic and ulcerative colitis in the elderly. *Geriatr Med Today* 1983;2(8):31–49.

36. Brandt LJ, Boley SJ, Goldberg L, Mitsudo S, Berman A: Colitis in the elderly: A reappraisal. *Am J Gastroenterol* 1981;76:239–245.

37. Brandt LJ, Boley SJ, Mitsudo S: Clinical characteristics and natural history of colitis in the elderly. *Am J Gastroenterol* 1982;77(6):382–386.

38. Boley SJ, Agrawal GP, Warren AR, et al: Pathophysiologic effects of bowel distention on intestinal blood flow. *Am J Surg* 1969;117:228–234.

39. Kozarek RA, Earnest DL, Silverstein ME, Smith RG: Air-pressure-induced colon injury during diagnostic colonoscopy. *Gastroenterology* 1980;78:7–14.
40. Diner WC, Patel G, Texter EC Jr, Baker ML, Tune JM, Hightower MD: Intraluminal pressure measurement during barium enema: Full column vs. air contrast. *Am J Roentgenol* 1981;137:217–221.
41. Brandt LJ, Katz HJ, Wolf EL, Mitsudo S, Boley SJ: Simulation of colonic carcinoma by ischemia. *Gastroenterology* 1985;88:1137–1142.
42. Toghill PJ, Benton P: Ulcerative colitis in elderly patients. *Gerontol Clin (Basel)* 1973;15:65–73.
43. Ritchie JK, Powell-Tuck J, Lennard-Jones JE: Clinical outcome of the first ten years of ulcerative colitis and proctitis. *Lancet* 1978;1:1140–1143.
44. Diethelm AG, Nickel WF, Wantz GE: Ulcerative colitis in the elderly patient. *Surg Gynecol Obstet* 1968;126:1223–1229.

15

Hepatitis and Immunization

Geoffrey C. Farrell

1. INTRODUCTION

Hepatitis is always a topic of great interest to health workers, not least because they are at risk of acquiring this infection from their patients. Hepatitis B, the most dangerous of the three known hepatitis viruses, is now preventable by immunization. Eradication of the disease on a world scale presents a continuing challenge but should be possible in the future. Hepatitis A is a benign enteric viral infection for which there is every prospect of an effective vaccine in the near future. On the other hand, control of non-A, non-B hepatitis awaits identification of the causative agent.

Most of this chapter will be devoted to the prevention of hepatitis B with particular attention to the present commercially available vaccine, its nature, indications, effectiveness, and possible limitations and to the prospects for new (cheaper) hepatitis B vaccines.

2. BACKGROUND

2.1. Global Importance of Hepatitis B

The discovery of Baruch Blumberg 20 years ago of an unusual precipitin in the blood of an Australian aboriginal quickly led to recognition

---

Geoffrey C. Farrell ● The University of Sydney and Gastroenterology Unit, Westmead Hospital, Westmead, NSW, Australia 2145.

Table 1. Geographical Variation in HBV Markers[a]

Country	HB$_s$Ag (% positive)	Anti-HB$_s$ (% positive)
Senegal	10.8	—
Romania	10.8	43
Greece	9.4	36
Thailand	9.3	42
Turkey	9.2	—
Uganda	7.2	50
U.S.S.R.	4.2	50
Japan	2.1	16
U.S.A.	0.9	—
Canada	0.7	3.8
Australia	0.3	2.9
U.K.	0.1	2.7

[a]Data modified from Sobeslavsky.[1]

of the hepatitis B virus (HBV). It was then readily appreciated that HBV was responsible not only for the discomfort and mortality of acute hepatitis B, but also for chronic liver disease and primary liver cancer. An unusual property of the HBV is its propensity to persist in a significant proportion of infected humans. This property underlies the problem of endemicity and transmission. A second property of the virus is its tendency to program the host liver to synthesize an excess of viral coat protein, known as hepatitis B surface antigen (HB$_s$Ag). This property has provided a novel opportunity for the development of a protective vaccine.

There are striking geographical and regional variations in HBV carrier rates (Table 1). In Asia, sub-Saharan Africa, southeastern Europe, parts of the Middle East, Oceania, and parts of South America carrier rates for HBV exceed 10%.[1] It has been estimated that there are at least 200 million carriers of HBV in the world. Carrier rates are much lower (<1%) in predominantly Anglo-Saxon Western societies such as North America, United Kingdom, and Australia. Even so, hepatitis B is a growing problem in these countries. This is probably due to such factors as recent immigration patterns, a subculture of intravenous drug addiction, and societal attitudes permitting greater promiscuity in certain groups. Thus, although hepatitis B is less of a general public health problem in Australia and Canada than in Sudan, Cambodia, or Papua New Guinea, there are groups in these populations who are at risk of acquiring hepatitis B by virtue of their intimate exposure to individuals who are HBV carriers. These high-risk categories are listed in Table 2. Because the strategy

Table 2. High-Risk Groups for HBV in Western Society

1. Indigenous races: Australian aboriginals, Alaskan eskimos
2. Immigrants from hyperendemic countries
3. Nonmedical use of needles: Intravenous drug addicts, tattooing, acupuncture
4. Promiscuous life-style: Male homosexuals, prostitutes
5. Inmates of institutes: Mentally retarded, prisoners
6. Health care workers: Dental, medical, laboratory personnel, students
7. Patients: Renal dialysis patients, recipients of blood/blood products
8. Families of HBV carriers: Especially sexual partners and infants born to HBV-positive mothers

of any program to eliminate hepatitis B must be aimed at reducing the pool of HBV carriers, these high-risk groups are the prime target for immunization.

The three commonest "events" that occur with HBV infection, inapparent infection, acute viral hepatitis, and chronic "healthy" carrier state, are all relatively benign. However, three other sequelae are associated with a considerable morbidity and mortality. Hepatitis B is more likely than hepatitis A and non-A, non-B hepatitis to result in lethal fulminant hepatic failure. Some possible exceptions are sporadic non-A, non-B hepatitis in the very young, very old, and pregnant patient and δ-agent infection. Chronic HBV infection is the most common cause of chronic active hepatitis and cirrhosis in most parts of the world and is second only to alcoholism as a cause of cirrhosis in affluent countries. Finally, HBV is almost certainly oncogenic and the major causative factor in hepatocellular carcinoma (primary liver cancer, PLC). The evidence for the etiological role of HBV in PLC is detailed in Table 3. In all countries, males are more likely than females to become carriers of HBV and are thus at greater risk of developing the complications cited.

Table 3. Evidence for Etiological Role of HBV in Primary Liver Cancer (PLC)

1. Geographical incidence correlates with HBV carrier rate
2. HB_sAg-positive rate in PLC much greater than in controls, e.g., Taiwan, 80% versus 10%; South African black, 90% versus 20%
3. In low-prevalence area, high rate of anti-HB_c in PLC patients, e.g., 70% in London, Los Angeles
4. Longitudinal studies of HBV carriers: Risk of PLC is up to 1000 times that of controls
5. Relationship of chronic HBV infection to cirrhosis and of cirrhosis to PLC
6. Demonstration of HBV-DNA in genome of PLC cells
7. Analogy with woodchuck and Pekin duck hepadna viruses

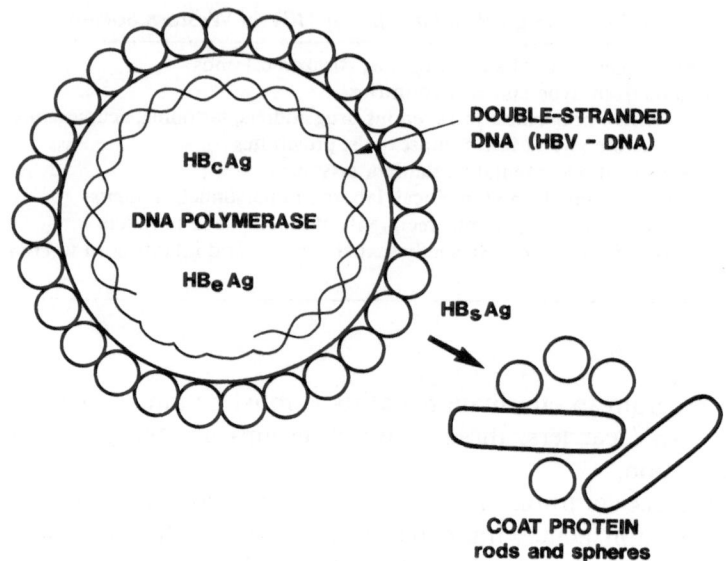

Figure 1. The Dane particle.

2.2. Properties of the Hepatitis B Virus

The hepatitis B virion was first visualized under electron microscopy by Dane and is often referred to as the Dane particle. This distinguishes the complete 42-nm viral particle from other, smaller structures (20-nm spheres and 20 × 150-nm tubules) which circulate in blood in great excess and are the empty lipoprotein coat (HB$_s$Ag) of the HBV.[2] It is now known that HBV is one of a newly recognized group of hepadna viruses, so called because they are DNA-containing hepatotrophic agents.[2] Other members of the hepadna virus group infect such diverse hosts as Pekin ducks, Eastern woodchucks, and Beechey ground squirrels, but evidence that they are more widespread in native and domestic fauna is tenuous. Study of the hepadna viruses in other species is providing useful information about their biology, including their role in oncogenesis.

A diagram of the HBV is presented in Fig. 1. The core of the virus contains an incomplete circular ring of DNA (HBV-DNA) and at least three proteins including the hepatitis B core antigen (HB$_c$Ag), the hepatitis B e antigen (HB$_e$Ag), and hepatitis B specific DNA–polymerase. An understanding of the biology of the HBV and the relationship with its human host forms the basis for development of effective hepatitis B vaccines.[2]

Only intact hepatitis B virions are infectious. The course of events following inoculation of hepatitis B virus has been studied carefully in human subjects. After an incubation period of 6–12 weeks during which virus is presumably replicating in the liver, HB_sAg is detectable in the circulation. Three to six weeks later the onset of illness occurs, heralded by a precipitate rise in the serum transaminases (e.g., alanine aminotransferase, ALT). The current concept concerning the pathogenesis of hepatocellular necrosis is that T lymphocytes attach to infected liver cells, the site of recognition being viral antigens (most likely HB_cAg or HB_eAg) incorporated into the hepatocyte plasma membrane. One to two weeks after the appearance of HB_sAg in the circulation, HB_eAg also appears, and, shortly after this, antibodies directed against HB_cAg (i.e., anti-HB_c) are detectable in the bloodstream. HB_eAg is positive for a variable period. Sometime during recovery it becomes undetectable, and a few weeks later anti-HB_e appears. Similarly, and usually following clinical and biochemical resolution of acute hepatitis, HB_sAg disappears. The appearance of anti-HB_s signifies not only complete recovery but acquisition of effective immunity against all subtypes of HBV (see Section 2.3). In contrast, anti-HB_c remains positive even in the 10% of patients who become carriers.

The HBV chronic carrier state is indicated serologically by positive HB_sAg (usually), negative anti-HB_s, positive anti-HB_c, and variably positive HB_eAg or anti-HB_e. In rare instances (5–10%) of HB_sAg-negative HBV carriers, the only serological indicator is anti-HB_c. It is relevant to note that anti-HB_s is negative in this situation. Hence, anti-HB_c does not correlate with HBV clearance and, of itself, anti-HB_c appears unlikely to confer protection against hepatitis B infection.

2.3. Hepatitis B Subtypes

Four antigenic subtypes of HBV have been recognized, indicating a degree of heterogeneity in HB_sAg polypeptides. The major group antigen is termed "a" specificity and appears to be common to all HBV subtypes. The two other pairs of subtype-specific antigens have been called the d/y and w/r systems, respectively, so that the four major antigenic subtypes of HBV are adw, adr, ayw, and ayr. Of these, ad is common in the United States, Europe, Asia, and Oceania and ay in drug addicts and renal dialysis units and also in the Middle East, Africa, some areas of Eastern Europe, and Australian aborigines. Fortunately, infection with one subtype appears to confer immunity against each of the other types.[2]

2.4. Mode of Transmission of HBV

HBV is spread by parenteral and sexual transmission (Table 4). Blood and some bodily secretions including semen and saliva contain intact HBV-DNA and are infectious. The screening of donor blood for

Table 4. Transmission of Hepatitis B Virus

Mode	Examples	Risk
Sexual	Male homosexual	Lifetime 80%
	Spouse of HBV carrier	50%
Vertical	Mother acute hepatitis B in third trimester	70%
	Mother HB$_e$Ag positive carrier	Approx. 100%
	Mother anti-HB$_e$ positive carrier	<5%
Family spread	Sexual, vertical	As above
	Other, e.g., children of HB$_s$Ag-positive father, HB$_s$Ag-negative mother	20%
Contamination of needles	i.v. drug addicts	80%
	Acupuncture, tattoos	0–20%
Occupational (blood/serum contact)	Dentists, surgeons, laboratory technicians, dialysis units	10–30% 10–50%
Institutes for mentally retarded		30–50%

HB$_s$Ag has eliminated most cases of posttransfusion hepatitis B, although occasional cases are encountered because HBV carriers may rarely be HB$_s$Ag negative. A continuing risk of needle transmissions is related to intravenous drug abuse, tattooing, acupuncture, and occupational exposure by health care workers (Table 4). Health care workers are also at risk by having contaminated blood or perhaps saliva enter breaches in their skin.

One of the most important pathways of hepatitis B infection is by vertical transmission, that is, passage of virus from a mother to her baby at or about the time of delivery. Vertical transmission is most likely if the mother has acute hepatitis B during the third trimester of pregnancy, or if she is an HB$_e$Ag-positive HBV carrier. Hence, the risk of vertical transmission is related most closely to the HB$_e$Ag status (or infectivity) of the mother (Table 5).[3,4] The virus is most likely to be passed from mother to

Table 5. HB$_e$Ag and Vertical Transmission of HBV from Asymptomatic Carrier Mothers[a]

	Baby's serum	
Mother's serum	HB$_s$Ag (+)	HB$_s$Ag (−)
HB$_e$Ag positive (25)	25	0
Anti-HB$_e$ positive (59)	0	59

[a]Data from Miyakawa and Mayumi.[3] Values are number of individuals studied.

baby at the time of delivery, but in rare instances true transplacental spread may occur. The greatest significance of vertical transmission is that it facilitates the chronic carrier status. Ninety percent of male infants who acquire HBV at the time of birth become chronic HBV carriers.[4]

Vertical and sexual transmission are not the only means by which HBV is spread within families and do not explain spread within closed communities such as institutions for the mentally retarded. The presence of an HBV carrier in a household allows the possibility of so-called horizontal transmission of hepatitis B to nonsexual contacts. Sharing of toothbrushes, razors, toys, and the like provides an obvious risk for inoculation of HBV. The infectivity of blood from an HB_eAg-positive HBV carrier may be very high, the infectious dose being as small as 10^{-6} ml. Episodes of percutaneous contact may not be obvious, and it seems likely that most horizontal transmission is by inapparent transcutaneous inoculation promoted by close personal contact. The risk of acquiring hepatitis B under these circumstances is inversely related to age, young children being at greatest risk. The high risk of a child (or staff member) acquiring hepatitis B upon entering an institute for the mentally retarded is related to the large pool of carriers, especially Down syndrome patients, who have a high hepatitis B carrier rate, and to behavioral aspects such as biting, skin trauma, and drooling.

A summary of important modes of hepatitis B transmission and the related risk of experiencing an HBV event is given in Table 4. Hepatitis B is a sexually transmitted disease, and this accounts for a large component of intrafamilial spread.[5,6] Sexual contacts of drug addicts and of prostitutes are at increased risk of acquiring hepatitis B. One of the highest risk groups is male homosexuals in whom the risk is more closely related to the number of sexual contacts and perhaps to immune suppression rather than to the method of sexual activity.

3. APPROACHES TO DEVELOPING A HEPATITIS B VACCINE

It has not so far proved possible to grow HBV in tissue culture, and animal hosts are confined to a small number of primates including chimpanzees and marmosets. However, the propensity of human HBV carriers to have an overwhelming excess of circulating empty viral coat protein (e.g., 10^{10} particles/ml) compared with infectious intact virions, together with the size discrepancy of the infectious and noninfectious particles, provides the opportunity to isolate a purified preparation of HB_sAg particles from human blood. As discussed in Section 4.2, this approach has led to the present immunogenic and highly protective inactivated subunit HBV vaccine which was released commercially in 1982.

Modern biotechnology has provided tools for designing alternative hepatitis B vaccines. One line of approach is to produce purified polypeptide subunits of HB_sAg either synthetically or biosynthetically by gene-cloning techniques. The entire structure of HB_sAg has now been sequenced, and gene probes for several regions have been cloned.[7,8] Preliminary data concerning the immunogenicity and protectiveness of the resultant putative HBV vaccines are discussed in Section 6.

Another exciting approach, which also exploits molecular biology, is the cloning of the HB_sAg gene into eukaryotic cells (in this case a yeast) with subsequent harvesting of the biosynthesized HB_sAg.[9] The HB_sAg gene can also be inserted into a "benign pathogen" such as the vaccinia virus.[10] The way in which this agent might be laden with multiple virus antigen-producing genes may be the ultimate in vaccine development from the conceptual as well as the economic and logistic viewpoint.

4. RESULTS OF HEPATITIS B VACCINES

4.1. Historical Background

In studies conducted in 1970–71, Krugman and his colleagues demonstrated that when heat-inactivated (98°C for 1 min) serum from a HBV carrier was injected into volunteers, it protected approximately 70% of them against subsequent challenge with live virus.[11] Such immunity was associated with development of anti-HB_s. Although this approach to developing a vaccine was crude, it did establish the principles of heat inactivation of HBV and of HB_sAg as a protective vaccine.

Subsequent attempts to prepare a HBV vaccine employed more sophisticated biophysical and biochemical techniques to separate the noninfectious HB_sAg subunits from whole HBV particles and to inactivate any potentially contaminating infectious agents. Several groups, including Purcell and Gerin at the National Institutes of Health, Maurice Hilleman and co-workers at the Merck Institute, and the late Philippe Maupas and his colleagues at the Pasteur Institute in Paris, began work on highly purified HB_sAg subunit vaccines.[12–14] Two of these vaccines (produced, respectively, by Merck, Sharp and Dohme and the Pasteur Institute) have been extensively tested for safety and efficacy and have been licensed for human use.

Since the Merck vaccine (Heptavax-B) is the currently available commercial hepatitis B vaccine in Australia, the steps involved in its preparation will now be discussed. The Pasteur Institute vaccine is prepared in a similar way and differs principally in being bivalent (ad/ay) rather than monovalent (ad).

4.2. Preparation of Hepatitis B Subunit Vaccine (Heptavax-B, Merck, Sharp and Dohme)

The vaccine, consisting of purified HB_sAg (subtype ad), is derived from the blood of human HBV carriers.[15] The production and testing cycle takes 65 weeks. Plasma is collected from designated HBV carriers (HB_eAg negative) in several licensed centers in large U.S. cities. HB_sAg is concentrated by ammonium sulfate precipitation and purified by a two-stage centrifugation process using isopycnic banding in sodium bromide and rate-zonal sedimentation on a sucrose gradient. This preparation is digested with pepsin and treated with 8 M urea before further purification by gel filtration. The highly purified product is then exposed to 1:4000 formalin and incubated at 36°C for 72 hr. These processes inactivate all known viruses. The final product is adsorbed onto aluminum hydroxide (alum), and thiomersal is added as a preservative.[15]

4.3. Safety Testing

Initial safety tests were performed in chimpanzees and human volunteers (executives of the Merck, Sharp and Dohme Company).[12,13] In these tests, and in subsequent field trials involving over 20,000 individuals who have been followed for up to 7 years, no untoward effects have been observed other than occasional arm soreness at the injection site. Each new batch of vaccine is subjected to potency checks and to safety tests designed to detect the presence of bacterial or viral contaminants, human serum proteins, blood group substances, or pyrogens. In addition, it is injected into chimpanzees to demonstrate the absence of live HBV. There have been no instances of non-A, non-B hepatitis following administration of Heptavax-B, and results also show clearly that the vaccine is devoid of the risk of transmitting hepatitis B. Concern that the causative agents of the acquired immune deficiency syndrome (AIDS) might be transmitted by the vaccine has been allayed by extensive observation of male homosexuals (and others) receiving the vaccine. Among 10,000 placebo-treated individuals, five developed AIDS whereas only two vaccine recipients developed AIDS. No case of AIDS has been seen after hepatitis B vaccination in a nonsusceptible individual.[16]

4.4. Immunogenicity

4.4.1. Healthy Subjects—Results, Dose, and Injection Course

Both the Merck and Maupas vaccines were demonstrated in chimpanzees to be highly immunogenic. After the injection of three doses of Heptavax-B, animals developed anti-HBs and were protected against intravenous challenge with approximately 1000 infectious doses of live virus of the same and different antigenic subtypes. Early studies of Heptavax-B in humans used 40-μg doses administered intramuscularly at 0, 1, and 6 months.[15] Following the second dose, 77% of subjects (at 2 months) had a detectable anti-HB$_s$ titer, and after the third dose 96% of subjects had detectable antibodies with the majority experiencing a sharp rise in titer after the third inoculum.

More recently, similar results have been obtained with a 20-μg dose.[17] Almost identical results have been obtained with a 5-μg dose of the Maupas vaccine.[18] It is important that the vaccine is injected into the arm rather than the buttock.

4.4.2. Low-Dose Vaccination

Several recent observations have indicated that lower doses of inactivated subunit HB$_s$Ag vaccines may provide effective immunization. Using a heat-inactivated subunit vaccine prepared by the Netherlands Red Cross Blood Transfusion Service, Coutinho et al. demonstrated that three 3-μg doses of vaccine given 1 month apart were effective in stimulating anti-HB$_s$ formation in 89% of male homosexuals at 4 months.[19] Desmyter and co-workers showed that four 3-μg injections of the same vaccine induced antibodies in 88% of patients and 100% of staff in a hemodialysis unit.[20] More recently, in a study from Washington and the Center for Disease Control, it was observed that a 2-μg dose of the Merck vaccine given intradermally on three occasions resulted in 83% of recipients developing anti-HB$_s$, usually of moderate to high titer.[21] Further trials of low-dose vaccination are being carried out. This approach is extremely attractive as it promises to ameliorate the two greatest problems with the present vaccine: cost and future availability of suitable donors.

4.4.3. Immunogenicity in Special Circumstances—Age, Renal
Failure, Immune Suppression

One of the most crucial times for interrupting transmission of the HBV is in the neonatal period (see Section 4.5). It is thus reassuring that results of vaccination in the first 6 months of life are similar to those in adults.[4,22] The usual dose regimen has been 10 μg given within the first 2 weeks, followed by similar doses at 1 month and 6 months.

It is important to note that many of the reported trials of hepatitis B vaccination have been in young subjects. There have been some reports of decreased immunogenicity in individuals over the age of 40 years, and this aspect requires further study.[23-25]

There is stronger evidence that the vaccine is less immunogenic in patients within dialysis units, most likely as a result of the suppressed immune state of such patients.[26] In a French study of 138 hemodialysis patients injected with the Institut Pasteur Production vaccine, immunization did reduce hepatitis B events significantly (from 45% to 21%), but only 60% of recipients developed anti-HB$_s$.[27] Moreover, the mean peak value of anti-HB$_s$ titers in hemodialyzed patients was 121 mIU/ml compared with 2433 mIU/ml in dialysis unit staff members. Similar results have been reported by the Maupas group.[28] The two French studies used a vaccine dose equivalent to 5 μg HB$_s$Ag (mixed subtypes ad and ay). Stevens et al. used the equivalent of 40 μg HB$_s$Ag in the Merck vaccine and obtained better results. An immune response after two or three doses was seen in 80%, and following a booster dose given 6 months later, this increased to 89%.[29] Finally, using a different heat-inactivated subunit vaccine, a Belgian and Dutch group have shown that 3 μg of HB$_s$Ag at 0, 1, 2, and 5 months produced anti-HB$_s$ in 88% of patients and 100% of staff in renal dialysis units.[20] It is now recommended that a double dose (40 μg) of vaccine be administered to patients with renal failure or other evidence of immune suppression.[26,30]

4.4.4. Vaccination Failures

About 4% of healthy individuals fail to respond to a standard course of Heptavax-B, and an additional 2–5% are hyporesponders (low anti-HB$_s$ titer after three injections). There is mounting evidence that failure to develop an adequate anti-HB$_s$ titer following a course of hepatitis B vaccination is genetically determined.[31] In one study, individuals with a low titer of anti-HB$_s$ responded adequately to a second course of vaccination. However, most nonresponders failed to respond even to a second full immunization course.[31]

The question arises whether the success of a course of hepatitis B vaccination should be assessed by determination of antibody titers. Since the bulk of evidence suggests that 96% of healthy subjects will have a satisfactory anti-HB$_s$ titer after a standard course of vaccination, and nonresponders are unlikely to ever respond to revaccination, the cost-effectiveness of such an assessment of efficacy could not be justified. However, should an individual be so assessed and anti-HB$_s$ titer be found to be low (<10 IU/liter) a further course of vaccination can be recommended since it has been demonstrated in chimpanzees that low anti-HB$_s$ titers can be overwhelmed by a massive inoculum of HBV.[2]

An unanswered question also relates to long-term efficacy of the vaccine. It is known that "naturally acquired" (i.e., from previous infection) anti-HB$_s$ titers do wane slowly over 10 years. The current vaccine has only been tested during the last 8 years so that data pertaining to long-term efficacy of the vaccine and the possible requirement for booster injections at 5- to 10-year intervals are still awaited.

4.5. Protection against HBV Infection

All the data so far indicate an excellent correlation between immunogenicity of the vaccine and protection against hepatitis B events. In the earliest study of the efficacy of a hepatitis B vaccine, Maupas et al. observed hepatitis B events only in nonresponsive vaccinees.[23] Although this was not a blinded or placebo-controlled study, it clearly demonstrated the effectiveness of hepatitis B vaccination in a renal dialysis unit setting.[23]

The effectiveness of hepatitis B vaccination was then examined more rigorously by Szmuness et al. in a double-blind, placebo-controlled randomized trial.[15,32] The vaccine was the Merck inactivated hepatitis B subunit vaccine (Heptavax-B), and the trial population was 1083 New York homosexual men. This was a particularly appropriate population to study since preliminary data indicated that 5.1% were HB$_s$Ag positive, 55% both anti-HB$_s$ and anti-HB$_c$ positive, and 8% only anti-HB$_c$ positive. The annual incidence of seroconversion was estimated to be 7.6% for HB$_s$Ag and 11.6% for anti-HB$_s$, and in approximately one-third of these cases, seroconversion was accompanied by an elevation in ALT. In the trial, 40 μg of the inactivated HB$_s$Ag subunit vaccine (ad subtype) or placebo was administered at 0, 1, and 6 months. An 85% follow-up was obtained. In placebo-treated controls, 35% experienced a hepatitis B event in 18 months, whereas only 7.6% of vaccine recipients had a hepatitis B event (Table 6). Among the 4% of vaccine recipients who failed to develop an antibody titer, the incidence of HB$_s$Ag-positive events was close to that found in the nonimmunized controls. When considered for the entire study period, the efficacy rate of vaccination was 92.3% in cases that met the criteria for hepatitis and 78.3% for all HBV events, including subjects who developed only anti-HB$_c$.

Table 6. Attack Rates for Categories of End Point in New York Hepatitis B Vaccine Trial[a]

End point	Placebo group		Vaccine recipients	
	No.	Rate	No.	Rate
Hepatitis B (ALT > 90)	45	18%	7	1.4%
All HB_sAg-positive events	70	24%	11	3.0%
All HBV events including anti-HB_c conversions	93	35%	29	7.6%

[a]Data from Szmuness et al.[15] All differences between vaccine and placebo group are significant, $p < 0.0001$.

No HBV infections occurred among subjects who received all three doses of vaccine and developed an immune response. Most of the hepatitis B events in vaccine recipients occurred in the first 4 months after receiving the vaccine suggesting that affected individuals had been exposed to HBV before the time of vaccination. However, even in the first 4 months after starting immunization, i.e., during the incubation period of HBV infections, there was a significant reduction of hepatitis B events in vaccinated individuals compared with controls.[32] This unexpected result was the first indication of the possibility that postexposure vaccination is at least partially effective.

In the New York trial, hepatitis B vaccine was equally effective in preventing subclinical infection, acute hepatitis B, and development of a chronic HBV carrier state.[15,32] Thus, vaccination prevents rather than attenuates HBV infection. This is in contradistinction to hepatitis B hyperimmune serum globulin (HBIG), which not only confers passive prophylaxis following acute parenteral, sexual, or vertical transmission, but is also associated with passive–active immunization with development of anti-HB_c and anti-HB_s.[33,34] The logical conclusion of these observations is that appropriate measures for preventing hepatitis B following acute parenteral (e.g., needle-stick) or sexual exposure are HBIG (within 48 hr) and vaccination starting immediately. It has been demonstrated that efficacy of hepatitis B vaccination is not diminished by HBIG, and coadministration of Heptavax-B and HBIG is not associated with any increased incidence of side effects.[35]

There have now been several trials, mostly controlled, attesting to the efficacy of hepatitis B vaccines in preventing HBV infection in susceptible populations.[4,12–15,17–29,32,36]

One of the strongest indications for hepatitis B vaccination is for the interruption of vertical transmission of HBV. Beasley and his colleagues

Table 7. Perinatal Transmission of Hepatitis B by HB$_e$Ag-
Positive Mothers in Taipei: Efficacy of Prevention with
HBIG and Hepatitis B Vaccine[a]

Treatment	HB$_s$Ag carrier rate of offspring	Efficacy of prevention
Placebo	90%	—
HBIG	26%	75%
Hepatitis B vaccine	20%	80%
HBIG + vaccine	6%	90%

[a]Data from Beasley et al.[4]

from Taiwan have assembled an impressive body of data which have a
bearing on the indication for and efficacy of such intervention.[4] In the
absence of any action to prevent vertical transmission, children of HBV
carrier mothers in Taiwan have a 40% risk of becoming HBV carriers
themselves (the risk may differ in other countries; for instance, it is 10%
in Greece).[3] The risk of vertical transmission of hepatitis B correlates
closely with the HB$_e$Ag status of the mother (Table 5). HB$_e$Ag-negative
mothers with anti-HB$_e$ rarely transmit.[3]

Beasley and co-workers found that hepatitis B vaccination of newborn infants was 80% protective against acquisition of hepatitis B.[4] The
timing of the initial dose of vaccine did not appear to be crucial, provided
it was within 28 days of delivery, but it seems pragmatic to give it within
the first week of life. Hepatitis B vaccination was about as protective as
HBIG given within 48 hr of delivery and followed by second and third
doses 3 and 6 months later.[34] However, there was synergistic benefit from
the combined administration of HBIG (given once) and hepatitis B vaccination (three injections) to the extent that 95% of babies so treated did
not become HBV carriers (Table 7).[4] The remaining 5% presumably
acquired hepatitis B by transplacental spread in utero. This study is one
of the most important in considering the question of hepatitis B prevention since it provides the best example of combined efficacy of HBIG and
hepatitis B vaccination in postexposure prophylaxis. In this and other
studies it has been shown that children up to 10 years respond well to
three doses of 10 μg of vaccine.[4]

4.6. Limitations of Current Vaccine

There are several logistic and theoretical problems concerning the
current inactivated HB$_s$Ag-subunit vaccine prepared from human HBV

carriers. These concern the duration and complexity of the preparative process, the consequent high cost of the vaccine, the necessity to have HBV carriers as a source of the vaccine, and the lack of acceptability of the vaccine to potential recipients because of fears about possible contamination with the AIDS-related virus and other infectious particles.

The cost of the present commercial vaccine, over $100 for a three-injection course, has considerably dampened institutional or governmental enthusiasm for introducing vaccination programs. In countries where vaccination of the entire population would seem desirable present cost would greatly exceed current per capita expenditure on health. In economically developed countries, the negligible risk of hepatitis B infection in the general population means that vaccination is not cost-effective except in high-risk groups.[37-40] However, there are still problems in obtaining a satisfactory acceptance rate of vaccination even when this is offered gratis to groups such as health workers.[41] This relates in part to the perceived risks associated with the origin of the vaccine from human blood. Although the possibility that any live particle could survive pepsin, 8 M urea, and formalin inactivation is remote, and it is well known that no cases of AIDS attributable to hepatitis B vaccination have been reported,[41] fear of this disease transcends rational debate and is a major reason why vaccination rates among health care personnel are poor even when the cost is met by the institution.

5. STRATEGIES FOR HEPATITIS B PREVENTION AND ERADICATION

5.1. Hyperendemic Countries

Countries with HBV carrier rates over 5% have the most to gain by eradication of hepatitis B because this strategy is likely to prevent the majority of deaths from cirrhosis and PLC. The most useful approach would be to vaccinate all children of HBV carrier mothers at birth and all other children within the first 3 years of life.[41,42] At present, this approach is not feasible because of the prohibitive cost of the commercially available vaccine and also because there would be insufficient production of this product to meet the needs of Third World populations. It is for these reasons that countries such as China, Singapore, Nigeria, and Japan are currently attempting to develop their own plasma-derived hepatitis B vaccines.

5.2. Low-Incidence Countries

In countries such as Canada and Australia where the overall carrier rate for HBV is well below 1% and the incidence of naturally acquired anti-HB$_s$ is 5–10%, it is unrealistic to vaccinate the entire population. The best approach appears to be to vaccinate high-risk groups within the population (3–5% of the population in Canada and Australia) and those who may be in intimate contact with HBV carriers.[37–40] Appropriate target groups for hepatitis B vaccination would include

1. *High-risk groups in the community,*[40,42,43] namely, sexual and other close contacts of patients with acute hepatitis B and chronic HBV carriers, male homosexuals, ethnic groups including aboriginals and recent immigrants, intravenous drug abusers, prostitutes, inmates and staff of institutions for the mentally retarded and penitentiaries, kindergartens and preschools containing children from ethnic groups with a high carrier rate.

2. *Selected groups of patients,* such as hemophiliacs, renal dialysis patients, patients receiving chemotherapy as well as other patients requiring frequent transfusions of blood or administration of blood products.

3. *Hospital, dental, and paramedical staff.* The risk of acquiring HBV infection varies greatly between hospital staff and for some groups, such as clerical staff and nursing administrators, is no greater than for the community as a whole. Because of the cost factor, most institutions have adopted a policy of selective vaccination of higher-risk groups, which includes dentists; surgeons; gynecological surgeons; nurses with hands-on patient exposure, especially in renal dialysis wards, intensive-care units and operating theaters; physicians in services such as nephrology and gastroenterology; laboratory staff and specimen collectors; medical, dental, and nursing students; mortuary attendants; and other staff in close contact with blood and blood products.[44,45] It is important to note that the time of greatest risk for a person in a high-risk occupation is during the initial exposure. Hence, the optimal time for vaccination is before or at the time of entry to the high-risk area. It is also relevant to note that the hepatitis B risk of particular hospitals varies greatly according to their role in the community and geographical location.

Because cost is a major concern of health authorities when consideration is given to instituting a hepatitis B vaccination program, the question of prevaccination screening tests arises. If one assumes the unit cost of one course of hepatitis B vaccine is $120 and the cost of a single screening test is $15, it will clearly not be cost-effective to screen a population if the incidence of HBV markers in that population is less than 12.5%. Since the incidence of HBV markers in hospital staff is about that figure, it is clearly not justifiable on cost-effective analyses to perform more than one screening test.

Even when not clearly cost-effective, screening may be requested on other grounds such as the individual wishing to avoid unnecessary vaccination. However, should institutions elect not to instigate screening prior to vaccination, there are data to reassure recipients that unwitting immunization of HBV carriers or individuals with natural immunity is not associated with any special risk.[22,46] The single test usually selected for prevaccination screening is the anti-HB$_c$ since this test will detect HBV carriers as well as individuals who are immune because of earlier exposure to the HBV. Determination of anti-HB$_c$ alone as a screening maneuver does raise the question of what to do with the person who has a positive result. The view of the author is that such individuals should have explained to them the two possible explanations for a positive anti-HB$_c$ and should then be allowed themselves to elect or refuse further investigations of HBV serology and liver function.

Cost-effectiveness analysis for the use of hepatitis B vaccine has been performed for various groups in the U.S. population.[37-41] When considering medical expenses alone, it was estimated that vaccination of susceptible persons will save health care costs for populations with an annual hepatitis B attack rate above 5% and may be cost-effective for populations with attack rates as low as 1–2% if other costs are taken into consideration. Screening followed by vaccination of homosexual men and vaccination *without* prior screening of surgical residents would each result in saving of medical costs to the community (social costs were not considered in this study).[37] For the general population, however, neither screening nor vaccination is justified in terms of communal cost-effectiveness strategy.

There are important political, ethical, and social issues concerning hepatitis B immunization programs that have not yet been fully addressed. One example is the question of vaccination of minority groups. Who is to pay? How is stigmatization of such groups to be avoided? In Australia a group in outstanding need of HBV immunization is the Australian aboriginal population, yet the cost of this program would exceed the current annual budget devoted to aboriginal health. At another level, the question of immunization of hospital employees in high-risk areas poses difficulties. Unfortunately, when freely offered, acceptance of hepatitis B vaccination has thus far been suboptimal.[41]

Should the responsible authorities have the right to institute policies of positive discrimination in favor of vaccinated individuals in an attempt to protect the health of their staff?

5.3. Contacts and Families of Patients with Hepatitis B

The interruption of spread of HBV is most urgent following sexual, percutaneous, or other close contact with a patient with acute hepatitis B or chronic HBV carriage. This also applies to the newborn offspring of similarly affected mothers.[4,38,42] The currently recommended treatment of such contacts is immediate (i.e., within 48 hr) HBIG and commencement of a course of hepatitis B immunization. In more equivocal cases of risk, such as household members who are not sexual partners and babies of HB_eAg-negative HBV carrier mothers,[3,42] the most reasonable approach is hepatitis B vaccination (following anti-HB_c screening in the case of family members of HBV carriers) without administration of the scarcely available HBIG. It is the view of the author that there is still need for physicians to adopt a more affirmative role in recommending hepatitis B vaccination for contacts of patients with infectious HBV diseases.

6. NEWER HEPATITIS B VACCINES

The need for cheaper vaccines and for products prepared from more acceptable and readily available sources than blood of chronic HBV carriers is evident from the preceding discussion. The theoretical approach to new vaccines was introduced earlier (Section 3), and the current status of such second- and third-generation hepatitis B vaccines will now be elaborated. This subject has recently been reviewed elsewhere.[47]

6.1. Alternative Sources of HB$_s$Ag

6.1.1. Cell Lines

It has been possible to harvest HB$_s$Ag from HBV carrier hepatocellular carcinoma (PLC) cell lines (Alexander cells). The resultant antigen was purified by several chromatographic steps and enzyme treatments and was formalin inactivated and formulated with alum along conventional lines.[47] The cell culture vaccine was equipotent to the human plasma-derived vaccine and has proved safe in tests in chimpanzees and human subjects with advanced malignancy.[48] The purification and DNA destructive processes were such as to delete any possible oncogenic DNA that might have been present in the starting fluid. Nevertheless, current licensing policies would have to be altered before such a vaccine would be acceptable for field studies.[30] Licensing authorities have, to date, banned production of vaccines in heteroploid cells.

6.1.2. Yeast Vaccine

The biosynthesis of the 25,000-molecular-weight polypeptide HB_sAg in prokaryotic or eukaryotic cells offers an alternative procedure to produce HB_sAg free from human proteins. Following the successful cloning of the HBV genome in *Escherichia coli*, determination of its primary structure allowed localization of the gene (gene S) coding for HB_sAg. Vectors carrying the DNA sequence for HB_sAg have been prepared, and the antigen has now been expressed both in *E. coli* and in the yeast *Saccharomyces cerevisiae*.[7–9] Expression of the gene in yeast has been much better than in *E. coli*. This has led to the development of a hepatitis B vaccine (subtype adw) of yeast cell origin.[9] Electron microscopy showed that the purified HB_sAg used for this vaccine exists as aggregate particles 20 nm in diameter and has morphological characteristics of free HB_sAg in infected plasma and of the purified antigen now used in plasma-derived hepatitis B vaccines. In contrast to HB_sAg from human plasma, the antigen produced by recombinant yeast is not glycosylated.[9]

The purified antigen in alum formulation stimulated anti-HB_s production in several animals including chimpanzees. Moreover, immunization with the vaccine fully protected chimpanzees that were challenged intravenously with either homologous or heterologous subtype adr or ayw HBV virus of human origin. The yeast vaccine was administered to 37 healthy adult volunteers (employees of the Merck, Sharp and Dohme company) each of whom received a 10-µg dose of HB_sAg at 0, 1, and 6 months.[49] The immunogenicity of the vaccine appears identical to that of the plasma-derived vaccine. At 1 month 27–40% of the recipients had anti-HB_s, at 3 months this rose to 80–100%, and large boosts in titer followed the third dose at 6 months. No serious reactions were attributable to the vaccine, and the most frequent complaint was transient soreness at the injection site.

6.2. Polypeptide Vaccines

The HB_sAg is made up of seven polypeptides of which two are glycoproteins.[2] The most antigenically active portions are located on a nonglycosylated peptide with a molecular weight of 25,000 and a glycosylated peptide with a molecular weight of 30,000. These polypeptides have been purified from human plasma and demonstrated to be free of viral DNA and other extraneous material. However, they are generally of low yield and poorly antigenic even though some studies have demonstrated safety and efficacy in chimpanzees.

As a result of recent developments in analyzing the gene coding for HB_sAg, it has been possible to determine the entire amino acid sequence of the antigenic 25,000-molecular-weight polypeptide. This has led to prediction of the antigenically active areas and has opened the way for their synthesis. Several polypeptides have now been produced and shown to stimulate the production of anti-HB_s.[47] Further studies examining the protectiveness of these synthetic vaccines are still under evaluation.

6.3. Live Vector Hepatitis B Vaccine: Recombinant Vaccinia Virus

Another potential application of recombinant DNA technology to vaccine development is the use of live virus vectors to express foreign genes. This approach has been adopted by a group at the National Institutes of Health (NIH). They inserted the coding sequence for HB_sAg (adw) into a silent region of the vaccinia virus genome under control of vaccinia virus early promoters.[10] Cells infected with these vaccinia virus recombinants synthesize and excrete HB_sAg of the glycosylated type. Rabbits vaccinated with the vector virus rapidly produced anti-HB_s antibodies. Two chimpanzees vaccinated with the live recombinant vaccinia virus were protected against hepatitis following challenge with HBV, although they did undergo conversion to anti-HB_s and anti-HB_c indicative of mild, inapparent infection.[50] The chimpanzees had little or no circulating anti-HB_s after vaccination but were immunologically "primed." Thus, the feasibility of using a recombinant vaccinia virus as a live hepatitis B vaccine has been demonstrated although more work is required to improve HB_sAg expression.

The campaign to eradicate smallpox has been the most successful mass vaccination program carried out in underdeveloped countries. Some reasons for this include the low cost of the vaccine, its stability, and the ability of medically unskilled personnel to administer it as a single dose on a mass scale. Since stable, infectious vaccinia virus recombinants may contain up to 25,000 base pairs of foreign DNA,[10] it may be possible to prepare polyvalent vaccines against a number of different infectious agents.

Recognized untoward reactions to vaccination that are associated with currently licensed strains include postvaccinial encephalitis, eczema vaccination, and vaccinia necrosum. There is thus a need to evaluate fully more attenuated strains of vaccinia that have recently been developed. However, even the low incidence of side effects of vaccination would be greatly outweighed by effective hepatitis B immunization in hyperendemic regions of the world.[10,47]

7. PROSPECTS FOR HEPATITIS A IMMUNIZATION

Hepatitis A is not associated with a chronic carrier state or late complications but is a significant public health problem justifying control by immunization. The first hepatitis A vaccine was prepared by formalin-inactivating live virus harvested from infected marmoset live.[51] Animals that had been immunized with inactivated partially purified virus were resistant to intravenous challenge with live virus. However, marmoset livers are not a practical source of virus from which to mass-produce a vaccine.

The hepatitis A virus is a small RNA virus which has now been grown in a variety of primary and continuous cell lines of primate origin. The two best studied strains are CR 326, originally isolated at the Merck Institute in a closed line of fetal rhesus monkey kidney cells, and HM 175, a strain obtained from a patient admitted to the Fairfield Hospital for Infectious Diseases, Melbourne, Australia. The latter strain was isolated in African green monkey kidney cells by workers at NIH. Viral isolates were slow growing at first but improved on passage. Specific viral antigen was detected in the cytoplasm of infected cells and, on later passages, in the supernatant fluid. Studies to define the optimal conditions for high virus yield are continuing.

After 20 or more passages in cell culture, both CR 326 and HM 175 appear to have become attenuated. When inoculated into chimpanzees, both strains produce infection and seroconversion without disease. It remains to be seen whether one or both strains are effective and safe in humans. If so, it should be possible to produce the vaccine in commercial quantities and have it licensed within 3–4 years.[52,53]

REFERENCES

1. Sobeslavsky O: Prevalence of markers of hepatitis B virus infection in various countries: A WHO collaborative study. *Bull Wld Hlth Org* 1980;58:621–628.
2. Robinson WS: Biology of human hepatitis viruses, pp 863–910, in Zakim D, Boyer TD (eds.): *Hepatology. A Textbook of Liver Disease*. Philadelphia, WB Saunders Co, 1982.
3. Miyakawa Y, Mayumi M: Characterization and clinical significance of HB$_e$Ag, in Vyas GN, Cohen SN, Schmid R (eds): *Viral Hepatitis*. Philadelphia, Franklin Institute Press, 1978, pp. 193–201.

4. Beasley RP, Hwang L-Y, Lee GC-Y, et al: Prevention of perinatally transmitted hepatitis B virus infections with hepatitis B immune globulin and hepatitis B vaccine. *Lancet* 1983;2:1099-1102.
5. Heathcote J, Gateau PH, Sherlock S: Role of hepatitis B antigen carriers in non-parenteral transmission of the hepatitis B virus. *Lancet* 1974;2:370-372.
6. Szmuness W, Much MI, Prince AM, et al: On the role of sexual behaviour in the spread of hepatitis B infection. *Ann Intern Med* 1975;83:489-495.
7. Burrell CJ, MacKay P, Greenway PJ, Hofschneider PH, Murray K: Expression in Escherichia coli of hepatitis B virus DNA sequences cloned in plasmic. pBR322. *Nature* 1979;279:43-47.
8. Charnay P, Gervais M, Louise A, Galibert F, Tiollais P: Biosynthesis of hepatitis B virus surface antigen in *Escherichia coli. Nature* 1980;286:893-895.
9. McAleer WJ, Buynak EB, Maigetter RZ, et al: Human hepatitis B vaccine from recombinant yeast. *Nature* 1984;307:178-180.
10. Smith GL, Macket M, Moss B: Infectious vaccinia virus recombinants that express hepatitis B virus surface antigen. *Nature* 1983;302:490-495.
11. Krugman S, Overby LR, Mushalwar IK, Ling C-M, Frosner GG, Deinhardt F: Viral hepatitis, type B. Studies on natural history and prevention reexamined. *N Engl J Med* 1979;300:101-106.
12. Purcell RH, Gerin JL: Hepatitis B vaccines: A status report, in Vyas G, Cohen SH, Schmid R (eds): *Viral Hepatitis.* Philadelphia, Franklin Institute Press, 1978, pp. 491-505.
13. Hilleman MR, Bertland AU, Buynak ER, et al: Clinical laboratory studies of HB$_s$Ag vaccine, in Vyas G, Cohen SN, Schmid R (eds): *Viral Hepatitis.* Philadelphia, Franklin Institute Press, 1978, pp. 525-537.
14. Maupas P, Goudeau A, Coursaget P, Drucker J, Bagros P: Immunization against hepatitis B in man. *Lancet* 1976;1:1367-1370.
15. Szmuness W, Stevens CE, Harley EJ, et al: Hepatitis B vaccine. Demonstration of efficacy in a controlled clinical trial in a high-risk population in the United States. *N Engl J Med* 1980;303:833-841.
16. Sacks HS, Rose DN, Chalmers TC: Should the risk of acquired immunodeficiency syndrome deter hepatitis B vaccination? A decision analysis. *JAMA* 1984;252:3375-3377.
17. Szmuness W, Stevens CE, Harley EJ, et al: Hepatitis B vaccine in medical staff of hemodialysis units. Efficacy and subtype cross-protection. *N Engl J Med* 1982;307:1481-1486.
18. Crosnier J, Jungers P, Courouce A-M, et al: Randomized placebo-controlled trial of hepatitis B surface antigen vaccine in French haemodialysis units; 1, medical staff. *Lancet* 1981;1:455-459.
19. Coutinho RA, Lelie N, Albrecht-Van Lent P, et al: Efficacy of a heat inactivated hepatitis B vaccine in male homosexuals: Outcome of a placebo-controlled double blind trial. *Br Med J* 1983;286:1303-1308.
20. Desmyter J, Colaert J, De Groote G, et al: Efficacy of heat-inactivated hepatitis B vaccine in haemodialysis patients and staff. *Lancet* 1983;2:1323-1327.
21. Miller KD, Gibbs RD, Mulligan MM, Nutman TB, Francis DP: Intradermal hepatitis B virus vaccine: Immunogenicity and side-effects in adults. *Lancet* 1983;2:1454-1456.
22. Maupas P, Chiron J-P, Barin F, et al: Efficacy of hepatitis B vaccine in prevention of early HB$_s$Ag carrier state in children. Controlled trial in an endemic area (Senegal). *Lancet* 1981;1:289-292.
23. Maupas P, Goudeau A, Coursaget P, Drucker J, Bagros P: Hepatitis B vaccine: Efficacy in high-risk settings. *Intervirology* 1978;10:196-208.

24. Szmuness W, Stevens CE, Harley EJ, Zang EA, Taylor PE, Alter HJ: The Dialysis Vaccine Trial Group. The immune response of healthy adults to a reduced dose of hepatitis B vaccine. *J Med Virol* 1981;8:123–129.
25. Lindsay KL, Herbert DA, Gitnick GL: Hepatitis B vaccine: Low postvaccination immunity in hospital personnel. *Gastroenterology* 1985;88:1675.
26. Bramwell SP, Tsakiris DJ, Briggs JD, et al: Dinitrochlorobenzene skin testing predicts response to hepatitis B vaccine in dialysis patients. *Lancet* 1985;1:1412–1415.
27. Crosnier J, Jungers P, Courouce AM, et al: Randomized placebo-controlled trial of hepatitis B surface antigen vaccine in French haemodialysis units: 11, Haemodialysis patients. *Lancet* 1981;1:797–800.
28. Maupas P, Goudeau A, Coursaget P, et al: Vaccine against hepatitis B—18 months prevention in a high-risk setting. *Med Microbiol Immunol* 1978;166:109–18.
29. Stevens CE, Szmuness W, Goodman AI, Weseley SA, Fotino M: Hepatitis B vaccine: Immune response in haemodialysis patients. *Lancet* 1980;2:1211–1213.
30. Gust ID, Lucas CR: Immunization against hepatitis B. *Aust Family Phys* 1983;12:657–660.
31. Craven DE, Kunches LM, Dienstag JL, et al: Analysis of nonresponsiveness to hepatitis B in health care workers. *Hepatology* 1984;4:1077.
32. Szmuness W, Stevens CE, Zang EA, Harley EJ, Kellner A: A controlled clinical trial of the efficacy of hepatitis B vaccine (Heptavax-B): A final report. *Hepatology* 1981;1:377–385.
33. Hoofnagle JH, Seeff LB, Bales ZB, Wright EC, Zimmerman HJ. The Veterans Administration Cooperative Study Group: Passive-active immunity from hepatitis B immune globulin: Re-analysis of a Veteran's Administration co-operative study of needle-stick hepatitis. *Ann Intern Med* 1979;91:813–818.
34. Beasley RP, Hwang L-Y, Lin C-C, et al: Hepatitis B immune globulin (HBIG) efficacy in the interruption of perinatal transmission of hepatitis B virus carrier state. *Lancet* 1981;2:388–393.
35. Szmuness W, Stevens CE, Oleszko WR, Goodman A: Passive–active immunization against hepatitis B: Immunogenicity studies in adult Americans. *Lancet* 1981;1:575–577.
36. Francis DP, Hadler SC, Thompson SE, et al: The prevention of hepatitis B with vaccine. Report of the Centers for Disease Control multi-center efficacy trial among homosexual men. *Ann Intern Med* 1982;97:362–366.
37. Mulley AG, Silverstein MD, Dienstag JL: Indications for use of hepatitis B vaccine, based on cost-effectiveness analysis. *N Engl J Med* 1982;307:644–652.
38. Chin J: The use of hepatitis B virus vaccine. *N Engl J Med* 1982;307:678–679.
39. Editorial, Costs and benefits of hepatitis B vaccination. *Lancet* 1982;2:1195–1196.
40. Coates RA, Rankin JG: Cost without benefit? The introduction of hepatitis B vaccine in Canada. *Can Med Assoc J* 1983;128:1158–1160.
41. Goldsmith MF: Crossing "threshold" of hepatitis B control awaits greater vaccine use. *JAMA* 1984;251:2765–2772.
42. Beasley RP, Hwang L-Y: Postnatal infectivity of hepatitis B surface antigen carrier mothers. *J Infect Dis* 1983;147:185–190.
43. Burrell CJ, Cameron AS, Hart G, Melbourne J, Beal RW: Hepatitis B reservoirs and attack rates in an Australian community. A basis for vaccination and cross-infection policies. *Med J Aust* 1983;2:492–496.
44. Jovanovich JF, Saravolatz LD, Arking LM: The risk of hepatitis B among select employee groups in an urban hospital. *JAMA* 1983;250:1893–1894.

45. Grady GF: Hepatitis B immunity in hospital staff targeted for vaccination. Role of screening tests in immunization programs. *JAMA* 1982;248:2266–2269.
46. Dienstag JL, Stevens CE, Bhan AK, Szmuness W: Hepatitis B vaccine administered to chronic carriers of hepatitis B surface antigen. *Ann Intern Med* 1982;96:575–579.
47. Purcell RH, Gerin JL: Prospects for second and third generation hepatitis B vaccines. *Hepatology* 1985;5:159–163.
48. McAleer WJ, Markus HZ, Wampler DE, et al: Vaccine against human hepatitis B virus prepared from antigen derived from human hepatoma cells in culture. *Proc Soc Exp Biol Med* 1984;175:314–319.
49. Scolnick EM, McLean AA, West DJ, McAleer WJ, Miller WJ, Buynak EB: Clinical evaluation in healthy adults of a hepatitis B vaccine made by recombinant DNA. *JAMA* 1984;251:2812–2815.
50. Moss B, Smith GL, Gerin JL, Purcell RH: Live recombinant vaccinia virus protects chimpanzees against hepatitis B. *Nature* 1984;311:67–69.
51. Provost PJ, Hilleman MR: An inactivated hepatitis A virus vaccine prepared from infected marmoset liver. *Proc Soc Exp Biol Med* 1978;159:201–203.
52. Anderson BN, Coulepes AG, Gust ID: Toward a hepatitis A vaccine. A review. *J Hyg (Lond)* 1984;3:269–276.
53. Jacobson IM, Dienstag JL: Viral hepatitis vaccines. *Annu Rev. Med* 1985;36:241–261.

16

Iatrogenic Aspects of Gastroenterological Practice

W. C. Watson

> A man went into hospital in Buenos Aires to have a bunion removed and ended up with a broken leg and collar bone, a heart attack and a ruptured stomach.
>
> Fearing the pain during the bunion treatment the patient asked for a general anaesthetic and this led to a heart attack. Doctors revived him by opening his chest and massaging his heart. He was put in an oxygen tent where he suffered a stomach contraction followed by a rupture of the stomach and peritonitis.
>
> Later the patient fell off a stretcher, broke a leg and collar bone, and suffered further damage to his heart. His bunion is still intact.
>
> —*Reuters News Report,* September 30, 1967

That is a graphic illustration of iatrogenic disease and is the report that first interested me in this subject.

In 1969 I defined iatrogenic disease as follows: "It is any worsening of a patient's condition which comes from seeking medical advice and which cannot be attributed to the natural history of the disease. It is something unpleasant which has happened to him because he has consulted a doctor and which was neither a necessary nor inevitable complication of his illness or its treatment."[1]

That definition has been adopted by a number of authors. Simply put, it is when the doctor makes you worse rather than better.

W. C. Watson ● Department of Gastroenterology, Victoria Hospital, London, Ontario, Canada N6A 4G5.

1. INTRODUCTION

Iatrogenic means "doctor caused," not just medicine or treatment caused. It is not new. Whether doctors have been trephining holes in the skull to release evil spirits, shedding blood to cleanse the body of toxins, or applying the most up-to-date scientific principles or mechanical gadgets, patients have always been at risk. If the ancients suffered from a lack of effective therapeutics, today's patient is as likely to suffer from their surfeit. Applied ignorance and misapplied knowledge are equally dangerous remedies.

The patient is at risk at every point in his relationship with the doctor. Risks are inescapable when such an encyclopedic subject as medicine is applied to such an unpredictable object as a human being. The obligation of the attending doctor is to reduce the degree of risk to the minimum. His best safety measures are skill (intellectual and manual) and restraint.

There are four main areas of risk:

1. Diagnostic procedures.
2. Treatment—medical/surgical/psychiatric.
3. Communication—misunderstandings, wrong advice, wrong diagnosis, misleading prognosis.
4. Clinical research.

In discussing this subject the standard of practice against which one judges error is the theoretical one of perfection, which may be tough, but can hardly be something less. Perfection, or something close to it, is presumably what we are striving for. Yet, having said that, some of the things that go wrong are not so much error as misadventure or just sheer bad luck. How else does one categorize mediastinal emphysema after rectal biopsy? Hemobilia after liver biopsy?[2]

In other words, although an iatrogenic event may imply culpability, as through carelessness, ignorance, or inexperience, it often does not. If the incidence of postpolypectomy bleeding is 5%, there is something badly wrong with the technique. If it is 0.5%, it is a reasonable statistical assumption that there is something about the 1 in 200 situations that is not the fault of the endoscopist but is rather part of clinical and biological variability and uncertainty.

However, it should be emphasized, especially for those who are involved in training programs, that complication rates are inversely related to experience. The first 50 cases get done the worst. Residents do not appreciate how much concealed anguish teachers endure as they look on at the first efforts of their trainees.

I want to make a somewhat subtle, but important point that attempts to distinguish between a straightforward, statistically acceptable complication and an iatrogenically dependent complication. Many of the drugs we prescribe—anticholinergics, steroids, H_2 blockers, to name a few—have recognized side effects. If a male patient gets gynecomastia from cimetidine or ranitidine when either of these drugs is prescribed for the proper reasons, that is a complication of therapy for which no one is to blame. But if a male patient gets gynecomastia from an H_2 blocker when he should never have been on it in the first place, that is an iatrogenic event. It is not the drug which is primarily responsible, it is the doctor. The same point can be made about the hypospermia of salazopyrin or the femoral head necrosis of prednisone. The latter example has been upheld by the courts as an iatrogenic rather than a therapeutic misadventure. It is important to be clear about this aspect of drug prescribing at a time when we have never had so many powerful and effective drugs at our disposal. A side effect from a drug given properly for the right reason is not an iatrogenic event, but an undesirable effect from a drug given improperly for the right reason or properly for the wrong reason is. An example of this that I would like to stress is the use of codeine and its analogs in management of the acute diarrhea of severe ulcerative colitis. That is the way to iatrogenically generated toxic megacolon.

Following is a discussion of events, in no special order, that can properly be regarded as iatrogenic.

2. SOME IATROGENIC EVENTS

Iatrogenic events reported in the gastroenterologic literature have included

- Bile gastritis after cholecystectomy[3]
- Esophageal perforation (most quoted)[4-6]
- Persistence of symptoms after cholecystectomy
- Accidental hepatic artery ligation
- Cardiac arrhythymias during endoscopy[7]
- Colonic obstruction after barium enema
- Intussusception caused by esophageal dilator thread[8]
- Bacteremia after upper gastrointestinal (GI) endoscopy[9-11]
- Bacterial enteritis after upper GI endoscopy

- Colonic explosion
- Inadvertent gastroileostomy[12]

All of these, in different ways, satisfy the definition of iatrogenic events of clinical importance. They are or lead to unpleasant outcomes which are not an integral part of the original disease. Most of them are due to direct doctor intervention. Some are avoidable. Some are not. They represent different kinds of doctor failure or none at all—only the fact that doctors, albeit with the best of intentions, did something.

Accidental hepatic artery ligation or ligation or transection of the common bile duct is a clear example of improper surgical technique, but not being cured by a cholecystectomy is a different matter. What does that represent? It seldom, if ever, means the surgery was done badly. It usually means that the wrong thing was done to begin with, which in turn means the wrong diagnosis. Not that we can always be expected to make the right diagnosis, but we should be expected to be conservative about diagnosing problem syndromes, especially when the treatments are invasive or risk-bearing. This is certainly an area where a second consultation may be warranted. What about investigative artifacts such as the mistaken interpretation of "cold nodules" in isotope liver scans? This can lead to unnecessary liver biopsies, wrong prognosis, and the unfortunate social and economic consequences that may follow.

Now let me discuss the GI tract and in a somewhat systematic way mention some well-known and not so well-known iatrogenic outcomes of management, whether due to drugs, instruments, the doctors who use them, or just bad luck—if there is such a thing. Since good luck is said to befall the individual who is prepared for it, a fair corollary must be that bad luck befalls the individual who is unprepared for it. The list will include examples of wrong diagnosis, procedural error, inappropriate therapy, and one or two other factors. I shall not mention things that, though important or serious from a clinical point of view, are an unavoidable outcome of certain investigative or treatment modalities at the present point of standard clinical experience. A good example of what I mean by this is the esophageal ulcer that follows variceal sclerosis.

2.1. The Esophagus

Tears of the esophagus are the most serious complications that can accompany instrumental procedures. These relate principally to the dilatation of strictures or the management of achalasia by pneumatic dilatation of the lower esophageal sphincter. The main reasons for tears are inexperience, carelessness, excessive boldness, and inappropriate instrumentation. Strictures are often accompanied by inflammatory damage to the wall or associated with diverticulae in which tips of bougies may lodge or, if they are due to carcinoma, are often associated with pathological weakness of the esophagus. Strictures need to be dilated carefully, only so much at a time, and whenever there is any doubt about the directional control of the dilator, it should be done over a guidewire. In this regard the new Savary bougies are a great advance.

Tears due to pneumatic dilatation of the lower esophageal sphincter are somewhat more unpredictable. This is a situation in which it is extremely important to warn the patient of the possibility of a tear. It is possible that with the new plastic vinyl water-filled dilators the possibility of a tear will be diminished, but unlikely that it will be eradicated completely.

Esophageal candidiasis usually occurs with the combination of impaired immunity and the presence of nasogastric tubes. The need for nasogastric intubation should always be assessed carefully. Such a tube is one of the most unpleasant things that patients endure and should never be left in position longer than is necessary. The main reason for impaired immunity leading to esophageal candidiasis is usually the administration of immunosuppressive therapy.

2.2. The Stomach

In my opinion, a management misconception that leads to unnecessary treatment is the too ready diagnosis of "gastritis" as a cause of symptoms. Too often inexperienced endoscopists feel obliged to provide a positive diagnosis when they really do not see anything wrong. Two main outcomes from erroneous attribution of a working diagnosis are, first, the search for the true diagnosis is deferred and, second, unnecessary treatment is introduced.

Unfortunately, one still sees malignant gastric ulcers that should have been diagnosed much earlier. Delay in the diagnosis of serious conditions when this could have been avoided by proper action is an iatrogenic occurrence, and the principal reason for it in the case of gastric ulcers is the radiological report which says in effect "this ulcer should be reviewed radiologically after so many weeks of treatment." Radiological review of gastric ulcers in those over the age of 40 is unacceptable.

Even when endoscopy is carried out, there is still the problem of how much biopsying to do. It appears that 12 biopsies will give a 95% probability of detecting carcinoma when present and six biopsies a 90% probability. Of course, the biopsies must be taken from the best sites, and these are usually around the rim or just under the lip of the ulcer. Biopsies from the base of the ulcer often provide nothing more than necrotic tissue. Provided the endoscopist is systematic in his biopsy technique, he cannot be faulted for the occasional failed diagnosis of carcinoma which will inevitably occur because of sampling inadequacy.

2.3. Endoscopic Retrograde Cannulation of the Pancreas (ERCP)

As with all new techniques, complication rates tend to fall off with experience. Pancreatitis due to introduction of too much dye seems to be less common nowadays. Duodenal penetration due to improper positioning of the cutting wire in the course of a sphincterotomy can only be reliably avoided by a radiological corroboration of the position of the wire. Post-ERCP infections seem to be not so much an iatrogenically related complication as a risk accentuated by preexisting pathology particularly when there is either cholestasis or the presence of pancreatic pseudocysts.

2.4. The Small Bowel

Not too much can go wrong in this area of the alimentary tract. It is seldom nowadays that we see stenosing ulcers of the small bowel due to administration of potassium chloride tablets. More important in my experience is the improper attribution of the diagnosis of celiac disease, with its lifelong implications, without small-bowel biopsy. The diagnosis of celiac disease on the basis of the response to gluten withdrawal alone is unacceptable. The social repercussions of the diagnosis of celiac disease are enormous, and patients are entitled to have this diagnosis properly confirmed.

2.5. The Gallbladder

The surgical ligation or tear of bile ducts in the course of a cholecystectomy is quite simply due to carelessness. The issue of unnecessary cholecystectomy, on the other hand, raises a different and interesting issue. The clue to unnecessary cholecystectomy is, of course, that the patient's preoperative symptoms persist after the surgery. Provided the symptoms are genuine, and the patient is not malingering, this sequence represents an erroneous preoperative diagnosis and the cholecystectomy becomes an iatrogenic occurrence. This is not to deny the difficulty of the correct diagnosis of right-upper-quadrant discomfort. My advice to the surgeon who is contemplating a cholecystectomy in a patient who does not have unequivocal evidence of gallbladder disease is to think of the so-called hepatic flexure syndrome and refer the patient to a gastroenterologist for another opinion.

2.6. The Pancreas

The main concern here is overtreatment of cancer of the pancreas. There is always the occasional case of early pancreatic carcinoma that has a good surgical result, but the majority of such carcinomas have a dismal prognosis, and unnecessary overtreatment of these patients simply adds a component of iatrogenic discomfort to their last days. Often this seems to be a situation in which the physician is treating either himself or the family usually by chemotherapeutic protocols that have no proven worth. This is not to deny the occasional value of certain palliative surgical procedures usually aimed at biliary decompression.

2.7. The Liver

Somewhat similar is the pointless investigation of liver metastases when these turn up unexpectedly in ultrascan examinations. Every physician should ask himself carefully what precisely can be achieved by the investigation of such a finding. Only if there is a useful palliative outcome should what often turn out to be exhaustive and exhausting investigations be set up. There is no merit in finding a small cecal carcinoma by colonoscopy unless the removal of such a lesion will prevent ongoing significant blood loss during the last weeks or months of the patient's life. If at some time in the future the eradication of metastatic disease becomes a reality, then this attitude may have to change.

The missed diagnosis of Gilbert disease leads to much unnecessary investigation and patient anxiety. The main reason for this is unfamiliarity with what is a relatively common disorder. Patients with this diagnosis should not have liver biopsies unless absolute corroboration of liver normality is required for, say, insurance purposes, there is a possibility of another, coincident liver pathology, or the patient insists on having it for his own peace of mind. The last has never arisen in my own experience.

Hepatic encephalopathy in the susceptible patient is too often unnecessarily induced because of physician unawareness of the adverse role of some therapeutic regimens. It is particularly important either to avoid or be careful in the use of diuretics, sedatives, hypnotics, and codeine and its analogs in the treatment of patients with underlying liver disease.

2.8. The Colon

A major philosophical management issue is what I regard as the overinvestigation of functional colonic disease. I concede that this is a controversial area that relates to personal practice philosophy, but in my opinion there is still too much unnecessary investigation carried out to make the diagnosis of functional bowel disease by exclusion. Tied in with this is the misdiagnosis of "colitis." To a large extent, this is a semantic misconception, but it also relates to inexperience with interpretation of sigmoidoscopic findings. This is another example in which a misattribution of an important diagnosis leads to unnecessary treatment, patient apprehension, and a potentially disadvantageous position relating to insurance risks.

Pseudomembranous colitis due to antibiotic use only qualifies as an iatrogenic effect if the antibiotics have been used inappropriately. This relates to a point I have made earlier in this chapter.

3. AVOIDING IATROGENIC EVENTS

The examples given illustrate the great variety of types of events that can have iatrogenically disadvantageous outcomes for patients.

What are we to do about the problem? Lapinsky comments somewhat colorfully,

> The normal symbiotic relationship between doctor and patient (pathogen and host) becomes disturbed by changes in the resistance of the host or by changes in the pathogenicity of the pathogen. Increased virulence of the physician is brought about by misdiagnosis, misinterpretation and overaggressive therapy among other factors. This illness [iatrogenic disease] can be prevented by increased knowledge, better judgment, a ceaseless consideration by the physician of each of his decisions and acts, and finally by the elimination of financial considerations from medical practice.

It is desirable, though perhaps not essential, to be up-to-date. The latest article in the *New England Journal of Medicine* is not the last word, and even the most elaborate multicentered trials can be wrong. Good judgment is virtually impossible to measure, but we seem to know those who have it and those who do not, and we are all familiar with those cleverest and extensively knowledgeable residents who have it least of all.

There is an inevitable time lag between the introduction of the new treatment of great promise or the diagnostic test of infallible accuracy and their proper assessment and evaluation. There are over 100 new laser units in the United States for the treatment of acute upper GI bleeding, but the leadoff paper at the first American Gastroenterology Association plenary session in New York last year showed that laser therapy was not better and perhaps even worse than standard conservative management.[13]

The matter of risk to the patient from equipment and procedural innovation is dealt with explicitly by Ellen Picard.[14] She writes, "The law must balance the desirability of promoting (technical) advances against resorting too readily to novel and untested treatment. The doctor need not employ the very latest tools to meet the standard of care, but neither can he ignore them once they have found their way into common use." There is a good legal precedent from the British House of Lords which maintains that a doctor is not expected to use the very latest equipment.

But since the practice of medicine and surgery is a progressive science, there must be innovation both in equipment and in the manner in which it is used. This, however, does not excuse the innovator from taking every precaution to foresee, anticipate, and minimize whatever risk to the patient may reside in the new activity. "The doctor who chooses to treat with the latest equipment or the newest techniques must meet a *higher* standard of care as must also the doctor who continues to use older methods after his more progressive colleagues have moved to new approaches."[14]

The doctor should get help and advice from colleagues who are familiar with new methods before he uses them himself, or he should attend courses on recent advances.

In my opinion, the degree of liability for an iatrogenic event has some relationship to necessity. For example, if variceal sclerosis is performed as an emergency procedure and the patient acquires an esophageal ulcer, that complication is acceptable when the immediate possible outcome was death. But the situation is different if sclerosis is done for prophylactic management of esophageal varices, where the threat to life is real but remote. This brings me back to the position that if the bad thing did not need to happen, it is iatrogenic.

But how bad is bad? What about "discomfort," avoidable or otherwise. At what point does a little extra discomfort while the residents do their first colonoscopies merge into iatrogenic discomfort. Fleming, in *The Law of Torts,* writes, "The skill demanded from beginners presents an increasingly difficult problem. While it is necessary to encourage them, it is evident that they cause more than their proportionate share of accidents."[15]

What guidelines can I suggest?

Get the appropriate training
—intellectual and manual, and in that order.

Get the simplest and safest equipment for the task in hand
—and maintain it properly.
Show restraint
—just because something *can* be done does not mean it *needs* to be
done or *should* be done.
Admit ignorance (to yourself)
—and if you have the wisdom to do that, other people will never find
out.

A final word of warning. It is possible to become unduly apprehensive about iatrogenic disease to the extent that the fear of making a mistake becomes inhibiting, leading to undue caution and intellectual inertia. Fortunate are the patients of the doctor who can advance with care and mark time on his toes.

REFERENCES

1. Watson WC: Iatrogenic disease or not quite what the doctor ordered. *Health Bull* 1969;27:1-2.
2. Ball TJ, Mutchnik MG, Cohen GM, et al: Hemobilia following percutaneous liver biopsy. *Gastroenterology* 1975;68:1297-1299.
3. Buxbaum KL: Bile gastritis occurring after cholecystectomy. *Am J Gastroenterol* 1982;77:305-311.
4. Ancona E, Semenzato M, Peracchia A: Iatrogenic perforation of the esophagus. *Acta Chir Belg* 1977;76:211-218.
5. Behnke EE, Gadlage R, Turner JS Jr: Instrumental perforation of the esophagus. *Laryngoscope* 1980;90:842-846.
6. Katon RM: Complications of upper gastrointestinal endoscopy in the gastrointestinal bleeder. *Dig Dis Sci* 1981;26:47-54.
7. Bough EW, Meyers S: Cardiovascular responses to upper gastrointestinal endoscopy. *Am J Gastroenterol* 1978;69:655-661.
8. Redmond P, Ambos M, Berliner L, et al: Iatrogenic intussusception: A complication of long intestinal tubes. *Am J Gastroenterol* 1982;77:39-42.
9. Byrne WJ, Euler AR, Campbell M, et al: Bacteremia in children following upper gastrointestinal endoscopy or colonoscopy. *J Pediatr Gastroenterol Nutr* 1982;1:551-553.
10. Cohen LB, Korsten MA, Scherl EJ, et al: Bacteremia after endoscopic injection sclerosis. *Gastrointest Endosc* 1983;29:198-200.
11. O'Connor HJ, Hamilton I, Lincoln CL, et al: Bacteremia with upper gastrointestinal endoscopy—A reappraisal. *Endoscopy* 1983;15:21-23.
12. Jay BS, Burrell M: Iatrogenic problems following gastric surgery. *Gastrointest Radiol* 1977;20:239-257.

13. Krejs GJ, Little KJ, Westergaard H, et al: Laser photocoagulation for the treatment of acute peptic ulcer bleeding: A randomized controlled clinical trial. *Gastroenterology* 1985;88:1457A.
14. Picard E: *Legal Liability of Doctors and Hospitals in Canada.* Toronto, Carswell Legal Publications, 1984.
15. Fleming JG: *The Law of Torts,* ed 6. Sydney, Australia, Law Book Company Limited, 1983.

17

The Development of Current Surgical Treatment of Inflammatory Bowel Disease

Donald J. Glotzer

1. INTRODUCTION

The current state of the art of surgery for inflammatory bowel disease (IBD) is best understood if viewed from the perspective of its historical development. Through the years medical and surgical treatment have been intertwined and interdependent as physicians and surgeons have attempted to understand and treat these often devastating diseases. Since the pathogenesis of IBD remains unknown, current treatment still emphasizes "art." Increasingly, however, scientific method has been used in exploring possible etiologies and in evaluating the results of various therapies including operation.

2. ULCERATIVE COLITIS

The historical account should begin with ulcerative colitis (UC) since it was a well-recognized entity a half-century earlier than was Crohn's disease (CD). Credit for the first clear description of UC is usually given

---

Donald J. Glotzer ● Departments of Surgery, Beth Israel Hospital and Harvard Medical School, Boston, Massachusetts 02115.

to Sir Samuel Wilks and Dr. Walter Moxon of Guy's Hospital in their *Lectures on Pathological Anatomy* published in 1875.[1] In a few brief paragraphs Wilks and Moxon described the pathological appearance of a severe colitis occurring in patients whose clinical course was characteristic and clearly different from that of "febrile epidemic dysentery" and other "morbid fluxes," as diarrheal diseases were known in that day. Subsequently Dr. William Hale-White, in a paper published in *Guy's Hospital Reports* for 1888, authored what is generally considered the first comprehensive clinical description of UC.[2]

A fascinating and entertaining account of how the physicians of the late-19th and early-20th centuries thought about and treated UC is provided in the *Proceedings of the Royal Society of Medicine* for 1909. In a comprehensive introductory lecture for a Royal Society symposium on UC, Sir William H. Allchin[3] described the turn-of-the-century state of the art. He recognized that UC was not due to the common intestinal pathogens and seemed to favor the theory that some endogeneous or exogenous luminal toxic product might make the mucosa susceptible to the resident intestinal flora. When Allchin states, "Numberless have been the drugs, astringents, antiseptics, and sedatives that have been administered by mouth with little or no assured benefit," it appears that he is far ahead of his time. He goes on to decry the value of enemas with diverse substances such as "tincture of hamamelis, adrenaline, boracic acid, nitrate of silver or the perchloride or pernitrate of iron." However, it seems clear that his disparagement of enemas was not because of prescience, but because of their presumed ineffectiveness in reaching all the surfaces of the inflamed bowel! In fact, as the ultimate treatment, the physicians sought help from their surgical friends to create "an artificial anus of the cecum or ascending colon which diverted the irritant and toxic ingredients" of intestinal contents and permitted "a very satisfactory irrigation of the colon with antiseptic solutions such as permangate of potash, boracic acid, creolin etc." Allchin concluded by giving dietary advice which often is well worth following today: "A small quantity of digestible solid food is to my mind preferable to a wholly slop diet!"

A surgeon at the Royal Society Symposium, Mr. G. H. Makins,[4] favored complete diversion of the fecal stream by proximal colostomy rather than the provision of access for irrigations, a view supported by Hale-White. Makins reported that in his hands diversion of the fecal stream by ileosigmoidostomy had failed, and he recognized the futility of diverting the fecal stream into the area of most severe disease involvement.

The symposium on UC at the Royal Society for 1909 concluded with reports of experience with UC in the major London hospitals.[5] As summarized in Table 1, hospitalized patients with UC had an average mortality of over 50% at the turn of the century. This is perhaps not surprising considering the treatments given and that probably only the severest cases of UC were recognized.

Despite the early efforts by Makins and others to relieve UC by diversion of the fecal stream, the usual rationale of operation in the early 1900s was to allow access to the colon for irrigations with the various medications already mentioned. To this purpose the first regularly performed operation for UC was appendicostomy (or a valvular cecostomy in the absence of an appendix). This operation was first performed by Wier at Roosevelt Hospital in New York in 1902.[6] Appendicostomy subsequently gained great popularity on both sides of the Atlantic. Interestingly, as late as the 1940s, appendicostomy was still regarded by some very prominent surgeons as an effective operation for UC.[7]

J. Y. Brown of St. Louis is generally given credit for the first use of ileostomy for UC. He reported in 1913[8] that a number of different diseases of the colon, including one case of UC, were benefited by ileostomy, which put the colon to rest by completely diverting the fecal stream. Even at that, Brown hedged his bets by establishing a concomitant cecostomy for irrigation purposes.

By the 1920s and 1930s the therapeutic concept of bowel rest with diverting ileostomy had gained primacy, based on its observed success in relieving symptoms and in restoring health. However, it also gradually became evident that the colon usually did not heal sufficiently with diversion of the fecal stream to allow subsequent restoration of intestinal con-

Table 1. Mortality of Hospitalized Patients with Ulcerative Colitis in London, circa 1909[a]

	No. cases	No. died	Mortality rate
Guy's Hospital	55	40	73%
Royal Free Hospital	2	2	100%
St. Bartholomew's Hospital	24	21	88%
St. George's Hospital	19	9	47%
St. Mary's Hospital	19	8	42%
St. Thomas's Hospital	80	40	50%
University College Hospital	51	13	25%
Overall	250	133	52%

[a]Data abstracted from Ref. 5.

tinuity. Moreover, the awareness grew that the colon and rectum, even though excluded, were subject to a number of complications including ongoing or increased disease activity, perforation, remote manifestations such as arthritis or pyoderma, and the development of carcinoma. With the recognition that the colon was a continued liability, the dictum evolved "once an ileostomy, always an ileostomy."

Based on these considerations the therapeutic principle of extirpation of the diseased colon gradually gained favor. Ileostomy became, in effect, the first stage of a staged colectomy. The surgeons of the 1930s, 1940s, and even early 1950s removed the colon bit by bit, as progressively more distal segments were excised at each stage, including ultimately the rectum. By the 1950s, however, with developments in supportive care and anesthesia, several groups (Table 2) reported that they had performed single-stage abdominal colectomy and ileostomy with a 0–6% mortality rate even in patients who required an emergency or urgent colectomy. These figures were far superior to those for ileostomy alone, for which mortality figures of 50% were common. Some adventurous surgeons in the early 1950s had been able to perform elective panproctocolectomy and ileostomy in a single stage without mortality (Table 2).

Preliminary diversionary ileostomy was gradually abandoned during the 1950s as increasingly the principle of extirpation was accepted as feasible, safe, and more effective. Panproctocolectomy and ileostomy, which is usually done in a single stage, is currently the operation of choice for UC and is the gold standard to which all other operations must be compared.

Table 2. Results of Early Efforts at One-Stage Subtotal Colectomy and Ileostomy in Ulcerative Colitis

Author(s)	Year	Emergency operation		Elective operation		Comments
		No. cases	Mortality rate	No. cases	Mortality rate	
Bacon and Trimpi[9]	1950			22	0%	
Gardner and Miller[10]	1951	17	5.8%	52	3.9%	
Counsell and Goligher[11]	1952			14	0%	Also 4 elective panproctocolectomies, all successful
Ripstein[12]	1953	43	4.6%			Also 4 elective panproctocolectomies, all successful

Even though the ultimate goal of extirpative surgery in UC is removal of the rectum as well as the abdominal colon, surgeons often appear to feel unnecessarily compelled to remove the entire colon and rectum at a single "sitting." I believe that there is still a place for the staged operation in the sicker, more depleted patients.

The toxic megacolon syndrome represents a prime example of the type of case in which a staged operation should be considered. In fact, Turnbull and his colleagues have gone still further with their advocacy of a multiple-ostomy, venting procedure for toxic megacolon.[13] However, by resorting to a modern-day form of diversion, Turnbull and associates may have ignored some of the lessons of history. Probably as a result, fully 10% of Turnbull's patients undergoing the multiple-ostomy procedure required reoperation during the same hospitalization. The colon in toxic megacolon perforates because it is disintegrating and not because it blows out. With gentle handling of the dilated colon, subtotal colectomy or even a panproctocolectomy can be carried out expeditiously and with low mortality.[14] In my experience retention of the rectum has not been a problem except when massive bleeding is part of the indication for operation. In these instances the rectum is better removed, since on a few occasions proctectomy in the postoperative period has been required as an emergency because of massive bleeding from the rectal stump.

Concomitant with the development of the cure for ulcerative colitis by extirpation of the diseased organ, developments in the care of the ileostomy and its construction had a significant impact on patient morbidity and late mortality. The early ileostomates were provided with crude, nonadherent metal or plastic receptacles with which to attempt to keep the ileostomy effluent from digesting and excoriating the peristomal skin. The rigid appliances worked fairly well during the day when the patient was upright, but at night when the patient was supine, the leakage of discharges wreaked havoc on the peristomal skin. As a result, many of these patients were reduced to a state of chronic invalidism.

A major breakthrough that changed the ileostomy from an affliction to a manageable handicap was the invention of the cemented-on appliance.[15] Interestingly enough, this development came about largely through the efforts of an afflicted patient. Although the Chicago surgeon, Alfred Strauss, provided some conceptual advice and encouragement, it was his patient, Koenig, a student chemist, who devised a pouch with a faceplate and formulated a relatively nonirritating latex rubber cement with which to seal the appliance to the skin. The Strauss–Koenig type of appliance and its then contemporary analogs revolutionized the surgery of UC. These appliances were the prototypes of innumerable modern appliances that allow ileostomates to live comfortably and relatively care-free.

As humble a "development" as it would seem to be, the use of karaya gum represented another liberating factor for ileostomates.[16] This complex polysaccharide derived from the *Sterculia urens* tree of India was previously used as a bulk laxative and for cementing dentures in place. It is said, perhaps apocryphally, that Dr. Rupert Turnbull, in using this material for the latter purpose, accidentally dropped some on his moist skin and noted that it adhered tenaciously. He immediately appreciated the potential value of karaya to the ileostomate since he was aware of the need for a substance that would adhere to moist, irritated skin and yet be porous enough to allow healing beneath it. Karaya powder, wafer, and paste are invaluable in the care of ileostomies. Second-generation similar substances are now used as adherent backing for appliances, replacing the old plastic and rubber faceplates and latex cement.

Parallel with advances in the care of ileostomies, there were developments in their method of construction. It was recognized by patients and surgeons alike that the ileostomy discharges would be more easily collected if the stoma were protuberant and spoutlike. The innovative Dr. Lester Dragstedt, of vagotomy fame, proposed for this purpose the application of thickness skin grafts to the serosal surface of a long, protruding length of ileum.[17] However, this procedure had to be abandoned since the grafted squamous mucosa of this penislike arrangement was no less susceptible to digestion than the periileostomy skin.

An additional major source of morbidity after ileostomy, dysfunction of the ileostomy, must be mentioned. Ileostomy dysfunction occurred in two forms: an acute form, early on after operation, and a chronic form.[18] This syndrome was characterized by severe ileostomy diarrhea, abdominal cramps, dehydration, hypovolemic shock, and, at times, ulceration, inflammation, and even perforation of the ileum. Warren and McKittrick,[18] in the analysis of their experience with ileostomy, reported that fully 62% of their patients developed dysfunction. These workers and others began to realize that ileostomy dysfunction was the result of a functional small-bowel obstruction at the level of the stoma. The fact that the acute symptoms of ileostomy dysfunction could be immediately relieved simply by catheterizing the stoma was part of the evidence for this theory.

What was the pathogenesis of functional obstruction of the ileal stoma? Prior to the 1950s ileostomies were constructed by simply bringing the ileum to the surface and holding it there by one or the other means until it adhered to the abdominal wall. The ileum then underwent a process of "maturation," which took place over 4–6 weeks when ultimately the mucosa healed to the skin. During the process of maturation, the serosa, like any other nonepithelial surface exposed to the environment, became inflamed and was covered with granulation tissue, especially since it was constantly bathed in ileostomy discharges. Warren and McKittrick[18] recognized that this collar of granulation tissue or its chronic counterpart, a cicatricial scar at the level of the skin and subcutaneous tissue, was the cause of ileostomy dysfunction and described remedial operations. However, in 1954, Crile and Turnbull[19] presented the definitive elucidation of the pathophysiology of ileostomy dysfunction. In a now classical paper they also demonstrated that a mucosal grafted ileostomy (rather than split-thickness skin, which Dragstedt had used) eliminated the problem of ileostomy dysfunction by allowing primary healing to take place. The lasting contribution of Crile and Turnbull, however, was not in their technique of ileostomy construction but in the concept. Two years earlier[20] Mr. Bryan Brooke of Birmingham, England, had described his technique of ileostomy construction, which featured a full-thickness turnback of the ileum. Brooke did not propose his method specifically for the prevention of ileostomy dysfunction, but as a technique for constructing a protruberant, easy-to-manage ileostomy which avoided a number of different complications including stomal stenosis. In this publication Brooke was also one of the first to advocate suture of the ileal mesentery to the lateral peritoneum to prevent internal herniation, volvulus, and small-bowel obstruction.

The Brooke method is the currently accepted technique for primary maturation of the ileostomy, and "Brooke ileostomy" is the generic name used for conventional ileostomy. However, many surgeons, including myself, prefer the retroperitoneal ileostomy, a modification devised by Goligher[21] in which the ileum used for the ileostomy is brought under a tunnel of freed-up lateral parietal peritoneum. I believe this technique is superior to mesenteric suture to the lateral parietes because it virtually eliminates the potential for internal herniation of small-bowel loops between the ileostomy and the lateral abdominal wall. Furthermore, because of the obliquity of the course of the ileum, there may be less potential for prolapse (which used to be a common postoperative complication) and also paraileostomy hernia. Nor should there be any hesitation in using Goligher's technique for Crohn's disease of the colon. Even if a prestomal recurrence should develop and require reoperation, I have not seen problems in freeing the ileum from the tunnel beneath the peritoneum.

Because of the various complications of ileostomy and the difficulties associated with its care, there was, in the earlier experience, a progressive late patient mortality after colectomy.[22] However, with the developments discussed earlier, sources of later mortality and morbidity have essentially been eliminated. By 1968 Daly[23] reported that patients undergoing colectomy for UC uncomplicated by cancer and who survived the first postoperative year had the same observed late mortality as that expected in an age-and-sex-matched normal population. Devroede *et al.*[24] reported similar results in children in that the slope of the postcolectomy survival curve paralleled that of the normal population in contrast to the slope for unoperated patients, which continued to deviate progressively and significantly. Even some insurance companies are beginning to recognize that colectomy and ileostomy cures patients with UC, and therefore in many instances they have been willing to underwrite life and even disability insurance for these patients (A. Marcus, personal communication, 1985).

Colectomy for patients with UC can now be carried out with a less than 3% operative mortality rate, and late morbidity and mortality have been virtually eliminated. We must recognize, however, that this longevity and health after operation for UC have been achieved at the expense of a permanent stoma, which, although manageable, still represents a definite physical and psychological disability. A long-term goal of surgeons has been to develop satisfactory alternatives to conventional Brooke ileostomy, perferably one that includes preservation of the anal sphincters.

As early as 1953, Mr. Stanley Aylett reported using ileoproctostomy as his operation of choice for most patients with ulcerative colitis. By 1966 he had performed this procedure in over 300 patients and reported excellent results in 83%.[25] Aylett also claimed that the diseased rectum usually healed after operation. Others have not achieved such spectacular success, and as a result, the Aylett operation has never gained great popularity, especially in North America. However, some independent observers have reported reasonable success with this procedure. For example, Watts and Hughes[26] surveyed patients after the Aylett operation performed by another surgeon, Hughes, and concluded that the results in about half were "satisfactory" and another 25% were "satisfactory-with-reservations." In a few highly selected patients with mild inflammation of the rectum and short duration of disease, so that the future development of carcinoma was not a major worry, I have had excellent results with this procedure. However, I think that most North American surgeons would agree that the majority of patients needing operation for UC are not candidates for the Aylett operation.

A much more recent development is that of the continent ileostomy pioneered and developed by Nils Kock of Goteborg, Sweden.[27] In its current version this ileostomy features (1) a pouch constructed by connecting adjacent loops of terminal ileum with long side-to-side anastomoses,

(2) an all-important nipple valve made by a reverse intussusception of the prestomal ileum, and (3) a flush, nonobstrusive stoma, which is placed in the pubic hair line. The patient covers the stoma with a small dressing to protect the clothing from mucus (hence the so-called "Bandaid ileostomy") and empties the pouch three or four times per day by catheterization with a large-bore tube. Various technical modifications have been somewhat successful in improving the initial results in terms of the percent of patients who are totally continent for both feces and gas. However, failure of the nipple valve has been a significant problem with this procedure, leading to incontinence or inability to catheterize the stoma. Failed valves can often be salvaged by revisions, but multiple reoperations may be necessary and they are not always successful. In this regard the development of stomal occlusive devices[28] to maintain an external pouchless state in some of these patients speaks for itself. "Pouchitis" (presumably secondary to overgrowth of Bacteroides species) is another not uncommon problem and is reminiscent of the old days of ileostomy dysfunction and inflammation. "Pouchitis" usually responds to antibiotics and nipple valve problems can be dealt with by successive revisions or stomal occlusive devices, but there are other sources of morbidity and even some mortality which can be attributed to the construction of the Kock pouch per se. Depending on the point of view of the patient and surgeon, these risks may or may not be worth taking. I sense that the popularity of the continent ileostomy is waning. This is not just because of the problems cited, but largely because of the recent interest in ileoanal pull-through procedures.

The concept of the ileoanal pull-through operation was originally proposed by Ravitch and Sabiston in 1947[29] as a sphincter-saving operation for UC and familial polyposis. These workers denuded a short segment of rectum of its diseased mucosa, pulled the ileum through the muscular tube, and sutured it to the dentate line. After some initial success, Ravitch and Sabiston essentially abandoned the procedure. In the 1960s, with the hope of making the reconstructed rectum function more normally than it did with the Ravitch procedure, I and my associates developed a modification which employed a long, muscular tube of rectum lined by ileal mucosa from which the muscularis had been stripped.[30] Primarily because nocturnal continence was less than perfect, I was not happy with this procedure and it was not appealing to properly informed, potential candidates for the operation. Martin and associates revived interest in pull-through procedures with their 1977 publication of excellent results in children with UC.[31] The late Sir Alan Parks began using a S-shaped pouch (similar to the Kock pouch), which he pulled through a short, mucosally denuded rectal stump.[32] For reasons that are not completely clear (see next paragraph), 50% of Parks' patients were unable to defecate spontaneously and required catheterization *per anum* for evacuation of the pouch.[32]

In conjunction with this type of procedure, Utsonomiya and his colleagues[33] in Japan described a J-shaped pouch which seemed to obviate the problems with defecation that Parks had observed. This modification sparked interest in the ileoanal pull-through procedure, and large series of patients and rather glowing results have been reported.[34-36] In recent reports the S-shaped pouch seems to work as well as the J pouch in some hands,[35] perhaps because of the use of a shorter ileal spout. A pouch devised by Fonkalsrud,[36] which features a long, isoperistaltic, lateral anastomosis of ileum to ileum, also appears to function satisfactorily.

Careful perusal of more analytical reports[34] on this procedure does not lead me to the conclusion that we have finally achieved surgical cure of UC with preservation of near-normal physiology. The number of bowel movements may be excessive in some patients. "Pouchitis" can be as problematic as with the Kock pouch. Small-bowel obstruction is a not uncommon postoperative complication. Perhaps most important, fully 33% of patients appear to have at least some degree of nocturnal seepage and 12% have some degree of incontinence by day.[34] Moreover, pull-through procedures are contraindicated in patients with Crohn's colitis (with which UC may be confused) in which cases recurrence of disease in the pouch or the prepouch ileum is a definite possibility. If this occurs, sorely needed intestine will have been sacrificed in the construction of the pouch, as would be the case in the event of a failed pouch in UC.

The advisability of pull-through procedures must be regarded as *sub judice* at the present time. They may be indicated in the meticulously informed patient with UC who fully understands the problems and the potential benefits of the alternative forms of therapy. The candidate must be motivated enough to accept the additional risks and drawbacks, which include the required additional surgery and the possibility of complications as tradeoffs for the potential gain, which, however, can be considerable in some patients.

3. CROHN'S DISEASE

In 1932, more than a half-century after the first description of UC, Crohn, Ginsburg, and Oppenheimer described 14 cases of "regional ileitis" which they distinguished from other granulomas of the ileocecal region.[37] Regarding the question of priority of recognition, Fielding[38] and subsequently Kyle[39] have recently pointed out that in 1913 the Scottish surgeon Dalziel had described a chronic enteritis grossly "resembling an eel in a state of rigor mortis," which clearly was regional enteritis (RE).[40] There may well be other even earlier contenders. However, the eponym Crohn's disease is merited since his report focused the attention of the medical community on this disease. Because of its completeness and clarity the paper is well worth reading today.

At the time of the original report one of the 14 patients had already developed "an annular stenosis a short distance proximal to the new anastomosis," a happenstance that was attributed to the fact that the "resection had not been carried out sufficiently oral to the lesion completely to eradicate the disease." The belief that CD could, like cancer, be stamped out by sufficiently radical surgery persisted for a long time, particularly among surgeons. Even as late as 1951 Crohn believed that operation was the treatment of choice for severe cases of regional enteritis.[41] Gradually, however, it has become increasingly clear that postoperative recurrence is so common that it is almost a descriptive feature of CD.

In an important publication in 1967 Lennard-Jones and Stalder[42] pointed out the wide disparities in the rates of recurrence reported from different centers. This variation was attributed in part to the type of evidence used by different investigators to document recurrent disease, i.e., whether this was based on symptoms alone, on the requirement for reoperation, or on x-ray and/or pathological evidence. As vital as the rigorous definition of recurrent disease is for this endeavor, the introduction by Lennard-Jones and Stalder of actuarial methodology into the determination of the rate of recurrence in CD was even more important. As in cancer recurrence, *crude* rates of recurrence are rather meaningless because they do not take into consideration the factor of time. As shown in Fig. 1, Lennard-Jones and Stalder's data on the *cumulative* rate of recurrence published in 1967 are almost superimposable on recent data from a number of other centers, which are, in turn, similar to each other. It is generally agreed that rates of recurrence in RE amount to about 35% at 5 years, 60% at 10 years, and 75% at 15 years.

After the definitive description of RE it took about another quarter century before primary CD of the colon was accepted as an entity. Very soon after Crohn's seminal report it was realized that the same lesion could involve every part of the proximal gut including the jejunum, duodenum, stomach, and even the esophagus. However, it was believed for a number of years that, in the absence of prior operation, spontaneous CD of the colon did not occur and that the ileocecal valve was a barrier to the distal spread of CD.

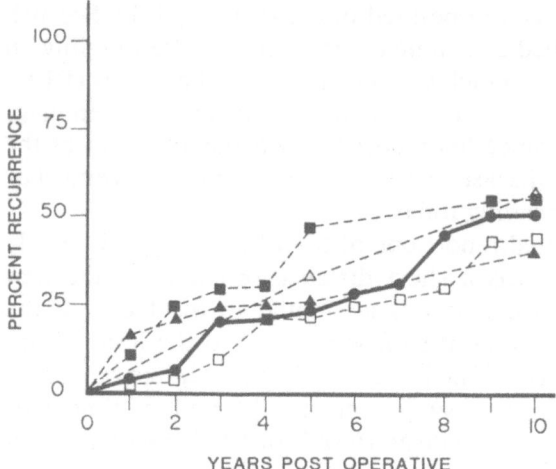

Figure 1. Plots of the cumulative rates of recurrence for ileitis in various series. Data taken from Lennard-Jones and Stalder, 1967[42] (●——●) are compared with those of several recent series [Cooke et al.,1980[78] (△- - - -△); Pennington et al., 1980[64] (■- - - -■); Trnka et al. 1982[59] (◻- - - -◻); and DeDombal et al., 1981[79] (▲- - - -▲)]. In marked contrast to earlier reports, there is a remarkable similarity of results from various centers now that actuarial methodology is used.

Although there were previous less comprehensive reports, the first clear recognition that colonic CD could occur as a primary process dates from publications from the late 1950s and early 1960s from St. Marks Hospital, London by Morson and Lockhart-Mummery.[43-45] Their work cleared up previous confusion about the nature of such entities as "right-sided UC," "UC with rectal sparing, "segmental UC," and RE and UC occurring in the same patient. It became evident that more than 50% of patients with colonic IBD previously diagnosed as UC in fact had CD of the colon (CDC).

With the general recognition and acceptance of CDC,[46,47] there arose controversy about the prognosis after operation, particularly in patients whose disease mimicked UC and who, therefore, required an ileostomy and colectomy to encompass the extent of their disease.[48-51] Because of a putative high rate of recurrence it was believed by some that operation in CDC should be performed only for complications or, if performed for intractability to medical management, postponed until much later than would be appropriate for a patient with UC.[46] Publications from different institutions indicated recurrence rates for CDC ranging from as low as 3%[51] to as high as 45%.[52]

The true rate of recurrence in CDC undoubtedly is substantially lower than the 46% and 33% rates reported from Mount Sinai Hospital in New York[52] and Birmingham, England,[53] respectively. These discrepancies appear to stem largely from a very elementary arithmetic principle: the calculation of a percent requires not only a numerator but a denominator. That is, the apparent percent recurrence depends not only on the number of patients having recurrence but also on an accurate assessment of the number of patients at risk. In the studies with very high rates of recurrence cited earlier, the clinical and pathological material on all patients with IBD was not reviewed. As a result, patients with CDC comprised only 11 and 12%, respectively, of the population of patients undergoing colectomy and ileostomy for IBD whereas this figure should be 50% or more. Therefore, many of the patients with CDC in the studies cited were considered to have UC and were not in the denominator of the fraction, *observed recurrences/patients at risk.* For this reason, I believe that the rates of recurrence were falsely inflated.[54]

During the 1940s exclusion bypass rather than resection was proposed by the Mount Sinai group as the operation of choice for RE.[41,55] This operation developed empirically as a result of experience with two-stage resections, namely, preliminary exclusion bypass to be followed by resection. It was noted that almost invariably the symptoms abated and signs of disease activity settled down after the first stage. Since the patients were already well after the first-stage operation, the second stage seemed superfluous and unwarranted. The bypass procedure was appealing because it was simpler and could be done with less morbidity and mortality than could resection. Moreover, it appeared that the rate of recurrence was lower, although there was great controversy among authorities about this latter point. In any event, during the 1950s exclusion bypass became the operation of choice for RE in many centers.

Improvements in supportive care and anesthesia gradually eroded the advantage of bypass over resection in terms of morbidity and mortality, and therefore, these factors became less and less relevant to the choice of procedure. Moreover, contrary to previous reports of superior long-term results with bypass, a number of recent publications have claimed that bypass is followed by a *higher* rate of recurrence than resection.[56,57] A number of investigators including ourselves[58,59] have not been able to confirm the latter claim despite the fact that in such retrospective analyses there could well be a selection bias in favor of resection. However, the bypassed segment may well be the site of future complications such as perforation or cancer, which also must be considered in the choice of operation.[59] It is well to remember that one-third or more of the reported small-bowel carcinomas complicating CD have occurred in bypassed segments.[60] Although the bypass operation is acceptable, resection is currently favored unless specifically contraindicated because of local, technical considerations.

The conduct of resection has changed over the years based on evolving understanding of the course of RE. Initially, resections for RE were performed in a manner similar to that of a standard right colectomy for carcinoma. This includes a wide removal of the mesentery to remove local lymph nodes, which mandates that the distal margin of resection will be in the right transverse colon. Removal of the enlarged mesenteric lymph nodes in RE has been recommended as a means of reducing postoperative recurrence,[61] a claim not supported by any comparative data. As a matter of fact, removal of all the enlarged nodes would often require resection of not only the right colon but also large segments of uninvolved small intestine because of the interruption of intestinal blood supply that would be necessary to accomplish this purpose.

With regard to the distal margin of resection it has long been recognized that recurrent disease usually involves the neoterminal ileum and usually stops just at the junction with the colon. A recent detailed analysis of our experience with anastomotic procedures in CD[59] confirmed this common clinical observation. Recurrent disease involved the neoterminal ileum 100% of the time in patients who had exclusively ileal disease initially and 85% of the time in patients with ileocolitis. Any colonic recurrence usually was of limited extent at the anastomotic site or was remote from the anastomosis, usually in conjunction with clinically more important ileal recurrence. Therefore, there is no need in the case of purely ileal or even right-sided ileocolic disease to resect the colon to the transverse colon and thereby sacrifice valuable water-absorbing colonic mucosa. For ileitis, the site of the distal anastomosis should be just beyond the caput of the cecum in the ascending colon. If there is colonic disease, a distal margin of resection just beyond the colonic involvement will suffice.

The opitmal proximal margin of resection has been the subject of much more ongoing controversy than has the distal margin. At one time Crohn and his surgeon colleague Garlock believed that 2 ft of normal bowel proximal to the diseased segment should be removed in order to minimize the rate of recurrence of disease.[41] The general principle that recurrent disease could be minimized by wide removal of normal intestine proximal to the disease has been espoused by many North American surgeons who often used frozen sections in order to verify inflammation-free margins. However, as far back as 1954 Van Patter et al.[62] reported that patients with close margins of resection fared as well vis-à-vis recurrence as those with wide margins. A number of more recent studies have shown that the length of the proximal margin of resection has no influence on the frequency of recurrent disease and how soon after operation this will occur.[59,63-66] In fact, patients with microscopic inflammation right at the margin of resection appear to have no higher rates of recurrence than those with microscopically normal margins.[63-66] Although there are still advocates of more radical resection in CD,[65-69] the weight of current opinion seems to favor lesser resections. This opinion is supported by a growing body of physiological, cytological, and electron microscopic data that suggest that CD may be universal or at least more widespread in the intestine than is evident on gross inspection or light microscopic study of operative specimens.[70–74]

A study by Rutgeerts et al.[75] sheds some further light on the postoperative behavior of the lesion of CD. Their data suggest that recurrence of disease occurs much more quickly than suggested even by the previously cited studies. These workers showed that patients who had undergone ileocolic resection for CD and were routinely colonoscoped within 1 year of operation had essentially the same frequency of recurrence as observed in groups of patients colonoscoped 1–3 and 3–10 years after operation. The only differences observed in these three groups of patients were that the lesions became more advanced and stenotic with the passage of time.

As a result of increased knowledge about CD and its response to operation, there has been a complete reversal in the philosophy of operation for RE and CDC amenable to anastomotic procedures. In times past, and still among a few diehards, the goal was cure of the disease by means of a radical extirpation. A growing number of authorities now advocate a conservative operation the purpose of which is to relieve otherwise unmanageable symptoms or to deal with specific troublesome or dangerous complications such as abscess, fistula, or stricture.

Perhaps the ultimate development in the concept of palliative surgery is strictureplasty, which some surgeons are now advocating particularly for multiple strictures in ileojejunitis. Short strictures are widened by longitudinal incision with transverse closure, analogous to Heineke–Mikulicz pyloroplasty. Longer strictures may be incised and closed by long, lateral–lateral anastomosis as in a Finney or Jaboulay pyloroplasty. In a somewhat limited number of patients there has been a surprisingly low rate of suture line complications and a high rate of success.[76,77] To be sure, many of the shorter, single strictures that were relieved by strictureplasty could have been handled just as well with a short resection. Strictureplasty further extends the current concept of limited palliative surgery in RE. This procedure may well achieve a definite place in the surgical armamentarium for this disease.

4. CONCLUSION

From the earliest recognition of IBD, physicians and surgeons have worked together to understand these diseases and bring relief to those suffering from them. As the concepts and the available treatments have changed, so have the operations and their indications.

Hopefully, in the future specific etiological treatment will be discovered that will make it unnecessary to cure colitis by such a destructive operation as panproctocolectomy and will spare the patient with CD the ever-present threat of postoperative recurrence.

REFERENCES

1. Wilks S, Moxon W: *Lectures on Pathological Anatomy*, ed 2. Philadelphia, Lindsay and Blakiston, 1875.
2. Hale-White W: On simple ulcerative colitis and other intestinal ulcers. *Guy's Hosp Rep* 1888;45:131–162.
3. Allchin WH: Ulcerative colitis: An address introductory to a discussion on the subject. *Proc R Soc Med* 1909;2:59–75.
4. Makins GH: Symposium on ulcerative colitis. *Proc R Soc Med* 1909;2:75–79.
5. Statistics of ulcerative colitis from the London hospitals, provided to form the basis for the above discussion. *Proc R Soc Med* 1909;2:100–156.
6. Corbett RS: A review of surgical treatment of chronic ulcerative colitis. *Proc R Soc Med* 1945;38:277–290.
7. Lockhart-Mummery JP: Discussion on the surgical treatment of idiopathic ulcerative colitis and its sequelae. *Proc R Soc Med* 1940;33:637–650.
8. Brown JY: The value of complete physiological rest of the large bowel in the treatment of certain ulcerative and obstructive lesions of this organ. *Surg Gynecol Obstet* 1913;16:610–613.
9. Bacon HE, Trimpi HD: The selection of an operative procedure for patients with medically intractable ulcerative colitis. *Surg Gynecol Obstet* 1950;91:409–420.
10. Gardner C, Miller GG: Total colectomy for ulcerative colitis. *Arch Surg* 1951;63:370–372.
11. Counsell PB, Goligher JC: Surgical treatment of ulcerative colitis. *Lancet* 1952;2:1045–1050.
12. Ripstein CB: Primary resection of the colon in acute ulcerative colitis. *JAMA* 1953;152:1093–1095.
13. Turnbull RB Jr, Hawk WA, Weakley FL: Surgical treatment of toxic megacolon: Ileostomy and colostomy to prepare patients for colectomy. *Am J Surg* 1971;122:325–331.
14. Binder SC, Patterson JF, Glotzer DJ: Toxic megacolon in ulcerative colitis. *Gastroenterology* 1974;66:909–915.
15. Strauss AA, Strauss SF: Surgical treatment of ulcerative colitis. *Surg Clin North Am* 1944;24:211–224.
16. Hill GL: *Ileostomy. Surgery, Physiology, and Management.* New York, Grune & Stratton, 1976, Chapter 1.
17. Dragstedt LR, Dack GM, Kirsner JB: Chronic ulcerative colitis: A summary of evidence implicating bacterium necrophorum as an etiologic agent. *Ann Surg* 1941;114:653–662.
18. Warren R, McKittrick LS: Ileostomy for ulcerative colitis: Technique, complications and management. *Surg Gynecol Obstet* 1951;93:557–567.

19. Crile G Jr, Turnbull RB: The mechanism and prevention of ileostomy dysfunction. *Ann Surg* 1954;140:429–466.
20. Brooke BN: Management of ileostomy including its complications. *Lancet* 1952;2:102–104.
21. Goligher JC: Extraperitoneal colostomy and ileostomy. *Br J Surg* 1958;46:97–103.
22. Bargen JA, Brown PW, Rankin FW: Indications for and technique of ileostomy in chronic ulcerative colitis. *Surg Gynecol Obstet* 1932;55:196–202.
23. Daly DW: Outcome of surgery for ulcerative colitis. *Ann R Coll Surg* Engl 1968;42:38–57.
24. Devroede GJ, Taylor WF, Sauer WG, Jackman RJ, Strickler GB: Cancer risk and life expectancy of children with ulcerative colitis. *N Engl J Med* 1971;285:17–21.
25. Aylett SO: Three hundred cases of diffuse ulcerative colitis treated by total colectomy and ileorectal anastomosis. *Br Med J* 1966;1:1001–1005.
26. Watts J Mck, Hughes ESR: Ulcerative colitis and Crohn's disease: Results after colectomy and ileorectal anastomosis. *Br J Surg* 1977;64:77–83.
27. Kock NG: Continent ileostomy. *Prog Surg* 1973;12:180–201.
28. Beahrs OH, Bess MA, Beart RW Jr, Pemberton JH: Indwelling ileostomy valve device. *Am J Surg* 1981;141:111–115.
29. Ravitch MM, Sabiston DC Jr: Anal ileostomy with preservation of the sphincter: A proposed operation in patients requiring total colectomy for benign lesions. *Surg Gynecol Obstet* 1947;84:1095–1099.
30. Glotzer DJ, Pihl BG: Preservation of continence after mucosal graft in the rectum and its feasibility in man. *Am J Surg* 1969;117:403–409.
31. Martin LW, LeCoultre C, Schubert WK: Total colectomy and mucosal proctectomy with preservation of continence in ulcerative colitis. *Ann Surg* 1977;186:470–480.
32. Parks AG, Nicholls RJ, Belliveau P: Proctocolectomy with ileal reservoir and anal anastomosis. *Br J Surg* 1980;67:533–538.
33. Utsonomiya J, Iwana T, Imajo M, et al: Total colectomy, mucosal proctectomy and ileoanal anastomosis. *Dis Colon Rectum* 1980;23:459–466.
34. Taylor BM, Beart RW Jr, Dozois RR, Kelly KA, Wolff BG, Ilstrup DM: The endorectal ileal pouch anal anastomosis. Current clinical results. *Dis Colon Rectum* 1984;27:347–350.
35. Rothenberger DA, Buls JG, Nivatvongs S, Goldberg SM: The Parks S-ileal pouch and anal anastomosis after colectomy and mucosal proctectomy. *Am J Surg* 1985;149:390–394.
36. Fonkalsrud EW: Endorectal ileoanal anastomosis with isoperistaltic ileal reservoir after colectomy and mucosal proctectomy. *Ann Surg* 1984;199:151–157.
37. Crohn BB, Ginzburg L, Oppenheimer GD: Regional ileitis: A pathologic and clinical entity. *JAMA* 1932;191:825–828.
38. Fielding JF: Dalziel's (Crohn's) disease: An historical review. *History Med* 1972;4:20–23.
39. Kyle J: Dalziel's disease—66 years on. *Br Med J* 1979;1:876–877.
40. Dalziel TK: Chronic interstitial enteritis. *Br Med J* 1913;2:1068–1070.
41. Garlock JH, Crohn BB, Klein SH, Yarnis H: An appraisal of the long-term results of surgical treatment of regional enteritis. *Gastroenterology* 1951;19:414–423.
42. Lennard-Jones JE, Stalder GA: Prognosis after resection of chronic regional enteritis. *Gut* 1967;8:332–336.
43. Morson B, Lockhart-Mummery HE: Crohn's disease of the colon. *Gastroenterologia* 1959;92:168–173.

44. Lockhart-Mummery HE, Morson, BC: Crohn's disease (regional enteritis) of the large intestine and its distinction from ulcerative colitis. *Gut* 1960;1:87–105.
45. Lockhart-Mummery HE, Morson BC: Crohn's disease of the large intestine. *Gut* 1964;5:493–509.
46. Lindner AE, Marshak RH, Wolf BS, Janowitz HD: Granulomatous colitis: A clinical study. *N Engl J Med* 1963;269:379–385.
47. Janowitz HD, Lindner AE, Marshak RH: Granulomatous colitis: Crohn's disease of the colon. *JAMA* 1965;191:825–828.
48. Glotzer DJ, Stone PA, Patterson JF: Prognosis after surgical treatment of granulomatous colitis. *N Engl J Med* 1967;277:273–279.
49. Glotzer DJ, Gardner RC, Goldman H, Hinrichs HR, Rosen H, Zetzel L: Comparative features and course of ulcerative and granulomatous colitis. *N Engl J Med* 1960;282:582–587.
50. Fawaz KA, Glotzer DJ, Goldman H, Dickersin GR, Gross W, Patterson JF: Ulcerative colitis and Crohn's disease of the colon—A comparison of the long-term postoperative courses. *Gastroenterology* 1976;71:372–378.
51. Nugent FW, Veidenheimer MC, Meissner WA, Haggitt RC: Prognosis after colonic resection for Crohn's disease of the colon. *Gastroenterology* 1973;65:398–402.
52. Korelitz BL: Recurrent regional ileitis after ileostomy for granulomatous colitis. *N Engl J Med* 1972;287:110–115.
53. Steinberg DM, Allan RN, Brooke BN: Sequelae of colectomy and ileostomy: Comparison between Crohn's colitis and ulcerative colitis. *Gastroenterology* 1966;68:448–452.
54. Glotzer DJ: Recurrence in Crohn's colitis: The numbers game. *World J Surg* 1980;4:173–182.
55. Garlock JH, Crohn BB: An appraisal of the results of surgery in treatment of regional ileitis. *JAMA* 1945;127:205–208.
56. Williams JA, Fielding JF, Cooke WT: A comparison of results of excision and bypass for ileal Crohn's disease. *Gut* 1972;13:973–975.
57. Homan WP, Dineen P: Comparison of the results of resection, bypass and bypass with exclusion for ileocecal Crohn's disease. *Ann Surg* 1978;187:530–535.
58. Mekhjian HS, Switz DM, Watts HD, Deren JJ, Katon RM, Beman FM: National cooperative Crohn's disease study: Factors determining recurrence of Crohn's disease after surgery. *Gastroenterology* 1979;77:907–913.
59. Trnka YM, Glotzer DJ, Kasdon EJ, Goldman H, Steer ML, Goldman LD: The long-term outcome of restorative operation in Crohn's disease. Influence of location, prognostic factors and surgical guidelines. *Ann Surg* 1982;196:345–355.
60. Greenstein AJ, Sachar DB, Pucillo A, et al: Cancer in Crohn's disease after diversionary surgery. A report of seven carcinomas occurring in excluded bowel. *Am J Surg* 1978;135:86–96.
61. Stahlgren LH, Ferguson LK: The results of surgical treatment of chronic regional enteritis. *JAMA* 1961;175:986–989.
62. Van Patter WN, Bargen JA, Dockerty MB, Feldman WH, Mayo CW, Waugh JM: Regional enteritis. *Gastroenterology* 1954;26:347–450.
63. Lee ECG, Papaioannou N: Recurrences following surgery for Crohn's disease. *Clin Gastroenterol* 1980;9:419–438.
64. Pennington L, Hamilton SR, Bayless TM, Cameron JL: Surgical management of Crohn's disease. Influence of disease at margin of resection. *Ann Surg* 1980;192:311–318.
65. Heuman R, Boeryd B, Bolin T, Sjodahl R: The influence of disease at the margin of resection on the outcome of Crohn's disease. *Br J Surg* 1983;70:579–621.

66. Hamilton SR, Reese J, Pennington L, Boitnott JK, Bayless TM, Cameron JL: The role of resection margin frozen section in the surgical management of Crohn's disease. *Surg Gynecol Obstet* 1985;160:57–62.
67. Karesen R, Serch-Hanssen A, Thoresan BO, Hertzberg J: Crohn's disease: Long-term results of surgical treatment. *Scand J Gastroenterol* 1981;16:57–64.
68. Bergman L, Krause U: Crohn's disease: A long-term study of the clinical course in 186 patients. *Scand J Gastroenterol* 1977;12:937–944.
69. Lindhagen T, Ekelund G, Leandoer L, Hildell J, Lindstrom C, Wenckert A: Recurrence rate after surgical treatment of Crohn's disease. *Scand J Gastroenterol* 1983;18:1037–1044.
70. Allan R, Steinberg DM, Dixon K, Cooke WT: Changes in the bidirectional sodium flux across the intestinal mucosa in Crohn's disease. *Gut* 1975;16:201–204.
71. Dunne WT, Cooke WT, Allan RH: Enzymatic and morphometric evidence for Crohn's disease as a diffuse lesion of the gastrointestinal tract. *Gut* 1977;18:290–294.
72. Ferguson R, Allan RN, Cooke WT: A study of the cellular infiltrate of the proximal jejunal mucosa in ulcerative colitis and Crohn's disease. *Gut* 1975;16:205–208.
73. Dvorak AM, Osage JE, Monahan RA, Dickersin GR: Crohn's disease: Transmission electron microscopic studies. III. Target tissues. Proliferation of and injury to smooth muscle and the autonomic nervous system. *Hum Pathol* 1980;11:620–634.
74. Dvorak AM, Silen W: Differentiation between Crohn's disease and other inflammatory conditions by electron microscopy. *Ann Surg* 1985;201:53–63.
75. Rutgeerts P, Geboes K, Van Trappen G, Kerremans R, Coenegrachts JL, Coremans G: Natural history of recurrent Crohn's disease at the ileocolonic anastomosis after curative surgery. *Gut* 1984;25:665–672.
76. Hawker PC, Allan RN, Dykes PW, Alexander-Williams J: Strictureplasty. A useful, effective surgical treatment in Crohn's disease. *Gut* 1980;24:A490.
77. Lee ECG, Papaioannou N: Minimal surgery for chronic obstruction with extensive or universal Crohn's disease. *Ann R Coll Surg Engl* 1982;64:229–233.
78. Cooke WT, Mallas E, Prior P, Allan RN: Crohn's disease: Course, treatment and long term prognosis. *Q J Med* 1980;49:363–384.
79. De Dombal FT, Burton I, Goligher JC: Recurrence of Crohn's disease after primary excisional surgery. *Gut* 1971;12:519–527.

18

Food Allergy and Adverse Reactions

Fergus Shanahan and Stephan R. Targan

1. INTRODUCTION

The concept of "food allergy" is not new.[1] Immunological responses to foodstuffs were demonstrated long before the modern era of sophisticated immunological investigative techniques.[1,2] Unfortunately, however, the subject has been shrouded in confusion and controversy for several decades, and in the minds of some physicians it has been relegated to the level of food faddism, cultism, and quackery. The problem has been compounded by the continuing presence of articles and advertising in the popular press which have, to a large extent, succeeded in giving many of their readers wild and exaggerated notions and expectations about the prevalence, spectrum, and investigation of putative food allergies.

Much of the confusion surrounding this subject has been created by the use of inappropriate terminology and by the tendency of some authors to cloud the issue by including all adverse food reactions under the general term *allergy*. Food allergy is only one of a multitude of possible adverse reactions to food contents and contaminants. Coupled with this problem has been a failure to appreciate the importance of carefully performed objective tests to minimize patient and observer bias in the investigation of suspected food reactions. Indiscriminate use of elimination and "hypoallergenic" diets based on vague symptoms without objective verification and/or the results of commercially advertised "food

Fergus Shanahan and Stephan R. Targan ● Division of Gastroenterology, University of California at Los Angeles School of Medicine, Los Angeles, California 90024.

allergy tests" is to be deplored and for some patients carries the very real threat of malnutrition.

Misconceptions and prejudice concerning the issue of food allergies and adverse reactions are still very prevalent, and the requirement for clarification and standardization of terminology has recently prompted independent reviews and recommendations by the American Academy of Allergy[3] and in England by the Royal College of Physicians.[4] The purpose of this chapter is to attempt to place the role of *true* food allergy as a cause of clinical illness in perspective for the practicing gastroenterologist, to discuss current concepts of its pathogenesis, and to highlight the difficulties and pitfalls in the investigation of patients with suspected adverse reactions or allergies to food.

2. CLASSIFICATION AND TERMINOLOGY

Adverse reactions to foods may be separated into two broad categories, depending on whether the immune system contributes to the abnormal reaction (Table 1). The terms *food hypersensitivity* and *food allergy* may be used interchangeably but should be restricted only to those reactions which have conclusively been shown to be mediated by the immune system.[3,4] Immunologically triggered reactions to food antigens may be *early* (IgE-mediated) or *delayed* (late-phase IgE-mediated responses, immune-complex-mediated, and possibly cell-mediated). With the excep-

Table 1. Adverse Reactions to Food

Nonimmunologically mediated
Idiosyncrasy
Gastrointestinal, e.g., alactasia
Systemic, e.g., glucosé 6-phosphate-dehydrogenase deficiency
Pharmacologic, e.g., caffeine, tyramine, serotonin, alcohol, histamine
Toxic, e.g., aflatoxins, botulism, mushroom toxins
Infectious, e.g., salmonellosis
Other contaminants and additives
Antibiotics, pesticides
Dyes, e.g., tartrazine
Flavorings and preservatives, e.g., monosodium glutamate (Chinese restaurant syndrome), sulfites, benzoate, nitrites, and nitrates
Gastrointestinal disorders, e.g., peptic ulcer, cholelithiasis
Psychological, e.g., phobias, distaste, pseudofood allergy
Immunologically mediated
Early, IgE mediated
Delayed, immune complexes/cell mediated immunity, e.g., celiac disease, ? others

tion of gluten-sensitive enteropathy, delayed immunologically mediated reactions to foods are not well defined. In this chapter we shall focus mainly on IgE-mediated food allergy, and the reader is referred elsewhere for reviews of the immunological basis of putative delayed immunological reactions to food antigens.[3,5,6]

Nonimmunologically mediated adverse reactions to food have multiple possible mechanisms (Table 1). They may closely mimic acute allergic reactions and, with increasing use of additives, preservatives, and processing in the food industry, are now a major diagnostic consideration in all cases of food-induced symptoms. It is important to note that a given food may produce an adverse reaction by multiple mechanisms. For example, intolerance to milk may be due to disaccharidase deficiency, penicillin allergy, or fat intolerance associated with cholelithiasis, in addition to immunological reactions to milk proteins. Immune responses to milk proteins are also probably heterogeneous.[7]

3. FOOD ALLERGY—REAL OR IMAGINED?

The actual incidence of adverse food reactions is not known, but it is probably much less common than believed by the lay public. Community studies in the United States[8] and in England[9,10] indicate that 20–40% of adults believe they have some form of adverse reaction to certain foods. These self-diagnoses have almost certainly been influenced by the recent barrage of publications[11] and advertisements aimed at the lay public which attribute a diverse number of symptoms to food allergies. When tested objectively using double-blind food challenges, the majority of complaints of possible food allergies cannot be reproduced.[12–14]

Nonimmunological mechanisms (Table 1) almost certainly account for the majority of confirmed food reactions, but accurate figures for their incidence and prevalence are not available.[3,4] Immunologically mediated reactions triggered by foods (true food allergy) are considerably more common in children than in adults[3,15] and not surprisingly are more common in atopic individuals.[3,4,15] Allergy to cow's milk is probably the most frequently diagnosed form of such reactions and has been estimated to affect up to 7–12% of all infants.[16] Its incidence declines with age and is uncommon in adults. A study of the natural history of confirmed food allergy in children has shown that the later the onset, the less likely it will be "outgrown."[17]

It has been estimated that approximately 1 in 10 atopic adult patients claiming to have a possible food allergy will have a reproducible, immunologically mediated adverse reaction to foods.[15,18] The majority of adult patients whose belief that they have a food allergy cannot be verified objectively appear to have a psychological basis for their symptoms.[13,18,19] Pearson *et al.*[20,21] have studied patients attending an allergy clinic who claimed to have a wide variety of symptoms supposedly due to food allergy. A specific adverse reaction to food substances was confirmed using double-blind provocation tests in 4 of 23 patients. One of the four patients had salicylate sensitivity, and the other three had IgE-mediated allergic reactions. None of the four patients had psychological problems. However, a high incidence of psychiatric disorders was found in patients whose belief that they had a food allergy could not be objectively confirmed. The most common psychiatric disorder found was depression.

The precise role of food allergies and adverse reactions as a cause of symptoms in adult patients referred to gastroenterology clinics has received limited study. A recent report found that only 3 of 49 patients referred with unexplained gastrointestinal symptoms in whom the diagnosis of food intolerance was considered could be shown to have specific food-related symptoms.[22] These authors have suggested that although some adult patients clearly have gastrointestinal symptoms due to verifiable adverse reactions to foods, the majority of such referrals have symptoms attributable to psychogenic factors.

4. THE MUCOSAL "BARRIER" AND ITS DEFENSE MECHANISMS

Only a single layer of epithelium covering the gut mucosa separates the internal milieu from the outside environment. Through this we must interact with our environment and absorb digested nutrients and yet exclude potentially harmful exogenous infectious, toxic, and antigenic agents. A variety of nonimmunological and immunological defense mechanisms operate to preserve the integrity of this mucosal barrier.[3,23-25]

Nonimmunological protective mechanisms include the normal intestinal flora, gastric acid and pancreatic digestive enzymes, gut motility, and mucus secretion. Collectively, these nonspecific defenses limit the presentation of antigenic material to the intestinal mucosa. Their importance may be appreciated in conditions such as achlorhydria and the blind-loop syndrome, which have been associated with increased mucosal penetration by exogenous antigens and the generation of circulating immune complexes to such antigenic material.[25,26] The continual cell turnover and renewal of the mucosal epithelium is also a critical inherent defense mechanism, and anything that interferes with this is associated with increased permeability to exogenous macromolecules.[25,27]

It is now well established that the local mucosal immune system represents a protective apparatus which functions largely independently of the systemic immune system, and its humoral and cellular limbs are uniquely adapted to respond to antigenic stimuli at the mucosal surface.[24] Thus, its major secretory immunoglobulin (IgA) has a unique selective transport system through the epithelial cells and is packaged with secretory component to render it resistant to lumenal digestive enzymes. One of the many functions of secretory IgA[23,24,28] is the prevention of absorption of dietary antigens (immune exclusion). This phenomenon of immune exclusion is well illustrated clinically in patients with selective IgA deficiency, many of whom have been shown to develop high titers of antibodies to milk and other food antigens.[29] Absorption of excessive amounts of milk antigens, such as casein, β-lactoglobulin, and bovine albumin, from these "leaky" mucosae may lead to the generation of antibodies of IgM and IgG classes and the generation of immune complexes in some individuals within an hour of drinking a glass of milk.[30] Although the majority of such patients are symptom-free, there is an increased incidence of atopy and immune-complex-mediated and autoimmune diseases associated with IgA deficiency.[31]

In addition to excluding exogenous antigens at the intestinal epithelial surface, it has been suggested that IgA may also provide an important backup system for eliminating circulating gut-derived immune complexes.[28] Thus, IgA is selectively transported across other mucosal surfaces including the biliary tract, and this route might provide a clearance mechanism for IgA–dietary antigen complexes. In addition to the biliary excretion of immune complexes, the liver has an important backup role in the immunological defense system of the gut. This includes the filtration function of the Kupffer cells and the downregulation of immune responses to dietary antigen absorbed into the portal circulation.[32]

5. ANTIGEN UPTAKE

Despite the presence of multiple defense mechanisms, there is a large body of evidence[25,33] which indicates that antigenic macromolecules and even particulate matter of no nutritional significance, but perhaps of immunological significance, can penetrate the epithelial surface and reach the systemic circulation under normal circumstances. There is evidence that even asbestos particles in drinking water may pass through the normal adult human gut mucosa and be eliminated in the urine.[34] Of particular relevance to the discussion of food allergy is the recent demonstration that small amounts of dietary antigens may be detected in breast milk.[35] This implies that absorbed dietary antigens may be transported from the gut to other mucosal sites, including the breast, and thus, babies, even if exclusively breast fed, may be exposed to multiple dietary antigens.

Uptake of antigenic material may occur through two routes: (1) through or between the columnar epithelial cells or (2) through the specialized lymphoepithelium or M cells overlying lymphoid aggregates. Antigen transport across the columnar epithelium occurs by an energy-dependent endocytotic mechanism. Although much of this is digested within the intracellular phagolysosome, a fraction of the ingested antigenic material escapes into the intercellular space by exocytosis at the basolateral membrane.[25,33] The clinical significance of this macromolecular absorption is unclear although it is known to be greater in premature and newborn infants than in adults and is also increased in the injured intestine.[25]

In contrast to the columnar epithelium, M cells appear to be specifically adapted to sample the antigenic environment within the gut lumen and to present it to the underlying gut-associated lymphoid tissue.[36] This appears to be the preferred route of absorption for lower (perhaps physiological) levels of antigenic load.[36]

6. IMMUNE RESPONSE TO DIETARY ANTIGENS

When certain dietary antigens are presented to the local mucosal immune system, two contrasting responses occur. Thus, the positive immune response at the gut (IgA antibody secretion and cell-mediated immunity) is paralleled by the induction of a state of systemic hyporesponsiveness (or tolerance), which is antigen-specific.[24,37] This phenomenon, sometimes termed the Sulzberger–Chase phenomenon, has been known for over a century, and its occurrence depends on several factors, including the prior immune status of the host to the specific antigen and the concentration, frequency of administration and molecular nature of the antigen. The mechanism(s) responsible for tolerance and its regulation is not known, although it probably involves active suppression. However, the induction of systemic hyporesponsiveness to ingested antigens clearly has important implications for food allergies. Thus, an active local immune response limiting mucosal penetration of dietary antigens may serve as the host's "first line" of defense. A state of systemic tolerance to the same antigens might act as the "second line," protecting the host from potentially destructive immune reactions to small amounts of antigen which succeed in evading immune exclusion and gain access to the systemic circulation.

7. PATHOGENESIS OF FOOD ALLERGY

Some of the most convincing and imaginative studies demonstrating food allergic phenomena *in vivo* were performed over a half-century ago. Brunner and Walzer[2] injected the serum of fish-sensitive subjects into the skin of human subjects who, upon ingestion of raw fish, subsequently developed wheal-and-flare reactions at the sensitized skin injection sites. This modified Prausnitz–Kustner reaction[38] demonstrated two phenomena. First, the absorption of undigested antigenic proteins occurs in the majority of humans, and second, a serum factor (now known to be IgE) exists in subjects sensitive to such proteins, which, when passively transferred, may locally sensitize nonallergic individuals.

Penetration of the intestinal mucosal barrier is the first step in the sequence of events leading to food allergic reactions. Sensitization to certain proteins may occur during the neonatal period when permeability to antigens is increased.[33]

Subsequent reexposure in later life may permit sufficient quantities of dietary allergen to be absorbed, resulting in allergic reactions (Fig. 1A and B). The majority of such reactions are IgE-mediated.

A long list of foods has been incriminated in causing IgE-mediated reactions, but the most commonly implicated are milk, eggs, nuts, fish, crustaceans, mollusks, soybeans, and wheat. Closely related foods may contain common or cross-reactive allergens. In some instances a specific allergenic component of the culprit food substance has been clearly identified.[39-42]

Sensitized subjects have IgE antibodies specifically against these allergenic molecules bound to the surface of mast cells in the gut mucosa and other tissues. Recognition of allergen by IgE on the mast cell surface is followed by binding and bridging of two IgE molecules, which, in turn, triggers the degranulation of mast cells (Fig. 1B). These events may be confined to the gut mucosa or may involve cutaneous and pulmonary mast cells also. Well-documented acute systemic anaphylaxis has also been described with systemic mast cell and basophil release of diverse and highly potent inflammatory mediators. These mediators include both preformed vasoactive amines, such as histamine, and newly generated secondary mediators, such as prostaglandins and leukotrienes.[43] The local intestinal inflammatory reaction leads to increased mucosal permeability, which may then facilitate the passage of more dietary macromole-

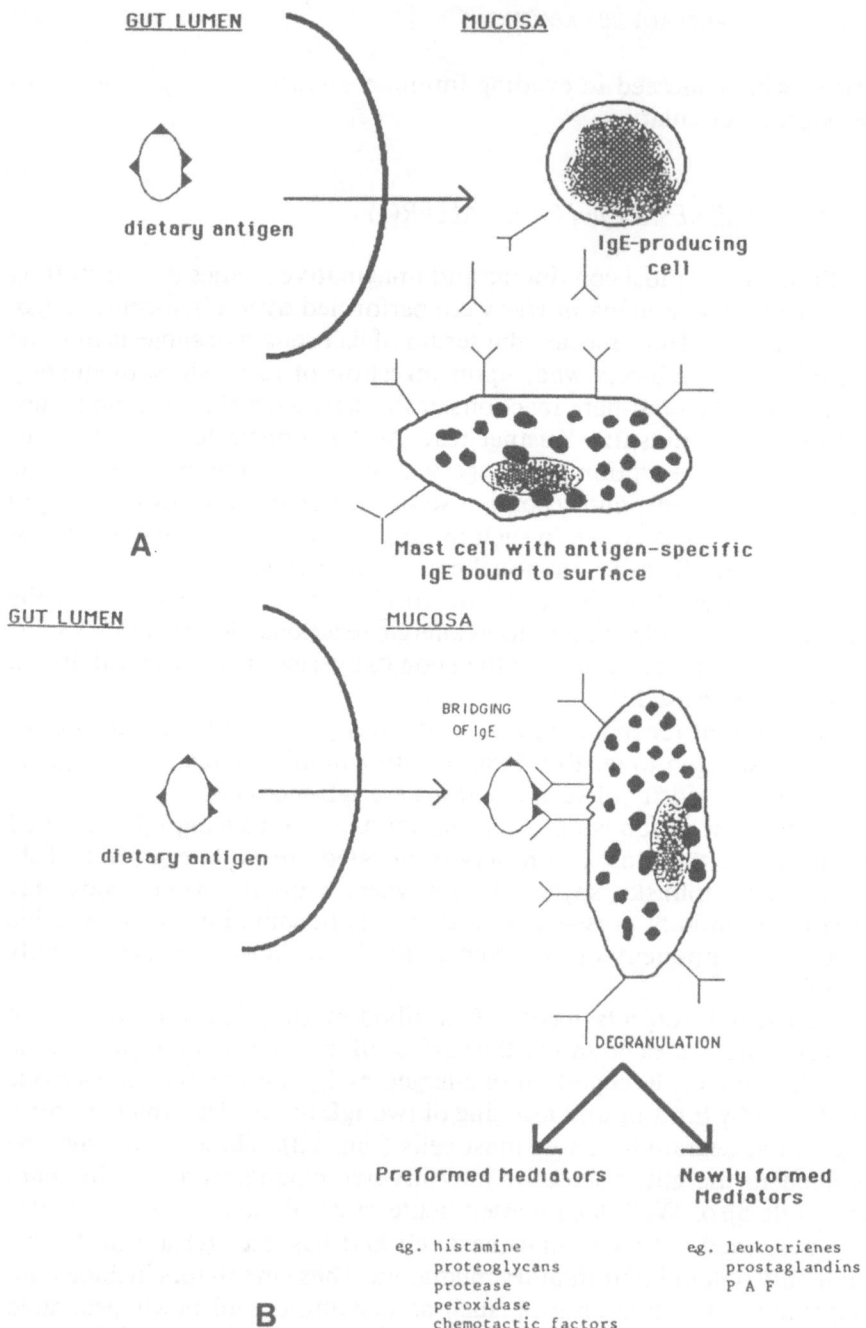

Figure 1. (A) Sensitization to food allergen. (B) Food allergic reaction.

cules across the mucosa and, thus, propagate the symptoms. Uptake of nonspecific dietary antigens may then stimulate an IgG response and immune complex formation leading to further exacerbation of disease.[25,33]

Mast cells are present in every layer of the intestinal wall and occur in large numbers at every level of the gastrointestinal tract.[44] However, they require special fixation and staining procedures for their demonstration.[45] Recent studies in rodents have suggested that intestinal mucosal mast cells differ morphologically, cytochemically, and functionally from mast cells at other sites.[45–47] Whether similar mast cell heterogeneity exists also in humans is not clear,[48] although there is histochemical evidence for distinct subpopulations of mast cells in the human gut also.[49] This is an area of intense research and may have implications for the therapy of food allergy since the intestinal mucosal mast cell differs from nonmucosal mast cells in its responsiveness to various antiallergic agents.[50]

8. CLINICAL FEATURES

Although nonimmunologically mediated adverse food reactions may mimic acute allergic phenomena, the clinical picture is variable and depends on the nature of mechanism involved. Details of specific adverse reactions may be found elsewhere.[3,4]

The symptoms associated with true food allergic reactions occur immediately or within 1–3 hr of ingestion. The organs primarily affected are the gastrointestinal tract, the skin, and the respiratory tract (Table 2). Systemic anaphylaxis has also been described.[3] Gastrointestinal symptoms are nonspecific and range from edema and pruritus of the lips, buccal, and pharyngeal mucosa, to vomiting, cramping, and diarrhea, depending on the level of the gut primarily affected. A variety of enteropathies have also been associated with delayed or apparently non-IgE-mediated immunological reactions to food antigens.[3,6] These are best exemplified by gluten-sensitive sprue[5] but may also include some cases of

Table 2. Common Clinical Features of Food Allergic Reactions

Gastrointestinal
   Early: Edema and pruritus of lips, buccal and pharyngeal mucosa, vomiting, abdominal
      pain
   Delayed: Diarrhea, bloating, steatorrhea
Extragastrointestinal: Anaphylaxis, urticaria, angioedema, eczema, asthma, rhinorrhea,
      arthralgia

---

eosinophilic gastroenteritis[3,6] and some cases of cow's-milk colitis.[7] Skin and respiratory manifestations of food allergy for which there is good evidence include urticaria, angioedema, eczema,[51] and asthma.[14] There is at present no good evidence to support claims that a wide range of neuropsychological symptoms such as tension–fatigue, depression, or childhood hyperkinesis may be induced by pharmacological or allergic reactions to foods.[3,4]

In a given individual, symptoms may be variable and not always reproducible. This variability may be partly dependent on the amount of food allergen ingested, partial denaturation by cooking, and extent of digestion before absorption. In addition, other factors, such as exercise[52] and the coincidental ingestion of salicylates,[53] may have a profound modulatory effect on the clinical expression of food allergic reactions.

9. INVESTIGATION OF THE PATIENT WITH SUSPECTED FOOD ALLERGY

It is clear that the differential diagnosis of food-related symptoms is wide and complex (Table 1). Yet, all studies point to the existence of a subset of patients, albeit small in the adult population, with genuine and reproducible adverse reactions to specific foods. The correct identification of this minority of patients is the major challenge. This requires a careful and objective assessment of supposed food-induced reactions, if one is to avoid missing a preventable illness in some patients and inappropriate and potentially harmful dietary restriction in others.

A careful physical examination and detailed history is essential and will in many cases suggest which of the multiple possible causes of adverse food reactions (Table 1) are responsible for the patient's symptoms. Particular attention should be paid to the quantity of food required to induce an attack; the severity, frequency, and timing of attacks in relation to ingestion of food; the nature and mode of preparation of the implicated food(s); and the presence of flavorings, preservatives, and other additives. Any relationship of symptoms to other factors such as exercise and coincidental aspirin ingestion should also be determined.

It cannot be assumed that symptoms suggestive of an IgE-mediated reaction such as acute urticaria or asthma are diagnostic of true (immunologically mediated) food allergy. Thus, several commonly ingested, nonimmunological trigger factors, particularly sulfites and salicylates, may very closely mimic IgE-mediated events and must first be excluded as a cause of symptoms. The diagnosis of food allergy requires, by definition, the demonstration (1) that ingestion of the implicated food can reproducibly induce the patients symptoms and (2) that an immunological mechanism is involved.

9.1. Food Challenge

The double-blind, placebo-controlled food challenge championed by May and Bock[54-56] is the most objective and unbiased way to confirm or refute a patient's belief that symptoms are related to a specific food. The challenge may be performed by nasogastric intubation, by masking the suspected food within other foods, or by using encapsulated dried food. Tartrazine-free opaque gelatin capsules are widely available, and most of the foods commonly implicated in food allergies are readily available in dried, powdered form. Full details of the procedure have been described in several publications.[3,12-14,54-56] Despite the objectivity of the double-blind challenge, the results of such tests should be critically assessed for potential pitfalls.[19] Thus, the conditions of the test do not precisely mimic natural ingestion, the appropriate quantity and preparation of food used may be critical, and for patients with subjective symptoms or those with frequent spontaneously fluctuating symptoms, the test, if positive, must be repeated several times with placebo control.[19] It should be noted that *any* form of *in vivo* provocation test (oral challenge or skin test) is unnecessary and dangerous and should never be performed in a patient with a history of food-related anaphylaxis.

When food allergy is considered to be a possible cause of symptoms, yet no particular food or food group has been implicated, a diet/symptom diary or an elimination diet may be helpful in identifying the culprit. Several elimination dietary regimens have been described.[3] These should be used for diagnosis only and not for long periods of time and should never jeopardize the nutritional status of the patient.

9.2. Demonstration of Immunological Mechanism

For practical purposes, the demonstration that an adverse food reaction is immunologically mediated involves the demonstration of IgE antibodies that have specificity for the implicated food allergen. At present, little is known about delayed immunologically mediated food allergic reactions. Jejunal biopsy is required for diagnosis of celiac sprue and other forms of enteropathy, but *in vitro* tests for cellular immunity to food antigens and food antigen–immune complexes are still under investigation and are not recommended as routine diagnostic procedures at present.

Several *in vivo* and *in vitro* tests have been developed to determine whether an adverse food reaction is IgE-mediated.[3,6,15] The risk of hepatitis, unfortunately, precludes the use of the Prausnitz–Kustner (passive cutaneous sensitization) test today. Direct skin testing, if properly performed with appropriate allergenic extracts and controls (details in refs. 3, 54–56), is a simple, reliable, and sensitive method of detecting specific sensitizing, cutaneous, mast cell-bound IgE antibodies. However, positive results must not be overinterpreted and do not necessarily imply that clinical food allergy exists. Many individuals have "asymptomatic hypersensitivity,"[54] do not develop symptoms on blind challenge with the test food, and do not require dietary restriction. Patients should, therefore, never be told that they have a food allergy on the basis of a positive skin test alone. Negative results correlate well with negative blind food challenges,[57] and it has been suggested that skin testing may be useful to screen patients with possible food allergy for subsequent provocation tests.[57,58] The sensitivity and specificity of skin tests will improve with better purification and standardization of allergenic extracts.[3]

When there is a risk of anaphylaxis with skin testing, or when extensive skin disease such as eczema exists, an *in vitro* test should be employed to demonstrate the presence of allergen-specific IgE. Reliable *in vitro* assays include the radioallergosorbent test (RAST), the enzyme-linked immunosorbent assay (ELISA), and the basophil histamine release assay. As with skin tests, positive results should be interpreted with caution.

The RAST is the most commonly used of these tests. The principles of the test are as follows: The suspected allergen is first bound to a solid-phase support such as a paper disk and then incubated with the serum being tested for the presence of allergen-specific IgE. The allergen-specific IgE, if present, will bind to the antigen on the solid support, and after washing to remove nonspecific binding, it can be demonstrated and quantitated by further incubation with radiolabeled anti-IgE. The ELISA is similar in principle, but the second antibody (anti-IgE) is enzyme linked and not radiolabeled. These tests are excellent research tools, but for clinical use they are expensive, time consuming, require close attention to technical details, and are no more sensitive than properly performed skin tests.[3,15,55] In contrast to the RAST and ELISA, which detect circulating allergen-specific IgE, the basophil histamine release assay demonstrates the release of histamine *in vitro* when allergen is incubated with the patient's basophils—presumptive evidence for the presence of allergen-specific IgE on the cell surface. This is used mainly as a research technique.

The "cytotoxicity food allergy test" so frequently advertised to the laity is based on the unsubstantiated claim that the incubation of allergenic food extracts with whole blood from supposedly food allergic subjects results in death of leukocytes. This and other controversial diagnostic techniques have recently been reviewed by the American Academy of Allergy and are not approved for clinical use.[59]

10. OVERVIEW

A general guideline to the investigation of possible adverse reactions to food is shown in Fig. 2. In practice, however, the approach should be individualized and will depend on several factors, including the age of the patient, compliance with challenge test protocols, and the severity and nature of symptoms. For patients with a clear history of objectively verifiable symptoms related to a specific food, an open food challenge may suffice. The patient with only episodic symptoms triggered by uncommonly encountered and nonessential foods should be instructed to avoid these and related substances and need not be challenged. The greatest diagnostic difficulty is posed by the patient with vague or subjective complaints, self-diagnosed as an adverse food reaction. In the adult population, and in particular the nonatopic individual, the likelihood of such symptoms being due to food allergy is very small. A psychological basis should be strongly considered, and a prolonged investigative workup beyond simple screening tests may not be appropriate or desirable for these patients. It is particularly important that these patients be tactfully dissuaded from using potentially harmful dietary restriction.

There is no controversy or confusion about the correct and only acceptable treatment of food allergy—avoidance of the offending food. Patient education is crucial, and expert dietary instruction and supervision is important to minimize inadvertent ingestion of food allergens and to ensure that the final diet is palatable and nutritionally adequate. Immunological and pharmacological therapeutic or preventive measures, reviewed elsewhere,[3] are of unproven value and are not acceptable alternatives to allergen avoidance.

11. CONCLUSIONS

Adverse reactions to foods represent an uncommon but definite clinical entity to adults. Much of the confusion surrounding this topic might be avoided if immunologically mediated mechanisms (food allergy) are

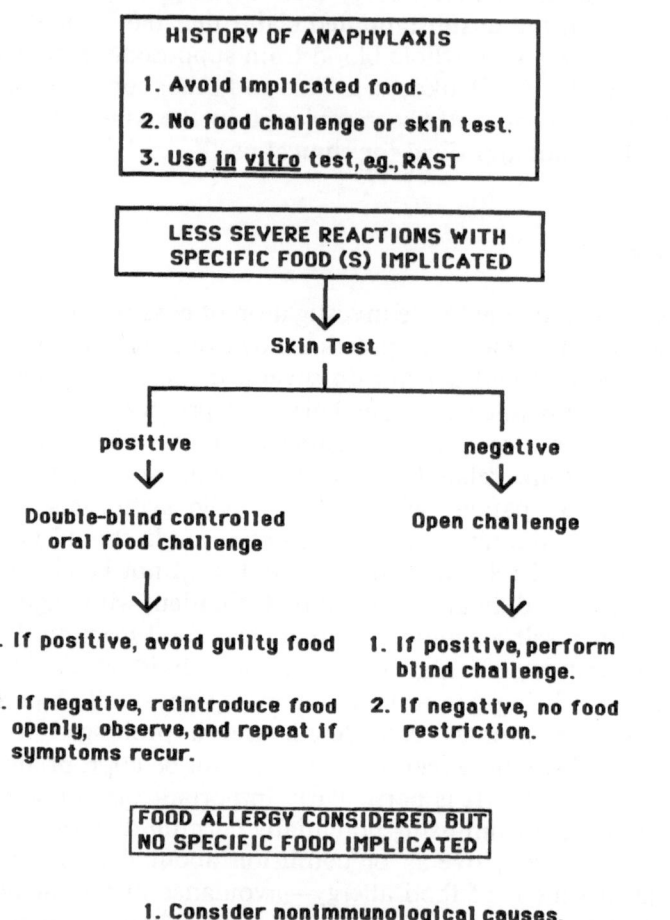

Figure 2. Approach to suspected food allergic patient.

distinguished from nonimmunologically mediated adverse food reactions and if an objective and unbiased approach is applied to the investigation of patients with claims of food allergies. Unless a scientific approach is widely adopted to the investigation of this problem, certain patients with an eminently preventable illness will go untreated, and a greater number of individuals taking restrictive diets for a misguided or self-diagnosis of food allergy will be at risk of malnutrition. The subject of food allergy need not be confused, controversial, or treated with suspicion. Rather, it offers exciting new fields of clinically relevant research. Much more needs to be known about the pathogenesis and diagnosis of delayed immunologically mediated food allergies and the normal control mechanisms preventing inappropriate immune reactions to the multitude of antigens in the normal diet. Other future research directions include the improvement of diagnostic tests by standardizing allergenic food extracts and the delineation of the optimal conditions for the performance of food challenges. In addition, the precise role of adverse reactions in foods in patients with unexplained gastrointestinal complaints needs more attention.

REFERENCES

1. May CD: Food Allergy: Lessons from the past. *J Allergy Clin Immunol* 1982;69:255–259.
2. Brunner M, Walzer M: Absorption of undigested proteins in human beings. *Arch Intern Med* 1928;42:172–179.
3. Anderson JA, Sogn DD (eds): *Adverse Reactions to Foods.* American Academy of Allergy and Immunology Committee on Adverse Reactions to Foods. Bethesda, MD, National Institute of Allergy and Infectious Diseases, Public Health Service, National Institutes of Health. NIH publication No. 84-2442, 1984.
4. Lessof MH, Gray JR, Hoffenberg R, et al: Food Intolerance and Food Aversion. A Joint Report of The Royal College of Physicians and the British Nutrition Foundation. *J R Coll Physicians London* 1984;18:83–123.
5. Strober W: Gluten-Sensitive Enteropathy—An abnormal immunologic response of the gastrointestinal tract to a dietary protein, in Shorter, RG, Kirsner JB (eds): *Gastrointestinal Immunity for the Clinician.* Orlando, FL, Grune & Stratton Inc., 1985, pp. 75–112.
6. Kulczycki A, MacDermott RP: Adverse reactions to food and eosinophilic gastroenteritis, in Shorter RG, Kirsner JB: *Gastrointestinal Immunity for the Clinician.* Orlando, FL, Grune & Stratton Inc., 1985, pp. 131–140.
7. Bahna SL: Pathogenesis of milk hypersensitivity. *Immunol Today* 1985;6:153–154.
8. Kerr GR, Wu-Lee M, El-Lozy M, McGrundy R, Stare FJ: Prevalence of the "Chinese restaurant syndrome." *J Am Diet Assoc* 1979;75:29–33.
9. Burr ML, Merrett TG: Food intolerance: A community survey. *Br J Nutr* 1983;49:217–219.
10. Bender AE, Matthews DR: Adverse reactions to foods. *Br J Nutr* 1981;46:403–407.
11. Mackarness R: *Not All In the Mind.* London, Pan, 1976.
12. Bock SA, Lee Y, Remigio LK, May CD: Studies of hypersensitivity reactions to foods in infants and children. *J Allergy Clin Immunol* 1978;62:327–334.
13. May CD: Food allergy—Material and ethereal. *N Engl J Med* 1980;302:1142–1143.
14. May CD: Objective clinical and laboratory studies of immediate hypersensitivity reactions to foods in asthmatics. *J Allergy Clin Immunol* 1976;58:500–515.
15. Metcalfe DD: Food Hypersensitivity. *J Allergy Clin Immunol* 1984;73:749.

16. Bahna SL, Heina DC: Cow's milk allergy. *Adv Pediatr* 1978;25:1–37.
17. Bock SA: The natural history of food sensitivity. *J Allergy Clin Immunol* 1982;69:173–177.
18. Lessof MH: Food intolerance and allergy—A review. *Q J Med* 1983;30:111–119.
19. Pearson DJ: Food allergy, hypersensitivity and intolerance. *J R Coll Physicians London* 1985;19:154–162.
20. Pearson DJ, Rix KJB, Bentley SJ: Food allergy: How much in the mind? A clinical and psychiatric study of suspected food hypersensitivity. *Lancet* 1983;1:1259–1261.
21. Rix KJB, Pearson DJ, Bentley SJ: A psychiatric study of patients with supposed food allergy. *Br J Psychiatry* 1984;145:121–126.
22. Farah DA, Calder I, Benson I, MacKenzie JF: Specific food intolerance: Its place as a cause of gastrointestinal symptoms. *Gut* 1985;26:164–168.
23. McNabb PC, Tomasi TB: Host defense mechanisms at mucosal surfaces. *Annu Rev Microbiol* 1981;35:477–496.
24. Bienenstock J, Befus AD: Mucosal immunology. *Immunology* 1980;41:249–270.
25. Walker WA: Mechanisms of antigen handling by the gut. *Clin Immunol Allergy* 1982;2:15–40.
26. Kraft SC, Rothberg RM, Knauer CM, Svoboda AC, Monroe LS, Farr RS: Gastric output and circulating anti-bovine serum albumin in adults. *Clin Exp Immunol* 1967;2:321–330.
27. Editorial. Intestinal permeability. *Lancet* 1985;1:256–258.
28. Bienenstock J, Befus AD: Some thoughts on the biological role of immunoglobulin A. *Gastroenterology* 1983;84:178–185.
29. Huntley CC, Robbins JB, Lyerly AD, Buckley RH: Characterization of precipitating antibodies to ruminant serum and milk proteins in humans with selective IgA deficiency. *N Engl J Med* 1971;284:7–10.
30. Cunningham-Rundles C, Brandeis WE, Good RA, Day NK: Milk precipitins, circulating immune complexes and IgA deficiency. *Proc Natl Acad Sci USA* 1978;75:3387–3389.
31. Ammann AJ, Hong R: Selective IgA deficiency: Presentation of 30 cases and a review of the literature. *Medicine* 1971;50:223–236.
32. Triger DR, Cynamon MH, Wright R: Studies on hepatic uptake of antigen. 1. Comparison of inferior vena cava and portal vein routes of immunization. *Immunology* 1973;25:941–950.
33. Kleinman RE, Harmatz PR, Walker WA: The gastrointestinal immune barrier: Its role in preventing antigen penetration of the intestine, in Shorter RG, Kirsner JB (eds): *Gastrointestinal Immunity for the Clinician.* Orlando, FL, Grune & Stratton Inc., 1985, pp. 23–32.
34. Cook PM, Olson GF: Ingested mineral fibers: Elimination in human urine. *Science* 1979;204:195–198.
35. Hemmings WA: First experience of dietary antigen. *Lancet* 1980;1:818.
36. Owen RL: Sequential uptake of horseradish peroxidase by lymphoid follicle epithelium of Peyer's patches in the normal unobstructed mouse intestine: An ultrastructural study. *Gastroenterology* 1977;72:440–451.
37. Bienenstock J, Befus AD: The gastrointestinal tract as an immune organ, in Shorter RG, Kirsner JB (eds): *Gastrointestinal Immunity for the Clinician.* Orlando, FL, Grune & Stratton Inc., 1985, pp. 1–22.
38. Prausnitz P, Kustner H: Studien uber die VeberempFindlichkeit. *Z Bakt Orig* 1921;86:160–168.

39. Elsayed S, Bennich H: The primary structure of allergen M from cod. *Scand J Immunol* 1975;4:203–208.
40. Moroz LA, Yang WH: Kunitz soybean trypsin inhibitor. A specific allergen in food anaphylaxis. *N Engl J Med* 1980;302:1126–1128.
41. Hoffman DR: The major heat stable allergen of shrimp. *Ann Allergy* 1981;47:17–22.
42. Sachs MI, Jones RT, Yunginger JW: Isolation and partial characterization of a major peanut allergen. *J Allergy Clin Immunol* 1981;67:27–34.
43. Wasserman SI: Mediators of immediate hypersensitivity. *J Allergy Clin Immunol* 1983;72:101–115.
44. Lemanske RF, Atkins FM, Metcalfe DD: Gastrointestinal mast cells in health and disease. 1. *J Pediatr* 1983;103:177–183.
45. Enerback L: The gut mucosal mast cell. *Monogr Allergy* 1981;17:222–232.
46. Bienenstock J, Befus AD, Pearce F, Denburg J, Goodacre R: Mast cell heterogeneity: Derivation and function with emphasis on the intestine. *J Allergy Clin Immunol* 1982;70:407–412.
47. Shanahan F, Befus AD, Denburg J, Bienenstock J: Mast cell heterogeneity. *Can J Physiol Pharmacol* 1984;62:734–737.
48. Fox CC, Dvorak AM, Peters SP, Kagey-Sobotka A, Lichtenstein LM: Isolation and characterization of human intestinal mucosal mast cells. *J Immunol* 1985;135:483–491.
49. Befus D, Goodacre R, Dyck N, Bienenstock J: Mast cell heterogeneity in man. 1. Histological studies of the intestine. *Int Arch Allergy Appl Immunol* 1985;76:232–236.
50. Pearce FL, Befus AD, Gauldie J, Bienenstock J: Mucosal mast cells. II. Effects of anti-allergic compounds on histamine secretion by isolated intestinal mast cells. *J Immunol* 1982;128:2481–2486.
51. Sampson HA, Jolie PL: Increased plasma histamine concentrations after food challenges in children with atopic dermatitis. *N Engl J Med* 1984;311:372–376.
52. Maultiz RM, Pratt DS, Schocket AL: Exercise-induced anaphylactic reaction to shellfish. *J Allergy Clin Immunol* 1979;63:433–434.
53. Cant AJ, Gibson P, Dancy M: Food hypersensitivity made life threatening by ingestion of aspirin. *Br Med J* 1984;288:755–756.
54. May CD, Bock SA: Adverse reactions to food due to hypersensitivity, in Middleton E Jr, Reed CE, Ellis EF (eds): *Allergy, Principles and Practice.* St. Louis, CV Mosby, 1978, vol 2, pp. 1159–1171.
55. Bock SA: Food sensitivity. A critical review of and practical approach. *Am J Dis Child* 1980;134:973–982.
56. May CD, Bock SA: A modern clinical approach to food hypersensitivity. *Allergy* 1978;33:166–188.
57. Metcalfe DD, Kaliner MA: "What is food to one . . . ?" *N Engl J Med* 1984;311:399–400.
58. Atkins FM, Steinberg SS, Metcalfe DD: Evaluation of immediate adverse reactions to foods in adult patients. 1. Correlation of demographic, laboratory, and prick skin test data with response to controlled oral food challenge. *J Allergy Clin Immunol* 1985;75:348–355.
59. Reisman RE: American Academy of Allergy position statements—Controversial techniques. *J Allergy Clin Immunol* 1981;67:333–338.

19

The Pathogenesis of Infectious Diarrhea

J. Richard Hamilton

1. INTRODUCTION

During the past decade much has been learned about the events that convert a peaceful state of coexistence between microbes and the gut into a diarrheal illness. Research into the pathogenesis of infectious diarrhea has been concerned with several aspects of the problem—the events leading to colonization of the intestine by pathogens and their attachment to or invasion of the intestinal wall, the mechanisms by which intestinal water and solute transport is distorted, leading to diarrhea, and finally, the factors that regulate shedding of offending organisms and repair of the damaged intestine. The effective application of new basic pathophysiology concepts to the care of patients with diarrhea has been widely publicized. Fortunately, infants and children in the developing world, for whom diarrheal diseases are so devastating, have been the major beneficiaries. Promoted by The Programme for Control of Diarrhoeal Diseases of the World Health Organization (WHO), treatment programs based on modern concepts of diarrhea pathogenesis have led to a dramatic reduction in mortality and morbidity in many Third-World countries.[1] Perhaps because of a lesser level of concern over the problem, physicians in developed countries have been relatively slow to take up these rational approaches to treatment.

J. Richard Hamilton • Division of Gastroenterology, Department of Pediatrics, University of Toronto and The Research Institute, The Hospital for Sick Children, Toronto, Ontario, Canada M5G 1X8.

Another less immediate fallout from research into the pathogenesis of diarrhea is the insight it brings to our understanding of normal gastrointestinal function, and, indirectly, the response of the gut to a variety of diseases. The global cost of diarrheal diseases, although less than it was 10 years ago, remains colossal. An essential basis for future improvements in care and consequent reductions in cost will continue to be contributed by basic and applied research. The following brief account of some current research activities in this field is intended to indicate that, indeed, the future is promising. This chapter emphasizes the gastroenterological, rather than microbiological and immunological, aspects of the subject. Before abnormal interactions between bowel and bugs are discussed, certain recently developed concepts of normal intestinal function will be reviewed.

2. THE NORMAL INTESTINE

The small intestine is the site of many enteric infections and the region where most of the intestinal absorption of salt and water occurs. Although deranged smooth muscle motility patterns,[2,3] altered neural function,[4] and abnormal vascular[5] and lymphatic flow could influence water and salt transportation in the gut, little is known about the response of these factors to enteric infection. What is clear is that the small intestinal epithelium and underlying lymphoid tissue are of central importance to the pathogenesis of infectious diarrhea.

2.1. Small Intestinal Epithelium

In the mammalian gut, epithelial proliferation is confined to the crypts. From proliferating undifferentiated crypt cells several cell types develop (Table 1). Some points relevant to the potential role of these cells in infectious diarrhea are the following.

Table 1. Small Intestinal Epithelial Cells

Membranous ("M") cells
Goblet cells
Paneth cells
Endocrine cells
Columnar absorptive cells

2.1.1. Membraneous (M) Cells

These cells are found in the dome epithelium overlying Peyer patches and may be confined to those sites. Owen's microscopic studies showed uptake of intact protein by M cells,[6] which, he suggested, may serve an antigen-sampling role. Certainly, their configuration is appropriate for this purpose. Studies in our laboratory used the Ussing chamber technique to quantitate macromolecular transport in piglet jejunal mucosa *in vitro* and demonstrated enhancement of horseradish peroxidase uptake across patch-containing segments compared with patch-free segments.[7] This process was partially inhibited by sodium flouride, suggesting that it was an active cellular phenomenon. Possibly the sparsity or absence of surface mucus or glycocalyx, the special properties of the overlying unstirred water layer, or increased porosity of the underlying basement membrane in the patches may play some part in this enhanced macromolecular absorption. Nevertheless, available evidence favors an antigen-sampling role for the M cell. Theoretically, these cells could influence interactions between intestinal microorganisms, dietary antigens, and the host immune system.

2.1.2. Goblet Cells

These polarized, mucin-secreting cells appear to arise from undifferentiated precursors in the crypts.[8] The quality and quantity of intestinal mucus probably exert an important influence on interactions between the gut and microorganisms too.[9] Quality varies depending on the rate of production, on the cosecretion of certain enzymes, and on the chemical structure of constituent glycoproteins, or mucins. As a viscous gel, the mucus barrier may trap microorganisms and dietary proteins in the lumen or enzymes and proteins released from the wall; as a fluid sol, mucus could exert a cleansing action in the lumen. Control of the amount and nature of secreting mucus is poorly understood.

2.1.3. Paneth Cells

Little is known of the function of these distinctive granulated cells, confined to the crypts and derived also from undifferentiated crypt cells. The presence of degenerating protozoa and bacteria in their lysozyme fractions suggests a possible involvement in regulating enteric flora.[8]

2.1.4. Endocrine Cells

At least 15 endocrine paracrine cells have been identified in the mammalian gut.[10] Most of them produce active peptides, many of which can alter intestinal transport function, but a role for these cells in infectious diarrhea has not been elucidated.

2.1.5. Columnar Absorptive Cells

The dominant cell type in the small intestine epithelium, the columnar absorptive cell, differentiates as it migrates up from the crypt to be shed from the tip of the villus.[11,12] This process of cell renewal is extremely relevant to the evolution of at least some, if not all, types of infectious diarrhea. Earlier studies demonstrated a range of enzymatic markers of enterocyte differentiation. Activities of the brush border membrane (BBM) disaccharidases and alkaline phosphatase and basolateral membrane Na-K-ATPase increase as enterocytes differentiate.[13] Based on studies of winter flounder small intestine, which lacks a crypt compartment, Field proposed that absorptive function might reside primarily in villus cells whereas secretory events reside in the crypts.[14] Using a reproducible experimental model, described in more detail in Section 3.2.2., we have characterized some transport properties of the crypt and villus compartments of the piglet small-intestinal epithelium. For these studies we have been using jejunal epithelium taken from piglets 40 hr after experimental infection with transmissible gastroenteritis (TGE) virus; at that stage of the disease the virus, after invading the mucosa, has been shed, leaving an epithelium composed of undifferentiated crypt-type epithelial cells.[15] Studies attempting to define pathogenetic mechanisms of a disease, and a veterinary disease at that, are teaching us about the function of the normal intestine!

Recent experiments in our laboratory have examined ion, glucose, and amino acid transport in piglet small intestine, comparing acute TGE-infected mucosa with normal controls. To assess ion transport, we exposed jejunal epithelium mounted in Ussing chambers to theophylline, which inhibits phosphodiesterase in normal intestine causing intracellular accumulation of cAMP,[16] inhibition of mucosa to serosal fluxes of Na and Cl, and a brisk secretion of Cl. TGE-infected tissue responds to theophylline with a normal accumulation of cAMP but no inhibition of NaCl absorption. This cryptlike epithelium shows a brisk Cl secretory response to theophylline, suggesting that secretory function does reside in the crypts. The failure of furosemide to inhibit NaCl absorption in TGE jejunum further supports the conclusion that this cryptlike epithelium lacks the capacity for electroneutral NaCl absorption at its luminal membrane.

Earlier marker perfusion experiments *in vitro* and Ussing chamber studies *in vitro* demonstrated impaired capacity of the TGE intestine to absorb glucose. Recent experiments used BBM vehicles to delineate distinctive features of D-glucose transport in this experimental preparation of crypt cells.[17] Initial rates for Na-gradient-dependent D-glucose uptake into vesicles prepared from TGE mucosa were reduced, and overshoot was blunted. To determine whether this blunted response in crypt-type cells was due to an actual defect in the BBM glucose transporter, or whether it was secondary to other factors such as an altered Na gradient indirectly affecting glucose transport, we undertook equilibrium kinetic studies using vesicles incubated in gramicidin to clamp transmembrane potential. Glucose uptake was linear for 5 sec under these clamped conditions, allowing us to measure stereospecific sodium-dependent D-glucose uptake over a range of D-glucose concentrations and analyze the results in an Eadie–Hofstee plot. In control tissue the plotted points were curvilinear, a least-squares analysis deriving a "best fit" for two distinct straight lines, one representing high-affinity sites, the second low-affinity sites. For the TGE vesicles, the same calculations derived a single straight line which did not differ from the low-affility line of the control vesicles but did differ significantly from the high-affinity line. We concluded that crypt cell luminal membranes lack an effective high-affinity D-glucose–Na cotransporter and assume that this high-affinity carrier appears as the cell differentiates during its migration along the crypt–villus axis.

We had expected that neutral amino acid–Na cotransport across intestinal luminal membranes would conform to a pattern similar to that described earlier for glucose transport. We were wrong. First, in Ussing chambers, we observed that 3-O-methyl glucose and L-alanine together had a greater stimulatory effect on net Na absorption than did either substrate alone, suggesting separate transporters for glucose and alanine in normal and TGE intestine.[18] Measuring initial Na-gradient-dependent L-alanine uptake rates into BBM vesicles, we found normal accumulation ratios in vesicles from TGE jejunum.[19] These *in vitro* data strongly suggest that neural amino acid–Na cotransport is intact in the luminal membrane of crypt cells, a pattern quite distinct from that for glucose.

From these studies of disease a picture of transport function in the normal poorly differentiated crypt cell and, by inference, in the normal mature villus cell emerges. Alterations in the balance between these types of cell in the mucosa and the regulation of cell renewal in the small intestine can be expected to be important determinants of the capacity of the intestine to conserve water and salts.

2.2. Gut-Associated Lymphoid Tissue (GALT)

Since the intestinal epithelium is not completely impermeable to potential antigens, this lymphoid tissue is probably an important component of the intestine's defenses. The GALT consists of lymphocytes and plasma cells in the lamina propira, intraepithelial lymphocytes, lymphoid nodule (Peyer patches), and mesenteric lymph nodes.

Two lines of antigen-sensitive lymphoid cells, T and B lymphocytes, have been characterized. The B lymphocyte can differentiate into plasma cells that synthesize and secrete immunoglubulins, the major portion of which is IgA; little is known of the role of IgE, IgM, or IgG in mucosal defense, but IgA is assumed to be important. Lymphoid populations in the gut are interrelated. Peyer patches appear to contain a precursor population of lymphocytes that can disseminate to the lamina propria and epithelium to participate in locul mucosal immunity. IgA produced in the lamina propria is transported through epithelial cells into intestinal secretions as a dimer linked by a J chain to which secretory component is attached. Intestinal T cells are less well characterized. Forty to seventy percent of Peyer's patch cells are B cells whereas most intraepithelial lymphocytes are T cells. Lymphoid cells of gut origin also migrate to extraintestinal sites, the mammary gland, genital tract, and bronchial tree, for example.

3. INTESTINAL RESPONSE TO ENTERIC PATHOGENS

3.1. Colonization by Pathogens

3.1.1. Attachment and Invasion

A number of nonspecific host factors, listed in Table 2, maintain a sparse flora in the stomach and small intestine of healthy people.[20,21] To

Table 2. Intestinal Defenses against Infection

Gastric acid
Lactoferrin
Enteric flora
Intestinal motility
Mucus
Immune factors
Passive—colostrum, breast milk
Active—local immune response

colonize the small intestine, organisms must first survive passage through a region of low intraluminal pH in the stomach. Additional nonspecific intraluminal protective factors include lactoferrins contained in human milk, other flora, and their metabolic products (e.g., short-chain fatty acids). Administration of antibiotics and dietary adjustments, particularly changes in fiber content, are two clinical situations in which a change in the balance of the normal flora can allow certain species to proliferate. Also, intestinal motility and perhaps villus motility are significant mechanisms for clearing enteric organisms. Small-bowel bacterial overgrowth is a well-known consequence of defective motility, and experimentally, inhibition of motility can be a requisite for creating models of enteric infection.[22] A possible role for the mucus gel layer has been discussed already. Several factors that may be associated with enteric pathogens, *Escherichia coli* and *Vibrio cholerae* enterotoxins, immune complexes, PGE_2, and perhaps bile salts may stimulate mucus release *in vitro*.

The M cells and a lack of surface mucus may render the dome epithelium relatively permeable to pathogens, which would then come quickly into contact with lymphoid tissue. Our preliminary collaborative studies of lapine rotavirus with Dr. Martin Petric indicate that although the virus does infect villus epithelium it is the patch epithelium that is particularly vulnerable to invasion by this virus.[23] Also, in the patches, virus antigen could be seen by immune fluorescence not only in the epithelium but also in adjacent lymphoid tissue, suggesting a process of invasion followed by an immunological response.

Certain properties of enteric organisms themselves can be important factors in determining their pathogenicity.[24] For example, the motility of *V. cholerae* probably enhances its penetration of the mucus layer, such patterns of propulsion being further enhanced by chemotactic properties of the bacterium. The importance to pathogenicity of various bacterial enzymes has been noted too; mucinase produced by *V. cholerae* and *Shigella flexneri*, glycosidase by a strain of *S. flexneri*, and *V. cholerae* protease are considered important determinants of pathogenicity.

Of great current research interest are the factors that determine a bacterium's capacity to attach to the intestinal surface.[25,26] If organisms succeed in overcoming the defensive strategies described earlier, they must attach to or invade the mucosa itself or its surface coat in order to colonize. *V. cholerae* and enterotoxigenic strains of *E. coli* cause no structural damage to the mucosa, but they colonize either the glycocalyceal coat or the brush border surface itself. Genetic studies have identified piglets with intestinal brush borders differing in their capacity to bind enterotoxigenic *E. coli*, and it has been suggested that these differences depend on glycolipids in the surface membranes. Other strains of diarrhea-producing bacteria, for example, the rabbit diarrhea *E. coli* (RDEC-1), attach to the mucosal surface, effacing microvilli; they may produce cytotoxins but they have not been shown to produce enterotoxins. Plasmid-associated fimbriae have been demonstrated on this latter organism. The initial site of their attachment, the M cells overlying lymphoid follicles rather than absorptive columnar cells, is fimbria mediated.

Some pathogens invade the epithelium and deeper structures of the bowel wall. Salmonellae are engulfed by an invagination of the apical membrane. The biochemical processes that regulate this uptake, like the factors involved in invasion of the small intestinal epithelium by viruses such as the rotaviruses and the TGE virus, are unknown. The fact that these pathogens preferentially invade villus cells suggests a role for brush border receptors in the differentiated columnar epithelium.[26,27] The existence of receptors is further supported by the relative consistency of the region of the bowel involved in a range of invasive enteric infections. The determinants of invasion of the deeper layers of bowel observed in several bacterial enteritides, while the above viruses are mainly confined to the epithelium, are not known.

3.1.2. Immune Response

The dome epithelium is not the only site, but it may be a preferred site for attachment or invasion by enteric pathogens, providing direct access to lymphoid tissue in Peyer's patches. Enteric immunization can prime or suppress both intestinal and extraintestinal immune responses.[28] A variety of enteric antigens are known to stimulate production of specific IgA antibody in the gut. The local nature and protective effect of this response has been clearly demonstrated in studies using attenuated polio virus given by mouth. To generate a significant IgA response, it appears that at least one enteric priming dose is needed. The status of the antigen also is an important determinant of the local immune response; for example, immune responses of the intestinal lymphoid tissue to cholera toxin and cholera toxoid vary greatly. Colostrum and milk also contain IgA antibodies[29]; like those released into the gut lumen, they are linked to a secretory component and therefore are relatively resistant to proteolytic degradation by digestive enzymes. Furthermore, the mucus gel on the epithelial surface may trap quantities of IgA, thereby concentrating it at the epithelial surface and enhancing its protective effect.[30]

3.2. Mechanisms of Diarrhea

Diarrhea is the state of excessive loss of fluid and electrolyte in stools. Many factors could contribute to its pathogenesis, but to date, most research has focused on epithelial transport.[31] Some organisms remain in the gut lumen or on the outer surface of the mucosa and alter transport via enterotoxins they produce. Others invade the mucosal wall directly to cause changes in epithelial function. Some invasive organisms also produce enterotoxins, but in many cases mechanisms are simply not understood. The pathogenesis of the diarrhea resulting from enteroadherent *E. coli* infections is still a mystery, for example.

There are two models of infectious diarrhea for which considerable pathophysiological data have been accumulated: toxigenic diarrheas as exemplified by cholera and certain *E. coli* infections, and invasive enteritides caused by human rotavirus (HRV) and piglet TGE virus.

3.2.1. Toxigenic Diarrhea

Studies elucidating the actions of choleragen, the toxin of *V. cholerae,* have provided an extremely important stimulus to research into mechanisms of all types of diarrhea.[32,33] Choleragen binds by its B subunits to specific GM_1 ganglioside receptors in the brush border; its A_1 subunit activates adenylate cyclase in the basolateral membrane leading to intracellular cAMP accumulation. The heat-labile toxin of *E. coli* (LT) closely resembles choleragen in its structure, its binding to the brush border, and its capacity to activate adenylate cyclase leading to cAMP accumulation. The heat-stable *E. coli* toxin differs from LT in its structure; it activates guanylate cyclase leading to cyclic GMP accumulation.[34] The end results are similar, although cAMP appears to exert a more potent effect than cGMP on ion transport.

In the differentiated columnar cells that populate villi described earlier, cyclic AMP or cyclic GMP inhibit NaCl absorption at the brush border membrane. The dissaccharidases, glucose–Na cotransport, and alanine–Na cotransport all are intact, as is the basolateral membrane Na pump, the Na-K-ATPase system. In the crypts, where proliferating, relatively immature cells are located, the response to cyclic AMP and presumably to cholera toxin is brisk Cl secretion.[16] Our preliminary data suggest that this secretion, which results from increased permeability of the luminal membrane to chloride, depends too on an intact Na^+-K^+-ATPase system and intact NaCl uptake across the basolateral membrane. The dramatic result is a secretory diarrhea that can be massive and life threatening. The stools rarely contain significant amounts of organic solute, and fecal Na and Cl concentrations are approximately those of extracellular fluid.

3.2.2. Viral Diarrhea

Our current understanding of viral diarrhea is based on studies of TGE, a reproducible, experimentally inducible piglet corona-virus enteritis.[15] The TGE virus differs from HRV, but the pathophysiological response to TGE is the same as that seen when piglets are infected with HRV.[35] At the height of diarrhea, 40 hr after oral inoculation of piglets with TGE virus, several defects in epithelial transport have been found.[17-19] Glucose–Na cotransport is blunted, and electroneutral NaCl absorption at the luminal membrane is not detectable in acute TGE jejunum. Although L-alanine-stimulated Na absorption is blunted, Na-gradient-stimulated alanine uptake is normal in TGE brush border membrane vesicles, suggesting that the suppression of alanine-stimulated Na absorption is not a brush border phenomenon. In Ussing chambers, neither dipeptides, susceptible to BBM hydrolysis nor those resistant to hydrolysis stimulated Na absorption more than individual amino acid.[36]

Impaired BBM Na-gradient-dependent glucose transport in TGE appears to result from the absence of a functional high-affinity BBM carrier. The basolateral membrane pump, Na-K-ATPase, is reduced in activity as are the brush border membrane disaccharidases. We suspect that reduced Na-K-ATPase activity is not an important factor limiting the response to glucose since the TGE epithelium does possess a normal secretory response to cyclic AMP. Disaccharidase activities are low, but clinical trials have suggested that reduced levels of these enzymes are unlikely to be important determinants of acute viral diarrhea. Perhaps in some cases, late in the course of their illness, dietary disaccharide can contribute to persisting diarrhea because of intestinal disaccharidase deficiencies.

The functional profile of epithelial function in TGE diarrhea is similar, if not identical, to that described earlier for normal immature crypt cells. The virus invades the epithelium within 12 hr of inoculation, after which epithelial proliferation is stimulated in the crypts, cells migrate up along the crypt–villus axis at an accelerated rate, and the infected cells are shed rapidly into the lumen. Diarrhea becomes severe when the epithelium is composed of poorly differentiated crypt cell-type cells, and apparently when most virus has been shed. In babies, HRV probably remains in the mucosa during the early stages of diarrhea since virus is detectable in diarrheal stools in the third and fourth days of the illness.[27] Similarly, our preliminary studies in rabbits suggests that lapine rotavirus persists in the mucosa during the early stages of infection.[23]

Rotavirus and TGE diarrheal stools contain concentrations of Na and Cl (45–55 meq/liter), considerably less than those seen in toxigenic diarrheas like cholera.[37]

Another consequence of viral invasion and distorted epithelial dynamics may be a structual lesion. Severe flattening of villi and hyperplasia of crypts are reported in babies with HRV diarrhea and in piglets with TGE. Reduced surface area with reduced epithelial mass in theory could contribute to reduced absorptive function in viral enteritis, but from piglet studies we know that severe impairment of function can occur without a measurable structural lesion.[38] We believe that surface area is a relatively insignificant factor in the pathogenesis of viral diarrhea.

3.3. Repair

Obviously, clinical recovery depends on reversal of the pathophysiological abnormalities that led to the diarrheal illness in the first place. Cessation of nausea, vomiting, cramps, and anorexia undoubtedly contributes to the patient's recovery, but reversal of the pathophysiological determinants of diarrhea is of central importance.

The relative importance of different mechanisms available for clearing pathogenic organisms from the gut is unknown, but peristalsis and the constant rapid turnover of the epithelium must be very important. Peristaltic activity may be increased in certain enteric infections,[2] and theoretically, secondary metabolic disturbances could also interfere with intestinal motility in the course of severe diarrhea. When organisms invade and injure the villus epithelium, at least in the case of a viral pathogen, crypt cell proliferation is stimulated, and cell shedding from the villi and migration of cells up from the crypts along the crypt–villus axis are accelerated.[15] Presumably, inhibitory factors emanating from normal villus cells are lost when the virus damages these cells. Goblet cell mucin discharge is increased also, but whether quantitative or qualitative changes in intestinal mucus actually contribute to clearing of pathogens remains to be determined. A local immune response occurs, but the relative importance of the various populations of lyphoid tissue is not known. Furthermore, the actual processes involved in clearance of organisms from the lamina propria are unknown although probably macrophages are involved.

Recovery of epithelial function involves more than shedding of organisms and replacement of shed cells with newly divided ones. Repair also involves the generation of an epithelium with adequate absorptive function; it is mature differentiated cells that must replace the villus enterocytes lost in the course of an infection. A consideration of mucosal repair, therefore, becomes a consideration of the determinants of epithelial proliferation and differentiation.

Several factors listed in Table 3 may regulate cell proliferation in the gut although their effect on differentiation is unclear.[39] Many of these fac-

Table 3. Factors Regulating Small Intestinal
Proliferation and/or Differentiation

Nutritional factors
  Chronic protein–calorie malnutrition
  Specific substrate deprivation (e.g., CHO)
  Trace element deprivation (e.g., Zn, vitamin B_{12})
  Intraluminal food
Normal flora
Hormones
  Adrenal corticoids
  Thyroxin
  Growth hormone/somatomedin
  Enteroglucagon
  Epidermal growth factor
Neural pharmacological factors
  α-Adrenergic
  β-Adrenergic

tors are of little relevance to repair after enteric infection. At present no major role for hormones or neural factors in repair after infection is apparent, but the known impact of chronic protein–calorie malnutrition on cell renewal is undoubtedly relevant. Chronic starvation has been shown, consistently, to reduce cell proliferation in crypts and to reduce cell migration along the crypt–villus axis.[40] Whether it is the deprivation of energy and protein that is the key determinant of this response or whether micronutrients like iron and zinc play a pivotal role is not known. Animal experiments suggest that oral nutrients may be particularly important in promoting intestinal epithelial repair.[41,42] Our animal studies indicate that chronic malnutrition has a powerful impact early in life when the normal postnatal development of enterocyte function is disturbed.[40] With these considerations in mind, we postulated that repair of the gut after injury might be inhibited in the malnourished host. In the piglet, experimentally infected with TGE virus, this postulate has proven to be true.[43] Structural and functional recovery of the mucosa after TGE infection was delayed in nutritionally deprived animals, an observation that could not be attributed to a particularly severe initial injury in the malnourished animal. However, it seems that it is only after a very extensive intestinal injury, such as that encountered in viral enteritis, that repair is significantly delayed by malnutrition. When we produced ischemic injury to a short intestinal segment in the malnourished rabbit, structural and functional repair was scarcely affected although epithelial turnover was delayed.[42,44] We conclude that separate mechanisms exist for the regulation of cell proliferation and cell differentiation as reflected by the independent response of these two variables to undernutrition. However, a potential "vicious cycle" contributing to persisting intestinal dysfunction and malnutrition becomes apparent. Enteric infection and attendant diarrhea and anorexia cause undernutrition, which in turn delays repair of the mucosal lesion.

To date experimental models of malnutrition have dealt mainly with generalized deprivation of both macronutrients and micronutrients; the impact on intestinal cell proliferation or differentiation of specific micronutrient deficiencies has not been assessed.

The cellular mediators that control proliferation and differentation are not completely understood.[39] Because villus cell damage leads to stimulation of crypt proliferation, mature villus cells are thought to contain "chalones" that inhibit cell proliferation. Under experimental conditions cAMP stimulates cell proliferation, and it has been suggested that mesenchymal and even lymphoid tissue in the villus core exerts some influence on epithelial renewal. Polyamines that may serve some role in mediating cell proliferation also are of considerable current research interest.[45] An important limiting role in polyamine metabolism is served by ornithine decarboxylase; this cytoplasmic enzyme is increased in activity when proliferative activity is increased in the gut after massive resection.[46] Our preliminary studies show marked increases in activity after viral invasion and after ischemic injury, again associated with heightened proliferative activity. The possibility that polyamines may play some regulatory role in gut epithelial renewal is appealing, but the observation of enriched activity along the villus rather than in the proliferative zone of the crypts does not support the hypothesis[47]; identification of isoenzymes in the mucosal epithelium should allow a more detailed study of this issue.[48]

4. TREATMENT

Preventive measures must be the first priority in dealing with a health problem that kills millions of the world's babies each year and a significant number of children and adults. For the young infant, a degree of protection is available in the form of breast feeding. Not only is mother's milk the most appropriate food for the baby, but also it contains elements known to confer some passive protection against enteric pathogens. Rotavirus IgA antibodies identified in human milk[49] can be expected to resist intraluminal digestion because of their attachment to secretory component. Fortunately, earlier trends away from the breast are being reversed in many developing countries, where high attack rates are a consequence of poor sanitary and hygenic conditions.

As more enteric pathogens are identified and more is learned about their interaction with the gut, efforts increase to develop effective vaccines. The goal is to develop attenuated live organisms capable of generating an effective local immune protection against pathogenic organisms. Ironically, the success of a vaccine also depends on the organism's capacity to bypass or overcome, at least in part, existing host defense mechanisms like gastric acid and breast milk IgA. Clinical trials will be required to determine whether bicarbonate administration or withholding of breast feeding is essential to the efficacy of various oral vaccines. The most promising contenders for human diseases, to date, are two rotavirus vaccines, one an attenuated calf virus, found to be safe and protective in limited trials.[50,51] An attenuated simian rotavirus also has been shown to protect, but to date it has been associated with an incidence of febrile reactions.[51] Progress has also been made in the development of vaccines against animal bacterial pathogens.[52] Programs are being directed at the development of vaccines for several human bacterial pathogens but none is ready for clinical use.

4.1. Fluid and Electrolyte Balance

The foremost consideration, particularly for the young patient, must be rehydration of the dehydrated baby or preservation of hydration for the child who is not dehydrated. The application of sound pathophysiology principles to oral fluid therapy of diarrhea is one of the important medical advances of the century. Formulation of a balanced, buffered isotonic mixture of glucose and electrolytes, an oral rehydration solution (ORS) (Table 4), promoted by a highly successful WHO Diarrheal Disease Control Program, has had a dramatic impact on mortality and morbidity from diarrheal disease in the developing world.[53] This formulation, usually dispensed in a cachet or tablet for dissolution in a standard vol-

Table 4. Oral Rehydration Solution (ORS)—
World Health Organization

	mM
Glucose	111
Na	90
K	20
Cl	80
Citrate	10

ume of water, provides a balance of solute and water to make the best possible use of any absorptive function that remains in the gut after infection.[53] Designed initially for patients with cholera, it has been found effective for all but the most severely affected babies with viral enteritis.[54] Certainly, ORS is a vast improvement over many traditional beverages used for infant diarrhea, such as fruit juices and soft drinks, all of which are highly hyperosmolar sugar solutions.[55] Pediatricians have worried about the 90-mM Na concentration in ORS since it exceeds stool concentrations in viral enteritis, but actually the solution has been used effectively to treat hypernatremic infants with viral enteritis.[56] It is strongly recommended that WHO ORS not be force-fed and that, for very young infants, it be given with 1 volume of water per 2 volumes ORS; for worldwide use WHO must advocate the use of a single oral rehydration fomulation.

Regrettably, medical practices in developed countries, particularly in North America, have lagged behind the developing world in instituting this very effective treatment technique. Although some extremely ill infants will require intravenous fluids and electrolytes, rational oral therapy is simple, effective, and a preferable approach for most.[56]

Several proposed modifications of oral fluid therapy based on pathophysiological considerations described previously appear promising. Many have speculated that additional organic solutes, amino acids, peptides, and even more complex carbohydrates might further enhance water absorption if incorporated into oral treatment solutions. Since even in viral enteritis our studies showed both an additive response of Na absorption to alanine and glucose and intact BBM alanine absorption, there is a theoretical basis for incorporating an amino acid like L-alanine into oral hydration solutions. Furthermore, *in vivo* studies suggest that amino acids are absorbed more efficiently when presented to the mucosa as dipeptides than when provided as amino acids alone.[57] Current clinical studies are evaluating dipeptides in ORS mixtures, but our *in vitro* data do not indicate that they will have a particular advantage.[35] It has been suggested too that polysaccharides might be provided as a source of glucose in ORS to provide extra carbohydrates at lower osmotic cost,[58] assuming that some digestive function is preserved in patients with enteric infections. These concepts tend to support the suggestion that some foods might serve as an appropriate source of organic solute for ORS solutions. These latter solutions, most of which have utilized cooked rice, might be suitable as a prepared product, but they might also lend themselves to preparation in the home. Field trials have shown that rice-based cereal ORS is effective in reducing diarrheal stool output.[59]

The appeal of all the various improved ORS formulations is their possible capacity to reduce diarrhea. Apart from the obvious beneficial impact on fluid balance, such solutions can be expected to improve acceptance of oral fluid therapy; failure to decrease stool output is probably a major factor blocking more widespread acceptance of the current ORS solution. Unless cost or palatability problems are significant deterrents, it is likely that an improved ORS formulation capable of actually decreasing diarrhea will become available in the near future.[60]

4.2. Drugs

In general, drugs have no place in the treatment of acute infectious diarrhea. Clearance of pathogens is swift, and in most cases antibiotics are not helpful; they may even harm. Of course, there are special situations in children with infectious diarrhea where antibiotics are needed, but these are rare. Even if viricidal agents were available, they are unlikely to benefit patients with viral diarrhea because by the time diarrhea is significant, little time for the virus remains in the mucosa because of accelerated natural shedding.

As the pathogenesis of infective diarrhea was elucidated, great hope was held for a pharmacological approach to correction of the transport defects identified. Many drugs have been shown to enhance absorption or decrease secretion *in vitro*,[61] but *in vivo* they have been either ineffective or toxic. Unfortunately, antidiarrheal drugs continue to be promoted for the treatment of acute diarrhea; in children at least, they should not be used.

4.3. Nutritional Treatment

Since recovery from viral enteritis, and presumably other invasive infections, depends on an epithelial repair process that in turn is influenced by nutritional status, it makes theoretical sense to provide nutrients to patients with diarrhea.[62] The digestive tract is the preferred supply route for these nutrients. If the patient is young with meager nutritional reserves, particularly if he is malnourished initially, food is particularly important. Unfortunately, it has been traditional in many societies to withhold food or limit intake for extended periods during diarrhea. Limited feeding studies indicate that at the worst early feeding does no harm,[63-66] and a recently published epidemiological study showed that diarrheal illness was relatively prolonged among patients who were malnourished.[66] The latter clinical observation might have been predicted from current concepts of pathogenesis.

The breast-fed baby should continue to receive mother's milk, although extra hydration fluid may be needed as well. The question then arises as to whether some foods may aggravate diarrhea. The answer is yes, but rarely is the aggravation significant in relation to the benefits of food. In the face of a viral enteritis, at least two possible mechanisms by which dietary constituents might increase diarrhea are worth consideration, sugar intolerance and dietary protein intolerance.

Disaccharidase activities are reduced, particularly lactase activity in viral enteritis.[67] Large dietary loads of disaccharides, therefore, may cause watery, sugar-filled stools in cases of severe, prolonged mucosal disease, but in most populations, disaccharide absorption is not a limiting problem contributing to infectious diarrhea. Lactose intolerance is particularly prevalent among older children and adults belonging to native groups in North and South America. In the latter populations it is reasonable to defer cow's milk feeds for a few days early in the course of an enteritis.

Another theoretical problem that might be induced by diet during enteric infection is milk protein intolerance. It has been postulated that the infected bowel is excesssively permeable to intact protein antigens.[68] Our *in vivo* studies of piglet TGE suggest that this is the case,[69] although *in vitro* experiments showed an increased uptake only during the very early phase of infection and only in non-patch-containing regions of the small intestine.[70] There are no findings yet to suggest that such an enhanced antigen absorption is of real immunological significance, and there are no data to support a general policy of withholding milk protein from patients recovering from infectious diarrhea.

5. SUMMARY AND CONCLUSIONS

A range of pathogenic organisms interact with the gut causing diarrhea by several distinct mechanisms. Until effective preventive measures are available, these patients should be treated aggressively with oral fluid based on an understanding of the pathophysiological disorders underlying their illness. Furthermore, early provision of adequate nutrients is highly desirable in order to promote quick recovery. Ongoing research, while providing important information about the normal intestine, should provide data on which to base new approaches to preventive and active therapy.

REFERENCES

1. Fourth Programme Report 1984–1985: *Program for Control of Diarrhoeal Diseases.* Geneva, World Health Organization, 1985.
2. Summers RW: Role of motility in infectious diarrhea. *Gastroenterology* 1981;80:1070–1071.
3. Mathias JR, Sninsky CA: Motility of the small intestine: A look ahead. *Am J Physiol* 1985;11:G495–G500.
4. Hubel EA: Intestinal nerves and ion transport: Stimuli, reflexes, and responses. *Am J Physiol* 1985;11:G261–G271.
5. Harper SL, Behlen HG, Granger DN: Vasoactive agents and the mesenteric microcirculation. *Am J Physiol* 1985;11:G309–G315.
6. Owen RL: Sequential uptake of horseradish peroxidase by lymphoid follicle epithelium of Peyer's patches in the normal unobstructed mouse intestine. An ultrastructural study. *Gastorenterology* 1971;72:440–451.
7. Keljo DJ, Hamilton JR: Quantitative determination of macromolecular transport rate across intestinal Peyer's patches. *Am J Physiol* 1983;244(*Gastrointest Liver Physiol* 7):G637–G644.
8. Trier JS, Madara JL: Functional morphology of the mucosa of small intestine, in Johnston LR (ed): *Physiology of the Gastrointestinal Tract.* New York, Raven Press, 1981, pp 925–962.
9. Forstner G, Sherman P, Forstner J: Mucus: Function and structure, in Boedecker E (ed): *Attachment of Gut Organisms to the Gut Mucosa II.* Boca Raton, FL CPC Press Inc., 1984, pp 13–21.
10. Solcia E, Capella C, Buffa R, Usellini L, Feocca R, Sessa F: Endocrine cells of the digestive system, in Johnston LR (ed): *Physiology of the Gastrointestinal Tract.* New York, Raven Press, 1981, pp 39–58.
11. Cheng H, Leblond CP: Origin, differentiation and renewal of the four main epithelial cell types in the mouse small intestine. I. Columnar cells. *Am J Anat* 1974;141:461–480.
12. Williamson RCN: Intestinal adaptation II mechanisms of control. *N Engl J Med* 1978;298:1444–1450.
13. Weiser MM: Intestinal epithelial cell surface membrane glycoprotein synthesis. I An indicator of cellular differentiation. *J Biol Chem* 1973;248:2436–2541.
14. Field M: Regulation of active ion transport in the small intestine, in Elliott E, Knight J (eds): Acute Diarrhoea in Childhood. Ciba Foundation Symposium 42 (new series). Amsterdam, Elsevier, 1976, pp 109–122.
15. Hamilton JR, Gall DG, Butler DG, Middleton PJ: Viral gastroenteritis: Recent progress, remaining problems, in Elliott E, Knight J (eds): *Acute Diarrhoea in Childhood.* CIBA Foundation Symposium 42 (new series). Amsterdam, Elsevier, 1976, pp 223–231.
16. MacLeod J, Hamilton JR: Absence of electoneutral NaCl transport in jejunal crypt type epithelium (abstr.). *Gastroenterology* 1984;86:1169.
17. Keljo DJ, MacLeod RJ, Perdue MH, Butler EG, Hamilton JR: Sodium dependent D-glucose in piglet jejunal brush border membranes. Insights from a disease model. *Am J Physiol* 1985;249:G751–760.
18. Rhoads JM, MacLeod J, Khan M, Hamilton R: Impaired amino acid-facilitated Na transport in acute viral enteritis. *Gastroenterology* 1984;86:1170.
19. Rhoads M, MacLeod J, Hamilton R: Preservation of brush border membrane alanine transport in acute viral diarrhea. *Pediatr Res* 1984;19:230A.

20. Boedecker E: Animal models for bacterial infection of the gastrointestinal tract: An overview, in Keusch G, Walstrom T (eds): *Experimental Bacterial and Parasitic Infections*. Amsterdam, Elsevier, 1983, p 234.
21. Dupont HL: Interactions of enteric pathogens with the intestines, in Field M, Fordtran JS, Schultz SG (eds): *Secretory Diarrhea*. Bethesda, American Physiology Society, 1982, pp 61-65.
22. King CE, Toskes PP: The experimental rat blind loop preparations: A model for small intestine bacterial overgrowth in man, in *Animal Models for Intestinal Disease*. Boca Raton, FL, CRC Press, 1985, pp 217-223.
23. Guzman C, Rhoads M, Petric M, Hamilton R: Experimental rabbit rotavirus enteritis. A model of viral diarrhea. *Pediatr Res* 1986; 20:310A.
24. Formal SB, Hale TL, Boedecker EC: Interactions of enteric pathogens and the intestinal mucosa. *Phil Trans R Soc Lond* 1985;303:65-73.
25. Gaastra W, de Graaf FK: Host-specific fimbrial adhesions of noninvasive enterotoxigenic *Escherichia coli* strains. *Microbiol Rev* 1982;46:129-161.
26. Pensaert M, Halterman EO, Burnstein T: Transmissible gastorenteritis of swine: Virus-intestinal call interations. I. Immunofluorescence, histophatology and virus production in the small intestine through the course of infection. *Arch Gesamte Virusforsch* 1970;31:321-324.
27. Middleton PJ, Abbot GD, Szymanski MT, Bortolussi R, Hamilton JR: Orbivirus acute gastroenteritis of infancy. *Lancet* 1974;1241-1245.
28. Kagnoff MF: Immunology of the digestive system, in Johnston LR (ed): *Physiology of the Gastrointestinal Tract*. New York, Raven Press, 1981, pp 1337-1359.
29. Hanson LA, Carlsson B, Cruz JR: The immune response in the mammary gland, in Ogra P, Dayton D (eds): *Immunology of Breast Milk*. New York, Raven Press, 1979, pp 145-157.
30. Clamp JR: The relationship between the immune system and the mucus in the protection of mucous membranes. *Biochem Soc Trans* 1984;12:754-756.
31. Dobbins JW, Binder HS: Pathophysiology of diarrhea: Alterations in fluid and electrolyte transport. *Clin Gastroenterol* 1981;10:605-621.
32. Carpenter CCJ: Clinical and pathophysiologic features of diarrhea caused by *Vibro cholerae* and *Escherichia coli*, in Field M, Fordtran JS, Schultz SG (eds): *Secretory Diarrhea*. Bethesda, American Physiology Society, 1982, pp 67-83.
33. Fishman PH: Mechanisms of action of cholera toxin: Events on the cell surface, in Field M, Fordtran JS, Schultz SG (eds): *Secretory Diarrhea*. Bethesda, American Physiology Society, 1982.
34. Hughes JM, Murad F, Chang B, Geurant RL: Role of cyclic GMP in the action of heat stable enterotoxin of *Escherichia coli*. *Nature* 1978;271:755-756.
35. Davidson GP, Gail DG, Butler DG, Petric M, Hamilton JR: Human rotavirus enteritis induced in conventional piglets. Intestinal structure and transport. *J Clin Invest* 1979;60:1402-1414.
36. Rhoads M, MacLeod J, Katena E, Hamilton R: Response of Na absorption to dipeptide in acute viral diarrhea. *Pediatr Res* 1985;19:230A.
37. Tallett S, MacKenzie C, Middleton P, Kerzner B, Hamilton JR: Clinical laboratory and epidemiologic features of a viral gastroenteritis in infants and children. *Pediatrics* 1977;60:217-223.
38. Klein RM, McKenzie JC: The role of cell renewal in the cytogeny of the intestine. II. Regulation of cell proliferation in adult, fetal and neonatal intestine. *J Pediatr Gastroenterol Nutr* 1983;2:204-228.

39. Guiraldes E, Hamilton JR: Effect of chronic malnutrition on intestinal structure, epithelial renewal and enzymes in suckling rats. *Pediatr Res* 1981;15:930–934.
40. Butler DG, Gall DG, Kelly MH, Hamiton JR: Transmissible gastroenteritis: Mechanisms responsible for diarrhea in an acute viral enteritis in piglets. *J Clin Invest* 1974;53:1335–1342.
41. Kottler DP, Levine GM, Shiau YF: Effects of luminal nutrition and metabolic staus on in vivo glucose absorption. *Am J Physiol* 1981;245:G432–434.
42. Levine GM, Deren JJ, Yesdimir E: Small bowel resection: Oral intake is the stimulus for hyperplasia. *Am J Dig Dis* 1976;21:542.
43. Butzner JD, Butler DG, Miniats OP, Hamilton JR: Impact of chronic protein-calorie malnutrition on small intestinal repair after acute viral enteritis: A study in gnotoiotic piglets. *Pediatr Res* 1985;19:476–481.
44. Guzman C, Hamilton R: Intestinal repair in chronic protein–caloric malnutrition. *Pediatr Res* 1985;19:221A.
45. Tabor CW, Tabor H: Polyamines. *Annu Rev Biochem* 1984;53:749–790.
46. Luk GD, Baylin SB: Ornithine decarboxylase in intestinal maturation and adaption, in Robinson, JWL, Dowling RH, Riecken, EO (eds): *Mechanisms of Intestinal Adaption.* Lancaster, MTR, 1982, pp 65–80.
47. Sepulveda FV, Burton EA, Clarkson EM, Syme G: Cell differentiation and L-ornithine decarbonxylase activity in the small intestine of rats fed low and high protein diets. *Biochem Biophys Acta* 1982;716:439–442.
48. Richards JF, Lit K, Fuca R, Bourqeault C: Multiple species of ornithine decarboxylase in rat tissues: Effects of dexamethasone. *Biochim Biophy Res Commun* 1981;99:1461–1469.
49. Simhon A, Mata L: Antirotavirus antibody in human colostrum. *Lancet* 1978;1:39–40.
50. Vesikari T, Isolauri E, Delem A, et al: Clinical Efficacy of the RIT 4237 live attenuated bovine rotavirus vaccine in infants vaccinated before a rotavirus epidemic. *J Pediatr* 1985;107:189–194.
51. Wright PF, Thompson J, Kokubun K, Kapikian AZ: Rhesus rotavirus vaccine in children. *Pediatr Res* 1985;19:307A.
52. Clark S, Cahill A, Stirpaker C, Greenwod P, Gregson R, Tzipori S: Prevention by vaccination. Animal bacteria, in Tzipori S (ed): *Infectious Diarrhea in the Young.* Amsterdam, Elsevier, 1985, pp 481–487.
53. Hirschorn N: The treatment of acute diarrhea in children: A historical and physiological perspective. *Am J Clin Nutr* 1980;33:637–663.
54. Santosham M, Daum RS, Dillman L, et al: Oral rehydration therapy of infantile diarrhea. A controlled study of well nourished children hospitalized in the United States and Panama. *N Engl J Med* 1982;306:1070–1076.
55. Wendland BE, Arbus GS: Oral fluid therapy. Sodium and potassium content and osmolality of commercial "clear" soups and beverages. *Can Med Assoc J* 1979;121:564–571.
56. Santosham M, Burns B, Nadkarni V, et al: Oral rehydration therapy for acute diarrhea in ambulatory children in the United States. A double blind comparison of four different solutions. *Pedatrics* 1975;76:159–166.
57. Mathews DM: Intestinal absorption of peptides. *Physiol Rev* 1985;55:537–608.
58. Sandhu BK, Jones BJM, Brooks CGD, Silk DBA: Oral rehydration in acute infantile diarrhoea with a glucose-polymer electrolyte solution. *Arch Dis Child* 1982;57:152–160.
59. Molla AM, Sarkar SA, Hossain M, Molla A: Rice-powder electrolyte solution as oral therapy in diarrhea due to *Vibrio cholerae* and *Escherichia coli. Lancet* 1982;1:1317–1318.

60. Mahalanabis D, Patra PC: In search of a super oral rehydration solution. Can optimum use of organic solute-mediated sodium absorption lead to the development of an absorption promoting drug? *J Diar Dis Res* 1983;1:76–81.
61. Powell DW, Field M: Pharmacological approaches to treatment of secretory diarrhea, in Field M, Fordtran JS, Schultz SG (eds): *Secretory Diarrhea*. American Physiology Society, Bethesda, 1980, pp 187–210.
62. Hamilton JR: Treatment of acute diarrhea. *Pediatr Clin North Am* 1985;32:419–427.
63. Chung AW, Viscorva B: The effect of early oral feeding versus early oral starvation on the course of infantile diarrhea. *J Pediatr* 1948;33:14–22.
64. Dugdale A, Lovell S, Gibbs V, Ball D: Refeeding after acute gastroenteritis: a controlled study. *Arch Dis Child* 1982;57:76–78.
65. Rees L, Brook CGD: Gradual re-introduction of full-strength milk after acute gastroenteritis in children. *Lancet* 1979;1:770–771.
66. Black RE, Brown KH, Becker J: Malnutrition is a determining factor in diarrheal duration but not incidence among young children in a longitudinal study in rural Bangladesh. *Am J Clin Nutr* 1984;39:87–94.
67. Blacklow NR, Cukor G: Viral gastroenteritis. *N Engl J Med* 1981;304:397–406.
68. Walker-Smith JA: Cow's milk intolerance as a cause of post-enteritis diarrhea. *J Pediatr Gastroenterol Nutr* 1982;1:163–173.
69. Keljo DJ, Bloch KJ, Block M, Arrighi M, Hamilton JR: Antigen absorption is enhanced during viral enteritis. *Pediatr Res* 1985;19:224A.
70. Keljo DJ, Butler DG, Hamilton JR: Altered jejunal permeability to macromolecules during viral enteritis. *Gastroenterology* 1985;88:998–1004.

20

Dilemmas and Decisions in Digestive Disease

Howard M. Spiro

1. INTRODUCTION

This volume has been concerned with the scientific basis of gastroenterology, but we must also think about the humanistic basis of gastrointestinal practice. Science, after all, is the means, not the end, of medicine. The purpose of medicine is the cure of disease and the relief of pain, and that involves thinking of men and women and not just of stomachs and livers. By humanistic I imply no specifically secular bias (as opposed to a religious one), but simply use the word to emphasize the human, personal side of medicine where our moral dilemmas and decisions lie. Parenteral nutrition, for example, makes it possible to keep alive for some months an anencephalic trisomy 13 newborn, if we do not ask why we are preserving a human form without a human brain. Every year it is easier to transplant a liver to give an alcoholic with cirrhosis a new life to drink away, if we do not ask how our reserves are to be used. What can be done is not necessarily what should done.

The major problems of the 1980s have to do with restraint of (1) financial costs and (2) the overuse of diagnostic technology. Both, I fear, arise from the fact that we physicians like to do much *to* patients, but we do not always think about what we can do *for* them. It is the difference

Howard M. Spiro ● Section of Gastroenterology, Yale University School of Medicine, New Haven, Connecticut 06510.

between the *person,* specific and identifiable, a human being before us, and the *case,* shorn of identifiable personal qualities, displaying its diseased malfunctioning parts.

In Canada and the United States, as well as in Europe, these financial matters will come under control even if that means wresting control from the medical profession. There is no great decision to be made to dispense only a limited amount of money for medical care. There is a much greater problem in deciding how to spend that money, in discussing how much given for liver transplants, for example, is taken away from hyperalimentation for children with regional enteritis.

Fundamentally more important dilemmas are those at the borders of life, "bringing alive" at the beginning and "keeping alive" at the end: (1) birth and conception achievements and (2) the aging of the population. They are technical victories which rarely impinge on gastrointestinal practice, yet they lead to entrancing ethical dilemmas. From the ovary of a woman whose tubes are blocked several ova can be extracted, and some, fertilized by her husband's sperm, can be placed in her uterus, while others, fertilized by the sperm of another man, can be put into the uterus of his wife. Let us suppose that the first woman suffers an abortion. Can she then turn to the other woman to claim the child raised in that uterus as her own? These questions are dramatic, packed with emotions, and seemingly new, but they are not, at least for the moment, meaningful in gastrointestinal disease.

Such matters and many others are basically technical dilemmas. In science at the moment, there is much discussion of whether science advances by "paradigms," the idea that Thomas Kuhn made so famous: a great man or woman is seized with a new idea which becomes the popular explanatory model for his time. Other lesser men follow that metaphor, to mine all that it supplies. A good example in the 1940s and 1950s was the visionary concepts of that great adopted Canadian Hans Selye. The "alarm reaction," the evidence that stress has its effects through the adrenal cortex, was a universal stimulus to research, and it was supported by the therapeutic wonders of adrenal steroids. Later, as the novelty of Selye's ideas waned, other models, more lately immunological ones, took over to give a new, but equally temporary, universal explanation. Lately, however, historians of science are coming to suggest that the "great man" notion has been overextended. They believe that the technology of the times may be just as important to the advances of science as the great man's vision. On that view, one espoused particularly by Derek Price at Yale, scientists depend on technology for their achievements. Galileo could not make his great observations about the solar system until the lens grinders had polished their art enough to provide him with the right lenses for his telescope. It is a fascinating question, whether the scientist or the technician is more important. I suspect that they work together. But whether medicine is technology or science, we who practice clinical medicine apply technology for the benefit of our patients and our dilemmas are largely technical ones.

2. THE PHYSICIAN'S TWO WORLDS

We physicians live in two worlds: The world of science provides us with our knowledge of disease, with the very real advances in gastroenterology that we have been examining today and with our ideals. But physicians also live, and it is especially true for gastroenterologists, in the world of people, persons with instincts, pain, suffering, hope, and joy. The first world is the realm of physics, where everything can be measured; the other, so neglected in medical training, is the world of poetry where we can assess but do not measure.

The training of physicians focuses largely on the first world of science and technology because physicians, along with members of most other learned professions, have accepted the idea that only the techniques of hard sciences give answers that are permanent, comparable, and true. Physicians have adopted a model for medicine which is a bioscientific mechanical one that does not take into account social, personal, or psychological contributions to getting sick.

That model is quite understandable. Most of us gastroenterologists treat persons in whom personal, social, and psychological factors influence the manifestations of disease that we call illness, but what we can do about those matters has changed very little over the past century. Advances in the understanding of humans or society are minor compared to the advances in knowledge of biology or genetics. What was written a thousand or two thousand years ago often seems as pertinent as what makes this week's best-seller list, and often it is more substantial. Surveying the social cataclysms of Europe and Asia over the past 50 years, physicians cannot be blamed for feeling that the social studies, any understanding of the human as a person, have made very small advance. We cannot be faulted for seeking the surcease of hard science. For when we turn to the study of disease, we are delighted at how vastly quantification and the techniques of science have improved our knowledge and what we can do for our patients. We talk to a patient with duodenal ulcer about his troubles very little differently from the way Osler might have, but if we applied Osler's treatments, the lawyers would soon be crowding outside our door. Psychiatry may have given us new visions of why a man gets an ulcer, but science gave us the H_2 blockers to treat him.

Science pushes medical practice so fast that the pharmacological and technical advice in a textbook of 15 years ago is outmoded. Yet, physicians could read Shakespeare or Auden, novelists, poets, and philosophers today with as much pleasure and benefit as men and women of their times. Poets exists in the same time, and for all time, but Heraclitus has only an archaic knowledge for us today. We know so much more, and can do so much more, about lupus than about lust that it is no wonder that physicians pour over their scientific journals and ignore novels and poetry. I know as much today about why an alcoholic wants to drink as I did 30 years ago, but now I can plumb his pancreas to lay out its ducts and outline its contour with computed tomography. It is much more satisfying to look for the "hard data" that images and endoscopies provide in our patients than it is to listen to what the patients want to tell us about themselves, or what the novelists can tell us about life. That every patient is his own poem makes no difference to the doctor who has CT scans.

Let us consider the dichotomy of science and intuition in medicine. Science is what is known by measurement and quantification; its knowledge comes only slowly and grudgingly. Intuition is what we grasp immediately, instinctively, without delay. Medical practice relies increasingly only on science, but physicians are not always aware of the selective and even biased nature of data gathering. Preexisting theory may help a scientist select data that he obtains much more than we physicians recognize, and theory helps clinicians see what they want to see. That is not fraud, or even selection bias, but simply the "scientific condition." Medawar put it well, "We cannot browse over the field of nature like cows at pasture." Scientists have to select what data they use. Clinicians need to recognize that we convert human problems into technical ones by our selective data gathering, as we look into the spastic colon of a man with pain from life and try to treat his motility. Humanism in medicine suggests the equal importance to medical practice of intuition, what leaps to the mind suddenly without measurement, the unguided but undeviating attention to the person.

3. MAJOR HUMANISTIC PROBLEMS

Three major humanistic problems, less than technical, bedevil medicine, and they all begin with F: (1) fraud, (2) fads, and (3) frenzy. They are important in both academic and clinical life, and I should like to spend the remaining pages on them.

Academic fraud, for example, is now very well publicized but not widely discussed. It is too uncomfortable for all of us so committed to fact gathering and to the scientific credo to accept the idea that fabrication of data is more than the work of one "bad apple." Admitting such fraud erodes the basis of our careers, but there has been too little continuing discussion. To be sure, each example of fraud has been formally aired at the medical school where it took place, but then matters are quickly dropped in public. Everyone is so rightly ashamed of this threat to our values that we may be too anxious to suppress any discussion about the pressures to succeed too fast, to publish and get grants, that the system generates. Everyone I know who talks about these matters is still depressed, and some have even left academic life. Safeguards have been introduced to prevent fraud, professors have been enjoined to go over data more closely than ever before, and algorithms have been put in place to deal with future fraud. Such safeguards may prove barriers to further conversations about the problem that might more comfort the young, and all of us.

Fraud may be too strong a word for the smaller faults that lie closer to home. Yet the preparation of abstracts for national meetings before the data are complete, claiming results that are not yet certain, is a kind of fraud. Writing a summary of a paper that claims more than the data reported permit is a kind of fraud. Discussions that conveniently ignore statistical significance of what has been stated in the data, making claims that are not supported, are a kind of fraud. No less fraudulent is the publicity about each new finding that raises hope in the newspapers to raise money for the laboratory. We should all be talking more about these matters.

Many of us clinicians are guilty of fraud in what and how we tell our patients about what we are doing to them. Telling the truth to dying patients or getting informed consent from research subjects has received a lot of illumination over the past decade, but telling the whole truth to our patients every day may provide just as much of a challenge. How often does the clinician confess how little he or she really knows rather than highlighting how much he does know. When, for example, we suggest a colonoscopy with biopsies every 6 months to uncover dysplasia in a patient with longstanding ulcerative colitis, or when we advise colonic resection for a patient with carcinoma in a polyp, we should ask whether we tell our patients of the disagreement between pathologists and of the uncertainty that attends such matters. When we propose to do our fourth or fifth papillotomy, few tell the patient who has not asked that we have done only three or four before. It is not easy for me to tell the difference between some patients and some subjects. Does the patient–subject enrolled in a controlled clinical trial know that someone, group or office or university, gets paid—gets a profit—for the trials that they undergo? "He's only interested in the numbers, not the patients," a cynical house officer said recently of a doctor well versed in clinical trials. As we lament frauds in medicine at high levels, we should think about the difference between patients and subjects in office and clinic.

The fads of medicine provide a second issue. It is easy enough for gastroenterologists to criticize the enormous growth of coronary-care units, at least in the United States, and to skim with skepticism studies that report attempts, for example, to limit the size of a myocardial infarct. It is easy to wonder whether a patient with chest pain in the coronary-care unit in the middle of the night can ever give "informed consent" to the trial of a new procedure, whatever he may sign. Yet gastroenterologists are little different. They just have fewer crises. One of my friends tells how he walked in on a research colleague struggling to force, "insert" was the word he used, a pressure catheter into the rectum of a semicomatose patient. The patient was resisting with all the subcortical might he could gather. When my friend remonstrated, his colleague replied, "But he signed an informed consent yesterday and I don't want to waste it." I doubt that patients in any crisis, whether obtunded by fear or by drugs, can make an informed decision about clinical trials when asked to do so by those taking care of them. Substituted judgment might provide one better approach, but these are matters that we should be talking about.

Gastroenterologists everywhere are injecting sclerosing agents into esophageal varices quite frequently at present. Usually it is the same agent we used 35 years ago, when we learned that the benefit of variceal sclerosis was only temporary. Fortunately paid for by third-party payers, the approach remains an experimental but profitable one, on whose long-term benefits trials do not yet agree. I am convinced, as I was 35 years ago, that acute bleeding can be stopped, but that on the long term the cirrhotic's life is probably not prolonged. We spare the blood banks by such an approach, and the patient runs a lesser risk of non-A,non-B hepatitis or AIDS, but that is all. When we repeat sclerosis on our outpatients, do we tell them of all the published doubts, that they will probably live no longer if we do this to them, and do we give them the choice between repeated sclerosis or the risks of transfusions? How many of us tell our patients that they are receiving an uncertain as well as an unpleasant form of therapy? We act out of a good-hearted attempt to help, but we gloss over the uncertain nature of the results to our patients.

Many touted triumphs turn out to be ephemeral medical fads, but let me move on to the final F, frenzy, for it distorts all that we do. By frenzy I mean trying to do too much in too short a time. Not too long ago a department chairman in the United States resigned under pressure because it was claimed, and he admitted, that he had unwittingly plagiarized some eight pages of material. The plagiarism was so frank and full that no one consciously intending to cheat could have been as foolish. His excuse in many ways underlined the common problem. He had too many other responsibilities, he said, he had been too busy to review the proofs of what he had written to realize what had happened. He had relied on others, now dead, to get the appropriate permissions and they had not. Discussion ceased upon his resignation for there was general agreement that there had been expiation enough. A chairman at another school had resigned some years earlier because one of his associates had put together false data. That chief had also been too busy, doing too much, traveling too far, even writing too much. A brilliant and dedicated man was engaged in so many activities that he did not have the time to oversee the activities of his associates. Busy, energetic, frenetic people make business enterprises succeed, but the energies of the chief executive officer were not always the attributes of a clinical departmental chairman. Most of us in academic life run too fast, take on too many obligations, and leave too little time for contemplation or wonder. But that frenzied pressure of academic medicine gets very little discussion.

Is clinical practice so different? A survey of patients with inflammatory bowel disease in Connecticut and New York suggested that patients wanted more time, not more services, from their doctors. Those of us in clinical practice may well smile at such a request and respond that we do not have time enough to treat them all as it is. If you schedule too many patients and too many procedures for a busy day, it is so much easier and more satisfying for everyone, patient and doctor alike, to have the reassurances of the latest computed tomography (CT) or radionuclide scan or even from some arcane endoscopy. It is so much easier to endoscope the patient, and more rewarding, than to listen to what he has to say. Physicians are trained to get the data that the eye can view rather than to listen to the patient and rely on his words. Our model is a biomechanical one.

A few recent anecdotes from my practice: Recently, I saw a 36-year-old woman who had undergone six operations over the preceding 12 years. These included the inevitable hysterectomy, oophorectomy, and cholecystectomy along with laparotomy for the resulting adhesions. During the year before I saw her she had also undergone two operations for "intractable" peptic ulcer symptoms, in another state. To be sure, her careful and competent gastroenterologist had first treated her abdominal pain with H_2 blockers and had endoscoped her only after she had not responded to that management. He had found a 2-cm ulcer in her antrum and had watched it over the next 12–14 weeks of therapy, had asked about alcohol and aspirin abuse, and had even checked out her serum gastrin and salicylate levels, all of which had proven normal. Grudgingly, I know, he had ultimately assented to a partial gastrectomy and vagotomy for the persistent antral ulcer because he feared that it might be a lymphoma or even a carcinoma hidden away from his biopsy forceps. Her pains were not assuaged by the first operation on her stomach and so somewhat later, when a revision seemed in order, the gastroenterologist repeated all the right procedures, looked at the ulcer again, and rebiopsied it, ordered a CT scan to clear her pancreas of endocrine tumors, recognized that serum gastrin levels might have been misleading the first time, and did a secretin stimulation test. The second operation also left her pain intact. No one seemed to take into account, as was disclosed later, that her alcoholic father had abused her as a child, that, married at 15, she had been beaten by her equally alcoholic husband, and that her second husband had taken her from her hometown to a far-off state in an area she detested. At the cost of several laparotomies, the gastric ulcer at least provided the stimulus for her return to Connecticut. What will happen to her I do not know. The doctors had looked at her stomach carefully and considerately. But they had not paid any attention to her.

Recently, a young woman of 28 with chronic abdominal pain had suffered through the usual big "fruit basket" of diagnostic studies we carry out for uncertain abdominal pain. Endoscopic examination of her pancreatobiliary tree (ERCP), laparoscopy, CT scan, porphyrin levels, and much more had proven fruitless. I asked her gastroenterologist, who had trained with me, whether he had also considered her social, psychological, and personal travails. A fine physician, to whom I would willingly turn for my own care, he replied, "That's your business, Howard. My job is to be sure that there is no real disease."

Let me tell you also of a 36-year-old engineer, a salesman for an aggressive, high-technology company in Connecticut. A few years ago he developed severe epigastric pain, which might have been pancreatic in character although it never occurred at night and was relieved by lying down. Characteristically, the pain came on after a heavy business lunch with a few drinks and a business discussion with his clients. He slept through the night quite well, but the daytime pain became so severe that it kept him from working. As all studies proved negative, except for evidence by barium studies, endoscopy, and a pH probe of reflux esophagitis, he underwent a repair of a small hiatus hernia. The pain resisting that operation as it had previously resisted ERCP and computed tomography, he had the added inconvenience of being unable to belch. He therefore sought help at a famous clinic where a skilled surgeon who has written much on revising antireflux procedures redid the operation to open up the gastroesophageal junction. The pain persisted nevertheless. I saw the patient when he was beginning to return to work, but had not yet returned to those business lunches. Frankly, I could make nothing more of his pain even if I suspected that it might have achieved the purpose of keeping him from business. But when I asked him whether, hindsight being what it is, if he had known all that was to happen, he would have undergone the first repair, his answer was precise. "Boy, I could have lived with my pain if only the doctors hadn't kept worrying me the way they kept on looking for something else. I wish they had told me that it wasn't anything serious. I could have lived with it."

We doctors don't do that anymore. Like scientists or detectives, we want to see all the answers. In the search for truth and for data that our training in science instills, we forget that second realm of people, persons who are sick.

What I have suggested to you is that (1) intuition, what the mind grasps at once without measuring, may be as important in clinical gastroenterology as science, what we can measure and quantitate; (2) gastroenterologists must put the findings of our technical equipment into the context of the patient's life; and (3) most important, most physicians, in practice and in academic life, are in too much of a hurry. Many of the faults that I have reviewed with you, the fads and the frauds of our time, come, I believe at least in part, from our unwillingness to take the time to think, to contemplate what we are doing, to reflect, and to discuss our doubts. We need to talk more with each other about the human condition and not just about technical matters. We certainly need to talk more with our patients. Most of all, we need to recognize that medicine is neither a religion nor a science, however much we may need our scientific basis.

Not all answers are yet possible nor will they ever be as well defined in medicine as the models of physics. But surely we can improve matters by having some conversations with poets and philosophers, novelists and artists, about what we mean by human life, by persons, by men and women. Surely we can improve our medical practice by such meetings as this, but also by talking about what we mean by health and disease, by recognizing that pain in the belly, or even in the chest, does not always need physical asesssment as much as it will yield to mental, even spiritual refreshment. We must remember that the practice of medicine is not a scientific discipline like physics, but rather that it is a human vocation and that we are taking care of people and not only of cells or organs.

Index